Review of
Pulmonary and
Critical Care Medicine

Review of
Pulmonary and
Critical Care Medicine

REUBEN M. CHERNIACK, M.D.

Professor of Medicine

University of Colorado

National Jewish Center for Immunology
and Pulmonary Medicine

Denver, Colorado

1996

B.C. Decker Inc. • Hamilton

B.C. Decker Inc.
4 Hughson Street South
P.O. Box 620, L.C.D. 1
Hamilton, Ontario L8N 3K7
Tel: 905-522-7017
Fax: 905-522-7839
E-mail: info@bcdecker.com

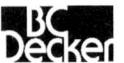

Printed in the United States of America

01 00 99 98 97 96 /EB/ 9 8 7 6 5 4 3 2 1

ISBN 1–55009–027–5

Notice: The authors and publisher have made every effort to ensure that the patient care recommended herein, including choice of drugs and drug dosages, is in accord with the accepted standard and practice at the time of publication. However, since research and regulation constantly change clinical standards, the reader is urged to check the product information sheet included in the package of each drug, which includes recommended doses, warnings, and contraindications. This is particularly important with new or infrequently used drugs.

Sales and Distribution

United States
Blackwell Science Inc.
238 Main Street
Cambridge, Massachusetts 02142
U.S.A.
Tel: 617 876 7000
Fax: 617 492 5263

Canada
Copp Clark Ltd.
2775 Matheson Boulevard E.
Mississauga, Ontario
Canada L4W 4P7
Tel: 905 238 6074
Fax: 905 238 6075

Japan
Igaku-Shoin Ltd.
Tokyo International P.O. Box 5063
1-28-36 Hongo, Bunkyo-ku
Tokyo 113, Japan
Tel: 81 3 3817 5680
Fax: 81 3 3815 7805

Australia
Blackwell Science Pty, Ltd.
54 University Street
Carlton, Victoria 3053
Australia
Tel: 03 9347 0300
Fax: 03 9349 3016

Outside of North America, Australia and Japan
Marston Book Services, Ltd.
P.O. Box 269
Abingdon
Oxon OX14 4YN
England
Tel: 44 01 235 465 500
Fax: 44 01 235 465 555

To
Edy
and
Karen, Mark and Mitch

Preface

Over the past decade a number of extremely valuable textbooks on pulmonary medicine have been published. These prove especially useful when one encounters a patient with a particular respiratory condition, or when preparing for examinations, such as the pulmonary boards. However, the ability to evaluate the extent of knowledge gained from such textbooks and to assess areas of weakness is only truly fulfilled when another such case is encountered or when tested by examination. The goal of the present book is to assist the "student" of pulmonary medicine in gaining an understanding of many aspects of pulmonary medicine through an interactive process. It is hoped that this will prove a valuable aid for those preparing for an examination and for those who wish to update their knowledge.

The book is organized into two main parts, namely multiple-choice questions and answers. Each part begins with basic principles and covers the gamut of pulmonary disorders and ends with critical care. For every answer I have provided a reasonably detailed rationale so that the reader will understand the underlying rationale, at least as I see it. Case problems are included in order to give the reader a feel for the clinical setting. More than 650 references are provided in an organized manner, from adenocarcinoma to yellow nail syndrome. The resulting book intends to serve as an inclusive review of the discipline so that the diligent reader will fare better in the board examination.

I am grateful to the many fellows in training in the Division of Pulmonary Medicine and Critical Care at the University of Colorado, who over the years have presented their interesting cases at the weekly Pulmonary Grand Rounds, and whose reviews of the literature have unwittingly formed the basis for many of the questions and answers in this book. I am also grateful to Dr. Marvin Schwarz, Head of the Division, for providing some of the radiographs.

RMC, Denver
August, 1995

Contents

QUESTIONS

1-1 Basic Principles

In all questions, one or more answers are correct.

B-1. The following statements pertain to the non-immune host:
   a. Phagocytosis is facilitated by natural opsonins present in the respiratory tract.
   b. Phagocytosis and particle inactivation by pulmonary phagocytes are augmented manifold by specific antibody secreted by effector B lymphocytes.
   c. The alternate pathway of complement activation can be triggered nonspecifically by microbial polysaccharides.
   d. Activation of the alternate complement pathway may stimulate the emigration of monocytes from the circulation.
   e. Effector T cells appear within hours after infection.

B-2. The following statements apply to immunodeficiency *except*:
   a. In X-linked hypogammaglobulinemia (Bruton's) there is a deficiency of all immunoglobulins.
   b. In ataxia-telangiectasia an IgA deficiency is common.
   c. Deficiency of all immunoglobulins can be associated with nephrosis.
   d. IgM deficiency is commonly associated with malignancies of the reticuloendothelial system.
   e. Phenytoins and penicillamine may be associated with selective IgG deficiency.

B-3. The following statements apply to the thymus gland and the immune reaction:
   a. The major role of the thymus gland is to provide mature B cells.
   b. The major effector cell in immunologically mediated resistance to bacterial infection are antibody-secreting B cells.
   c. The thymus gland selects and exports mature, antigen-specific T cells of appropriate specificities.
   d. IgM, IgE, IgG1, and IgG2 are involved in immune responses in the lung.
   e. The major *in vivo* role of suppressor CD 8 T cells is to function as cytotoxic T cells.

B-4. The following statements apply to the immune reaction:
   a. Cytotoxic T cells (CD 8+) recognize antigen in the context of class I MHC antigens.
   b Cytotoxic T cells (CD 8+) recognize antigen in the context of HLA-A, -B, and -C antigens.
   c. IL-1 is involved in T cell-mediated effects on macrophage function.
   d. T cells specific for a given antigen find the correct antigen-specific B cell because macrophages present antigen to both cells, causing them to interact.
   e. B cell help probably involves IL-1 and IL-3.

B-5. The following statements pertain to immune deficiency:
a. Complete absence of C3 is associated with recurrent *S. pneumoniae* infections.
b. Resistance to viral infections is usually normal in the immunoglobulin deficiency states.
c. Patients with primary or idiopathic neutropenia suffer from severe infection.
d. The majority of affected individuals with selective IgA deficiency are asymptomatic.
e. There is an inversion of the T4:T8 ratio in bronchoalveolar lavage in AIDS.

B-6. The following statements pertain to the immune process:
a. Specific T cells are involved in the initiation of the delayed hypersensitivity skin reaction to tuberculin antigen.
b. IgE triggers the release of soluble mediators of type II hypersensitivity.
c. Specific antibody and antibody-forming cells appear in lungs in hours in the previously unsensitized host.
d. Transudation of specific antibody or the influx of specific antibody-forming cells occurs rapidly in the immune host.
e. In the previously unsensitized host, sensitized effector T cells appear at the site of infection within days to weeks.

B-7. The following statements apply to the immune reaction:
a. Antigen-presenting cells must express class II MHC antigens.
b. Epithelial cells are capable of presenting antigen.
c. T cells are capable of presenting antigen.
d. T cells require interleukin-2 as a growth factor.
e. Interleukin-2 is a differentiation factor for some T cells.

B-8. The following statements pertain to pulmonary macrophages:
a. They arise from monocytes which begin in the bone marrow.
b. They live weeks to months.
c. They have surface membrane receptors for the Fc portions of IgG1, IgG3, and C3.
d. They present antigen to appropriate lymphocytes for induction of immune responses.
e. They serve as activated effector cells for specific T-cell immunity.

B-9. The following statements pertain to pulmonary lymphoid tissue:
a. Hilar lymph nodes and extrapulmonary lymph nodes are anatomically the same.
b. Hilar nodes contain higher concentrations of IgA than do other lymph nodes.
c. Hilar nodes contain lower concentrations of IgE positive cells than do other lymph nodes.
d. Lymphoid cells adjacent to bronchial glands contain all major classes of immunoglobulin.
e. BALT are nodules of lymphoid cells just below the bronchial mucosa.

B-10. The following statements pertain to hypogammaglobulinemia:
a. Severe combined immunodeficiency is an acquired immunoglobulin deficiency.
b. Common variable hypogammaglobulinemia is a congenital immunoglobulin deficiency.
c. Common variable hypogammaglobulinemia is characterized by a variable decrease in IgA, IgG, and IgM levels.
d. Common variable hypogammaglobulinemia is the immunoglobulin deficiency most often associated with bronchiectasis.
e. Lymphocytic interstitial pneumonitis is a manifestation of common variable hypogammaglobulinemia.

B-11. The following statements pertain to macrophages and the processing of antigen:
   a. They take up antigen and process it for presentation to lymphocytes.
   b. They display antigenic determinants on the surface membrane of the cell.
   c. They express surface membrane HLA-DR antigens.
   d. They secrete soluble mediators.
   e. A major function is to mediate delayed hypersensitivity and cellular cytotoxic reactions.

B-12. The following statements pertain to T lymphocytes:
   a. They arise from the bone marrow.
   b. They differentiate and mature after 10 days in the thymus gland.
   c. The distribution of phenotypes in blood is approximately T4, 35% and T8, 65%.
   d. T4 lymphocytes are helper cells for antibody-producing B cells and for cytotoxic T cells.
   e. Activated T cells mediate delayed hypersensitivity and cellular cytotoxic reactions.

B-13. The following statements pertain to polymorphonuclear leukocytes:
   a. They are normally present in large numbers in the interstitium.
   b. There are large numbers in the marginating pool in the pulmonary vascular bed.
   c. They are normally less phagocytic than macrophages.
   d. They die after phagocytosis and degradation of particles.
   e. They are ingested and digested by plasma cells.

B-14. The following statements pertain to lymphocytes in the lung:
   a. In delayed hypersensitivity reactions, polymorphonuclear phagocytes induce accumulation of lymphocytes.
   b. In delayed hypersensitivity reactions, lymphokines stimulate the influx of inflammatory cells.

   c. Viral antigens on the surface membranes of host cells are recognized by T4 lymphocytes.
   d. Natural killer (NK) lymphocytes mediate cytotoxic mechanisms directly.
   e. T8 cells promote antibody production by B cells and generation of cytotoxic T4 cells.

B-15. The following statements pertain to the immune host:
   a. Specific antibody and sensitized T cells are available immediately at the site of particle deposition.
   b. Antigen stimulates secretion of a variety of lymphokines by sensitized B lymphocytes.
   c. The interaction of antigen with either IgG or IgM results in the formation of immune complexes.
   d. Specific antibody secreted by effector B lymphocytes augments phagocytosis and particle inactivation by pulmonary phagocytes.
   e. Polymorphonuclear leukocytes move in and accumulate at exposure.

B-16. The following statements pertain to B lymphocytes:
   a. They arise from pluripotential stem cells and differentiate within the bone marrow.
   b. Mature B cells migrate to lymph nodes, spleen, and secondary lymphatic tissues.
   c. They proliferate and differentiate into plasmablasts and plasma cells after antigenic stimulation.
   d. Appropriately presented antigen triggers activation and clonal expansion.
   e. They recognize both antigen and HLA-DR on membrane surfaces of macrophages.

B-17. The following statements pertain to the immune process:
   a. Neutrophils engulf and process antigen for presentation to antigen-reactive lymphocytes.

b. Pulmonary lymphocytes coordinate cellular interactions and modulate responses by either enhancing or suppressing neutrophil proliferation and differentiation.

c. Macrophages are induced to accumulate at tissue sites of antigen deposition by the secretion of lymphokines.

d. Phagocytic and cytotoxic activities are enhanced by specific antibody.

e. Viral infections of the respiratory tract stimulate phagocytic and bactericidal activities.

B-18. The following statements apply to the immunosuppressed host:

a. Infection, commonly opportunistic, accounts for 50–75% of the diffuse pulmonary infiltrates.

b. It is necessary to use invasive procedures in the evaluation of these patients.

c. In AIDS patients bronchoalveolar lavage (BAL) is 80–85% sensitive in diagnosing *Pneumocystis carinii* pneumonia (PCP).

d. In the non–AIDS-immunosuppressed host the yield is highest in diagnosing malignancy.

e. In the non–AIDS-immunosuppressed host the yield is 83–96% in diagnosing viral pneumonia.

B-19. Which of the following statements are correct about eosinophilia and eosinophils?

a. Eosinophilia is found only in patients with allergic reactions.

b. The degree of eosinophilia parallels the intensity of airway obstruction in asthma.

c. Eosinophil major basic protein causes mediator release.

d. Eosinophil major basic protein can cause airway epithelial injury.

e. Polymorphonuclear leukocytes generate leukotrines to a much larger degree.

B-20. The following statements pertain to parasitic infections:

a. *Ascaris* can cause pulmonary infiltrations with eosinophilia.

b. *Strongyloides* can cause pulmonary infiltrations and pulmonary hypertension.

c. *Entamoeba histolytica* invades and obstructs the pulmonary vessels.

d. *Schistosoma* species can cause pulmonary infiltrations with pulmonary hypertension.

e. *Necator americanus* causes pulmonary infiltrations with pulmonary hypertension.

B-21. The treatment of tropical eosinophilia consists of:

a. Steroids.

b. Erythromycin.

c. Diethylcarbamazine.

d. Tetracycline.

e. Quinine.

B-22. The following pertain to tropical eosinophilia:

a. The disorder can be due to mosquito bites.

b. Hemoptysis may occur.

c. There may be an obstructive pattern on pulmonary function tests.

d. There may be a restrictive pattern.

e. Eosinophilia develops when microfilariae pass through the lungs.

B-23. In COPD, the following relationship between oxygen desaturation and pulmonary artery pressure elevation is true:

a. A 5% fall in oxygen saturation is associated with a 5 mm Hg increase in pulmonary artery pressure.

b. A 1% fall in oxygen saturation is associated with a 15 mm Hg increase in pulmonary artery pressure.

c. A 1% fall in oxygen saturation is associated with no increase in pulmonary artery pressure.

d. A 5% fall in oxygen saturation is associated with a 10 mm Hg increase in pulmonary artery pressure.

e. A 5% fall in oxygen saturation is associated with a 20 mm Hg increase in pulmonary artery pressure.

B-24. Correct statements about the respiratory muscles include the following:
a. The respiratory muscles are smooth muscles, made up of three different fiber types.
b. The diaphragm is the principal muscle of inspiration.
c. In the diaphragm half of the fibers are fast oxidative glycolytic (type IIA fibers), a quarter are fast glycolytic (type IIB fibers), and a quarter are slow oxidative fibers.
d. Contraction of the diaphragm primarily increases the volume of the thoracic cage in a vertical and transverse direction.
e. The descent of the diaphragm during inspiration raises the abdominal pressure and lowers the pressure in the lungs.

B-25. Correct statements about mechanics of breathing include the following:
a. Functional residual capacity is relatively constant because lung elastic recoil equals chest wall elastic recoil at FRC.
b. Airway resistance is lowest at FRC.
c. Compliance is the change in static pressure across the lungs divided by the volume change.
d. Compliance of the lungs varies, depending on the lung volume at which it is determined.
e. In fibrosis or lung congestion, lung compliance is reduced.

B-26. Correct statements about airway resistance include the following:
a. It is lung elastic recoil pressure/airflow.
b. It is (transpulmonary pressure-lung elastic recoil pressure)/airflow.
c. It is lowest at a high lung volume.
d. It can be calculated in a body plethysmograph from knowledge of the ratio

between plethysmograph and airway pressure and the airflow.
e. It is the reciprocal of conductance.

B-27. Correct statements about maximal expiratory flow (MEF) include the following:
a. MEF is effort-dependent at a high lung volume.
b. MEF is to a large extent effort-independent at a low volume.
c. MEF increases up to a point and then plateaus at low and mid lung volumes.
d. MEF is affected by upper respiratory obstruction at high volumes.
e. MEF is different from flows achieved in a maximum expiratory flow-volume curve at any volume.

B-28. Correct statements about maximal inspiratory flow include the following:
a. In normals, maximal inspiratory and expiratory flow rates are approximately equal.
b. In a variable lower airway obstruction, there is an initial burst of expiratory flow, with a plateau that ends abruptly, while inspiratory flow is only slightly reduced.
c. In a fixed airway obstruction, maximal inspiratory and expiratory flow are limited.
d. In a variable upper airway obstruction, maximal expiratory flow is limited more than inspiration.
e. In a carinal obstruction, maximal inspiratory flow is limited more than expiration.

B-29. Correct statements pertaining to gas exchange include the following:
a. An RQ greater than 2.0 is indicative of alveolar hypoventilation.
b. An abnormality of gas exchange may only become apparent during exertion.
c. The subject is in a steady state if the RQ is between .45 and .75.
d. With a constant minute ventilation, alveolar ventilation falls with a fall in respiratory rate.

e. In pure alveolar hypoventilation, the alveolar-arterial PO_2 difference ($P[A\text{-}a]O_2$) is elevated.

B-30. In healthy individuals, during normal breathing:
a. Pulmonary blood flow distribution is dependent on alveolar pressure.
b. The distribution of inspired air is greater at the bottom of the lung.
c. Ventilation and perfusion of alveoli are unequal at the top of the lung, ventilation being greater.
d. At the top of the lung, if pulmonary arterial pressure is greater than alveolar pressure, there is no flow.
e. At the bottom of the lung, alveolar pressure is greater than pulmonary artery pressure, but less than left atrial pressure.

B-31. Correct statements pertaining to diffusion include the following:
a. Diffusing capacity of any gas is calculated from the amount that disappears from the lung and the alveolo-arterial gradient for that gas.
b. Determination of D_LO_2 requires knowledge of the cardiac output.
c. D_LCO can be estimated by either a single or multiple breath technique.
d. Determination of D_LCO breathing different oxygen levels yields measurement of cardiac output.
e. D_LO_2 is calculated from the oxygen consumption/mean alveolocapillary gradient for oxygen ($P[\overline{A\text{-}c}]O_2$).

B-32. The amount of oxygen transported by hemoglobin, at a given oxygen tension, falls when:
a. The $PaCO_2$ falls.
b. The H+ ion concentration rises.
c. The temperature falls.
d. The pH falls.
e. The temperature rises.

B-33. A high ventilation-perfusion ratio implies:

a. Ventilation of poorly perfused alveoli.
b. Venous admixture-like perfusion.
c. Perfusion of poorly ventilated alveoli.
d. Reduced alveolar ventilation.
e. Dead space like ventilation.

B-34. All of the following statements about alveolar hypoventilation apply *except*:
a. In acute alveolar hypoventilation, pCO_2 is high, pH is low, bicarbonate and CO_2 content may be relatively normal.
b. In acute alveolar hypoventilation, alveolar ventilation is inadequate to cope with the carbon dioxide production.
c. In chronic alveolar hypoventilation, pCO_2 is high, pH is just below normal, and the bicarbonate and CO_2 content are elevated.
d. In chronic alveolar hypoventilation, pCO_2 is high, pH is above 7.45, and the bicarbonate and CO_2 content are elevated.
e. Alveolar hypoventilation cannot totally account for a low PaO_2 if the alveolo-arterial oxygen tension is elevated.

B-35. For a given minute ventilation, the $PaCO_2$ will rise when:
a. Respiratory rate falls.
b. Respiratory rate is increased.
c. CO_2 production is increased.
d. Tidal volume is increased.
e. Tidal volume is decreased.

B-36. Which of the following is applicable in assessment of acid-base status?
a. Bicarbonate can be calculated from $PaCO_2$ and CO_2 content.
b. Hydrogen ion concentration increases with ingestion of bicarbonate.
c. Bicarbonate is low in both respiratory alkalemia and metabolic acidemia.
d. Bicarbonate can be calculated from the pH and pCO_2.
e. A fall in $PaCO_2$ increases hydrogen ion concentration.

B-37. Eosinophilic infiltration of the alveolar structures occurs in all of the following *except*:
   a. Bronchiolitis obliterans and organizing pneumonia.
   b. Lymphoma.
   c. Pulmonary histiocytosis X.
   d. Idiopathic pulmonary fibrosis (IPF).
   e. Sarcoidosis.

B-38. Which of the following disorders has a predilection for the lower lobes?
   a. *Klebsiella* pneumonia.
   b. Postprimary histoplasmosis.
   c. *Haemophilus influenzae* pneumonia.
   d. Aspergillosis with mucoid impaction.
   e. Postprimary tuberculosis.

B-39. The following disorders have a predilection for the upper lobes *except*:
   a. End-stage sarcoidosis.
   b. Chronic hypersensitivity pneumonitis.
   c. Eosinophilic granuloma.
   d. Idiopathic pulmonary fibrosis.
   e. Ankylosing spondylitis.

B-40. Alveolar filling on chest roentgenograms is seen in the following *except*:
   a. Histoplasmosis.
   b. Chicken pox pneumonia.
   c. Lipoid pneumonia.
   d. Coccidioidomycosis.
   e. Bronchiolo-alveolar carcinoma.

B-41. The following are characteristic features of an alveolar filling process *except*:
   a. Air bronchograms in larger bronchi.
   b. Acinar rosettes with distal air bronchograms.
   c. Obliteration of heart borders.
   d. Silhouetting of diaphragm.
   e. Linear and nodular densities.

B-42. Which of the following disorders have a predilection for the upper lobes?
   a. Actinomycosis.
   b. Primary histoplasmosis.
   c. *Streptococcus pyogenes* pneumonia.
   d. Pulmonary A-V fistula.

   e. *Pseudomonas pseudomallei* pneumonia.

B-43. The following disorders with reticulonodular disease have increased lung volume *except*:
   a. Lymphangioleiomyomatosis.
   b. Eosinophilic granuloma.
   c. Chronic hypersensitivity pneumonitis.
   d. Aluminum pneumoconiosis.
   e. Diffuse panbronchiolitis.

B-44. The following apply to the bronchial circulation:
   a. In the adult the bronchial arteries usually originate from the aorta between T3 and T8.
   b. The bronchial arteries partly supply the esophagus.
   c. The bronchial veins empty into the azygos and hemiazygos veins.
   d. The distal bronchial venous plexus drains into the pulmonary veins.
   e. Approximately one third of the bronchial venous circulation returns to the right heart.

B-45. Number these causes of massive hemoptysis in order of frequency:
   a. Lung cancer. _____
   b. Chronic cavitary tuberculosis. _____
   c. Bronchovascular fistulas. _____
   d. Inflammatory lung disease. _____
   e. Lung abscess. _____

B-46. The following statements are true *except*:
   a. A right-sided pleural effusion may be seen in cirrhosis.
   b. Severe intrahepatic cholestasis may mimic primary biliary cirrhosis.
   c. Esophageal rupture can result from heavy lifting.
   d. Esophageal rupture can result from childbirth.
   e. In esophageal rupture pulmonary manifestations are usually right-sided.

B-47. Crohn's disease has been reported to be associated with:

a. Granulomatous lung disease.
b. Pneumonitis due to sulfasalazine.
c. Bronchiectasis.
d. Localized interstitial fibrosis.
e. Increased polymorphonuclears in BAL fluid.

B-48. The following statements apply to gastroesophageal function *except*:
a. Lower esophageal sphincter pressure is decreased by theophylline.
b. Lower esophageal sphincter pressure is increased by beta agonists.
c. Lower esophageal sphincter pressure is decreased by smoking.
d. The FVC and FEV1 are reduced with gastric but not duodenal ulcer.
e. Theophylline increases gastric acid secretion.

B-49. Gastroesophageal reflux can lead to the following *except*:
a. Pulmonary fibrosis.
b. Bronchospasm.
c. Recurrent pneumonia.
d. Sinusitis.
e. Laryngotracheal bronchitis.

B-50. The following statements apply to primary biliary cirrhosis:
a. Serum angiotensin-converting enzyme is elevated.
b. T8 lymphocytes are elevated in lavage.
c. Serum mitochondrial antibodies are positive.
d. The Kveim reaction is negative.
e. Focal biliary cirrhosis should lead to suspicion of cystic fibrosis.

B-51. The following statements apply to the trachea:
a. In normal subjects, the extrathoracic trachea is circular until it reaches the cricoid cartilage.
b. The trachea assumes a round or oval shape when it becomes intrathoracic.
c. Calcification of the tracheal cartilage is frequent in healthy people.
d. "Saber-sheath" trachea is coronal narrowing of the intrathoracic trachea at the thoracic inlet.
e. The great majority of patients with "saber-sheath" trachea are older men with COPD.

B-52. The following pertain to common variable hypogammaglobulinemia:
a. *H. influenzae* and *Pneumococcus* predominate in bronchiectasis associated with it.
b. The bronchiectasis is focal.
c. Patients are predisposed to noncaseating granulomas in the lungs.
d. Intramuscular immune globulin is more effective than the intravenous route in preventing infections.
e. Replacement therapy promotes normal growth in young patients.

B-53. The following apply to esophageal reflux:
a. Lower esophageal pressure decreases with inspiration.
b. Acid and pepsin secretion is not markedly increased in subjects with reflux esophagitis.
c. Reflux episodes are more frequent in patients with increased lower esophageal pressure.
d. Theophylline stimulates gastric acid secretion.
e. Cough may produce episodes of gastroesophageal reflux.

B-54. The following factors lower esophageal sphincter pressure:
a. Theophylline.
b. Reflux esophagitis.
c. Smoking.
d. Alcohol.
e. Beta agonists.

B-55. The following statements are true *except*:
a. Fulminant bronchitis and ulcerative colitis may be related.
b. Hypoxemia due to intrapulmonary shunting is present in hepatic failure.
c. Esophageal rupture can result from heavy lifting.

d. Esophageal rupture can result during forceful childbirth.

e. Pulmonary manifestations are usually right-sided in esophageal rupture.

B-56. In a patient with idiopathic pulmonary fibrosis and reduced exercise tolerance:
a. Maximum oxygen consumption may occur at a lower than expected work load.
b. Respiratory rate falls.
c. There is an inordinate increase in tidal volume.
d. Dead space/tidal volume ratio may increase.
e. The $Pa(A-a)O_2$ may be disproportionately elevated.

B-57. The following statements apply to roentgenograms of the chest:
a. In polyarteritis nodosa (PAN) consolidation is patchy and fleeting as in Löffler's syndrome.
b. Lymph node enlargement is common in Löffler's syndrome.
c. Pleural effusion is common in blastomycosis.
d. Chest wall involvement is common in blastomycosis.
e. Pleural effusion is common in *Haemophilus influenzae* infection.

B-58. Correct statements about obese individuals include the following:
a. VC is decreased.
b. TLC is reduced.
c. The pressure-volume curve of the lungs is shifted downward; the slope is reduced.
d. The most common abnormality in pulmonary function is a low expiratory reserve volume.
e. Breathing is slow and deep.

B-59. A low ventilation-perfusion ratio implies:
a. Ventilation of poorly perfused alveoli.
b. Venous admixture-like perfusion.
c. Perfusion of poorly ventilated alveoli.
d. Reduced alveolar ventilation.
e. Dead space like ventilation.

B-60. A low arterial CO_2 content and normal $PaCO_2$ are found in:
a. Metabolic acidosis.
b. Respiratory acidosis.
c. Metabolic alkalosis.
d. Respiratory alkalosis.
e. A mixed disorder.

B-61. Which of the following pertain to exercise?
a. The FEV_1 falls 5–15 minutes after cessation of an exercise load in very few patients with asthma.
b. There is often a refractory period after exercise in which another exercise will not result in bronchospasm.
c. Exercise-induced bronchospasm can be prevented in most cases by prior inhalation of steroids.
d. Exercise-induced bronchospasm can be prevented in most cases by prior inhalation of cromolyn and beta-2 agonists.
e. Exercise-induced bronchospasm will only develop if moist, warm air is inhaled, or if the subject breathes through the nose.

B-62. After endoscopic variceal sclerotherapy for esophageal varices:
a. Retrocardiac densities are due to paraesophageal inflammation.
b. Esophago-bronchopleural fistula is a late complication.
c. Barium swallow is indicated in suspected cases of esophagopleural fistula.
d. Use water-soluble contrast in suspected cases of esophagobronchial fistula.
e. If in doubt use barium swallow for diagnosis.

B-63. The following take place at the anaerobic threshold:
a. Carbon dioxide production rises disproportionately to the oxygen consumption.

b. Respiratory quotient and the pH fall.

c. Carbon dioxide production increases proportionately to ventilation.

d. Ventilation increases proportionately with oxygen consumption.

e. A metabolic alkalosis develops.

B-64. The following are part of the normal response to exercise:

a. Ventilation increases abruptly, primarily because of an increase in tidal volume.

b. Ventilation increases linearly with the work intensity, and then rises precipitously.

c. Cardiac output rises, primarily because of an increase in stroke volume.

d. Oxygen uptake increases to a point and then rises precipitously.

e. Blood flow is redistributed to exercising muscles.

B-65. The following apply to exercise testing in healthy individuals:

a. A cycle ergometer can be used.

b. A treadmill can be used.

c. Exercise should be stopped if tidal volume increases by 100%.

d. The efficiency during treadmill exercise is the ratio of power output to the caloric equivalent of the oxygen uptake.

e. The systolic blood pressure usually falls by 25 mm Hg during exercise.

B-66. At a given exercise work load in an individual who is physically unfit:

a. Heart rate is greater than expected.

b. Ventilation is greater than expected.

c. Carbon dioxide production falls.

d. Respiratory quotient rises above 2.0.

e. Arterial pH and lactate level may be low.

B-67. Hyperleukocytosis is associated with:

a. White blood cell count greater than 100,000.

b. Myeloproliferative or lymphoproliferative disorders.

c. Myeloblasts causing significant stasis in brain and lung capillaries.

d. Pulmonary leukostasis.

e. Marked hypoxemia, despite a relatively normal roentgenogram.

B-68. The following apply to pulmonary infiltrates in an immunocompromised patient:

a. Appearance in roentgenogram helps to rule out opportunistic infection.

b. Localized disease within 24 hours of treatment is usually opportunistic infection.

c. Localized disease late in treatment is usually noninfectious.

d. Diffuse disease occurring during treatment is usually noninfectious.

e. Bronchoscopy with lavage or biopsy in diffuse alveolar and interstial infiltrates within 48 hours of treatment has a low diagnostic yield.

B-69. The following statements apply to immune responses and resistance to infection:

a. Type II hypersensitivity diseases are caused by IgE antibodies binding to basophils and mast cells.

b. The disease process in tuberculosis is caused by B cell antibodies reacting against mycobacteria.

c. C-fixing bacteriolysins are important in antibacterial immunity.

d. The major types of immune responses involved in antiviral immunity are natural killer cells and antibody production.

e. The AIDS virus lowers resistance to mycobacteria by infecting CD 4+ helper T cells.

B-70. In pulmonary fibrosis:

a. Lung compliance is increased; flow rates are low; flow resistance is normal; FRC is reduced.

b. Lung compliance is decreased; flow rates are high; flow resistance is normal; FRC is reduced.

c. Lung compliance is increased; flow

rates are low; flow resistance is increased; FRC is reduced.

d. Lung compliance is reduced; flow rates are low; flow resistance is normal; FRC is reduced.

e. Lung compliance is decreased; flow rates are low; flow resistance is increased; FRC is reduced.

B-71. Which of the following is likely to be found in acute asthma?

a. The pressure-volume curve of the lungs is shifted upward; the slope is normal.

b. The pressure-volume curve of the lungs is shifted downward; the slope is reduced.

c. The pressure-volume curve of the lungs is shifted downward; the slope is normal.

d. The pressure-volume curve of the lungs is shifted upward; the slope is increased.

e. The pressure-volume curve of the lungs is shifted upward; the slope is reduced.

B-72. The most common abnormality in pulmonary function in obese patients is:

a. Low expiratory reserve volume.

b. Low vital capacity.

c. Low total lung capacity.

d. Low diffusing capacity.

e. Low inspiratory capacity.

B-73. In obese patients, there is generally:

a. Increased work of breathing.

b. Decreased carbon dioxide production and oxygen consumption.

c. Hypoxemia, normal or decreased carbon dioxide tension.

d. Decreased respiratory rate.

e. Increased lung volumes.

B-74. When there is nonuniform obstruction in the peripheral airways adjacent to the alveoli:

a. Total flow resistance may be little elevated.

b. Gas distribution is altered.

c. Peripheral unit time constants are nonuniformly distributed.

d. Maximal expiratory flow rates and FEV_1 can be normal.

e. Static lung compliance is altered.

B-75. Tests of airway hyperreactivity include:

a. Histamine or methacholine.

b. Exercise.

c. Specific allergenic or occupational agents.

d. Hot air inhalation.

e. Voluntary hyperventilation.

B-76. To definitely attribute alterations of arterial blood gases to a problem in gas exchange, one must examine:

a. PaO_2.

b. $PaCO_2$.

c. pH.

d. Steady state.

e. Minute ventilation.

B-77. The subject was in a steady state if the RQ was between:

a. .65–.95.

b. .45–.75.

c. .75–2.25.

d. .80–2.50.

e. .95–2.30.

B-78. The distribution of inspired air during normal breathing:

a. Is equal at the top and bottom of the lung.

b. Is greater at the bottom of the lung.

c. Is greater at the top of the lung.

d. Is equal to blood flow at the bottom of the lung.

e. Is greatest at the level of the pulmonary artery outflow tract.

B-79. The highest morbidity and mortality in asthma occurs from:

a. 8 a.m. to 11 a.m.

b. 11 a.m. to 6 p.m.

c. 6 p.m. to midnight.

d. Midnight to 6 a.m.

e. Is the same throughout the day.

B-80. At sea level, an increased right-to-left shunt in the heart or lungs can be ruled out if:
   a. The roentgenogram and hemoglobin are normal.
   b. $PaCO_2$ is greater than 50 mm Hg during exercise.
   c. PaO_2 is greater than 500 mm Hg on 100% oxygen.
   d. Oxygen saturation is 100% on 100% oxygen.
   e. PaO_2 is less than 500 mm Hg on 100% oxygen.

B-81. The following apply to orthodeoxia:
   a. Supine PaO_2 is lower than in the upright position.
   b. It is seen with pulmonary vascular abnormalities in chronic liver disease.
   c. It is seen with lung precapillary dilatations 15–160 microns in diameter.
   d. It is seen with true AV communications in the lower lung zones.
   e. It is seen with pleural based AV "spiders."

B-82. The diagnosis of liver-associated vascular abnormalities requires:
   a. Clinical diagnosis of chronic hepatic dysfunction.
   b. Preexisting condition known to cause liver disease.
   c. Hypoxemia.
   d. Demonstration of intrapulmonary vascular "shunting."
   e. Contrast-enhanced echocardiogram.

B-83. The following are features of hypereosinophilic syndrome (HES):
   a. Peripheral eosinophils are >1500/mm³.
   b. Significant allergy.
   c. Multi-organ system involvement.
   d. Eosinophilia is fleeting and lasts less than 1 month.
   e. Eosinophilic leukemia falls into this syndrome.

B-84. The following apply to hypereosinophilic syndrome:
   a. A female predominance.
   b. Mean age of onset is about 55 years.
   c. Urticaria/angioedema of the face and extremities.
   d. CVAs.
   e. Peripheral polyneuropathy.

B-85. The following are features of hypereosinophilic syndrome:
   a. Endocardial fibrosis.
   b. Progressive heart failure.
   c. Restrictive cardiomyopathy.
   d. Thrombosis of intramural coronary vessels.
   e. Thromboembolic events.

B-86. The following are cardiovascular features of hypereosinophilic syndrome:
   a. Mural thrombosis containing large numbers of eosinophils.
   b. Fibrotic thickening of the endocardium.
   c. Mitral insufficiency.
   d. Neutrophil infiltration of the myocardium.
   e. Aortic stenosis.

B-87. The following are hematologic features of hypereosinophilic syndrome:
   a. Large partially degranulated peripheral blood eosinophils.
   b. Polycythemia.
   c. The eosinophil count predicts the extent of organ damage.
   d. Immature WBCs.
   e. Teardrop-shaped RBCs.

B-88. The following are features of hypereosinophilic syndrome:
   a. Airflow limitation.
   b. Cognitive dysfunction.
   c. Pleural effusions.
   d. Pulmonary fibrosis.
   e. Therapy consists of prednisone and hydroxyurea.

B-89. The following are features of hypereosinophilic syndrome:
   a. Peripheral myeloblasts indicate a good prognosis.

b. Elevated LFTs and hepatomegaly.

c. Renal failure.

d. Cardiovascular disorders are very responsive to prednisone.

e. Prognosis is related to the degree of cardiac involvement.

B-90. A mixed apnea during sleep includes:

a. No airflow with varying effort.

b. No airflow with no effort.

c. No airflow with no effort and then increasing effort.

d. Marked reduction in tidal volume and respiratory rate.

e. No airflow with increasing effort.

B-91. Acute pulmonary edema can occur during sleep associated with:

a. Myocardial infarction.

b. Toxic fume inhalation.

c. Sleep apnea.

d. Asthma.

e. Interstitial disease.

B-92. The most common symptom of sleep apnea is:

a. Loud snoring.

b. Daytime somnolence.

c. Restless sleep (increased motor activity).

d. Decreased intellectual capacity.

e. Personality changes.

B-93. Which of the following may develop because of sleep apnea?

a. Systemic hypertension.

b. Pulmonary hypertension.

c. Mastocytosis.

d. Erythrocytosis.

e. Weight loss.

B-94. What percentage of sleep apneic patients are obese?

a. 40%.

b. 50%.

c. 60%.

d. 70%.

e. 80%.

B-95. What percentage of patients with the diagnosis of essential hypertension have sleep apnea?

a. 5%.

b. 15%.

c. 30%.

d. 40%.

e. 50%.

B-96. What endocrine abnormality is most commonly associated with sleep apnea?

a. Cushing's syndrome.

b. Hypothyroidism.

c. Acromegaly.

d. Hypogonadism.

e. Adrenal insufficiency.

B-97. In sleep apnea, REM sleep:

a. Is decreased to approximately 15% of total sleep.

b. Remains unchanged.

c. Is absent.

d. Decreases to approximately 20% of total sleep.

e. Increases to 40% of total sleep.

B-98. The level at which obstruction can occur in sleep apnea is:

a. Nasal.

b. Tonsillar.

c. Epiglottal.

d. Tracheal.

e. Carinal.

B-99. The nonsurgical treatment with the highest success rate in obstructive sleep apnea is:

a. Protriptyline hydrochloride.

b. Oxygen.

c. Nasal CPAP.

d. Weight loss.

e. Nasal pharyngeal airway.

B-100. The surgical treatment with the highest success rate in obstructive sleep apnea is:

a Uvulopalatopharyngoplasty.

b. Tracheostomy.

c. Tonsillectomy.

d. Mandibular advancement.

e. Adenoidectomy.

B-101. Treatment of central sleep apnea consists of:
a. Progesterone.
b. Carbonic anhydrase inhibitors.
c. Oxygen.
d. Tongue-retaining devices.
e. Lasix.

B-102. The most common cause of oxygen desaturation during sleep in patients with COPD is:
a. Apnea.
b. Hypopnea.
c. Right heart failure.
d. Paradoxical respiration.
e. Diffusion defect.

B-103. The most successful treatment of oxygen desaturation during sleep in COPD is:
a. Supplemental oxygen.
b. Progesterone.
c. Almitrine.
d. Protriptyline hydrochloride.
e. Carbonic anhydrase inhibitors.

B-104. Which of the following studies is most helpful in evaluating a patient's risk for a routine operative procedure?
a. History.
b. Physical examination.
c. Chest roentgenogram.
d. Electrocardiogram.
e. Liver function profile.

B-105. Following active immunization with tetanus toxoid injection, how often should a tetanus toxoid booster be given?
a. Every year.
b. Every 2 years.
c. Every 5 years.
d. Every 10 years.
e. Never.

B-106. The operative mortality risk is highest in patients with:
a. Serum creatinine levels of 2.5 mg/dl.
b. Atrial fibrillation.
c. Chronic obstructive lung disease with a pCO_2 of 45 mm Hg.
d. A history of subendocardial myocardial infarction (4 weeks ago).
e. A history of a stroke (6 months ago).

B-107. In elderly patients undergoing major surgery, the highest operative risk is associated with:
a. Pulmonary vascular disease.
b. Asthma.
c. Chronic obstructive lung disease.
d. Carcinoma of the lung.
e. History of a pulmonary embolus.

1-2 Airway Disease

A-1. The following apply to the Churg-Strauss syndrome:
a. HepS Ag is positive.
b. There is a history of allergic rhinitis/atopic disease.
c. The patient presents early as a difficult to control asthmatic.
d. Paranasal sinus disease occurs in >90%.

e. A vasculitic phase most commonly affects the kidney.

A-2. The following apply to the Churg-Strauss syndrome:
a. GI symptoms are present in the majority of cases.
b. Cerebral infarction is the usual cause of death.

c. Eosinophils are >10%.

d. Neuropathy is present in the majority of cases.

e. The ESR is usually normal.

A-3. The following apply to the Churg-Strauss syndrome:

a. Plasmapheresis is the mainstay of therapy.

b. The vasculitic phase usually remits before 1 year.

c. Intermittent steroids are adequate.

d. Refractory cases are usually managed with cyclophosphamide.

e. A short span between the first two phases and vasculitis carries a poor prognosis.

A-4. The Mounier-Kuhn syndrome is associated with:

a. Atrophy of the muscular support layer of the airways.

b. Tracheobronchomegaly.

c. Bronchial diverticulosis.

d. Weakness of the cartilaginous portions of the trachea.

e. Ballooning of the tracheobronchial tree balloons during expiration.

A-5. The Mounier-Kuhn syndrome is associated with:

a. Scalloped or corrugated appearance of the airways.

b. Marked honeycombing.

c. Pooling of secretions in the airways.

d. Pleural effusion.

e. Spontaneous pneumothorax.

A-6. Which of the following statements are true of Mounier-Kuhn syndrome?

a. Tracheobronchomegaly is present on the chest film (CXR) when the diameter of the trachea exceeds 15 mm in a transverse section.

b. Bronchomegaly is present on CXR if diameter of the right main bronchus is 11 mm.

c. Bronchomegaly is present on CXR if diameter of the right main bronchus is 12 mm.

d. Bronchoscopy is the procedure of choice for diagnosis of the Mounier-Kuhn syndrome.

e. CPAP is useful therapy for the Mounier-Kuhn syndrome.

A-7. Mounier-Kuhn syndrome:

a. Is an acquired condition secondary to chronic infections.

b. Is associated with congenital abnormalities of the heart.

c. Is associated with Ehlers-Danlos syndrome in adults.

d. Is more severe in patients who are frequent smokers.

e. Is associated with restrictive pulmonary function.

A-8. Correct statements when nonuniformly distributed obstruction in the peripheral airways are the only abnormality include the following:

a. Total flow resistance may be little elevated.

b. Gas distribution is altered.

c. Peripheral unit time constants are nonuniformly distributed.

d. Maximal expiratory flow rates and $FEV_{1.0}$ are reduced.

e. The static compliance of the lungs will be reduced.

A-9. Correct statements about airway hyperreactivity include the following:

a. Histamine and methacholine inhalation are nonspecific tests of airway hyperresponsiveness.

b. Inhalation of warm moist air frequently exaggerates exercise-induced bronchospasm.

c. In asthma, FRC is increased, the pressure-volume curve of the lungs is shifted upward, and the slope is reduced.

d. A fall of 20% of the $FEV_{1.0}$ following exercise is considered a positive response.

e. A fall of 35% of specific conductance following histamine or methacholine inhalation is considered a positive response.

A-10. Pancreatic insufficiency in cystic fibrosis patients can lead to which of the following deficiencies?
a. Vitamin A.
b. B vitamins.
c. Vitamin C.
d. Trace minerals.
e. Vitamin E.

A-11. The following statements apply to cystic fibrosis:
a. It is inherited as an autosomal recessive trait.
b. Siblings of affected individuals have a two out of three chance of carrying the cystic fibrosis gene.
c. There is a linkage of the cystic fibrosis gene with the serum enzyme paroxonase.
d. The cystic fibrosis gene has been mapped to chromosome number 7.
e. Infertility in men is due to maldevelopment of the sperm.

A-12. The following apply to bronchopulmonary fungal hypersensitivity:
a. In bronchopulmonary fungal hypersensitivity the fungus irritates the airways and produces asthma.
b. Fungal antigens are inducing the asthmatic response.
c. It is an invasive process.
d. Treatment of allergic bronchopulmonary aspergillosis (ABPA) consists of oral steroids following levels of blood eosinophilia and/or IgE.
e. Long-term sequelae include aspergilloma.

A-13. The following are diagnostic criteria for ABPA *except*:
a. Asthma and blood eosinophilia.
b. Immediate skin test reactivity, precipitating antibodies, increased IgE.
c. History of fleeting infiltrates.
d. Fibrosis.
e. Peripheral bronchiectasis.

A-14. The following statements pertain to alpha$_1$-antitrypsin deficiency:

a. It is an autosomal recessive disorder.
b. The alpha$_1$-protease inhibitor (A1PI) is coded for by a gene on chromosome 12.
c. In the null condition there is no detectable alpha$_1$-protease inhibitor in serum.
d. The alpha$_1$-protease inhibitor level may be normal but not function properly.
e. Alpha$_1$-protease inhibitor inhibits neutrophil elastase.

A-15. The following statements pertain to alpha$_1$-antitrypsin deficiency *except*:
a. The Z protein is easily secreted from the hepatocyte cytosol.
b. The function of the Z protein against neutrophil elastase is reduced.
c. The S protein has less activity against neutrophil elastase than does the Z protein.
d. Neoplasia raises serum levels of alpha$_1$-protease inhibitor.
e. All homozygotes are symptomatic by 50 to 60 years of age.

A-16. The following statements pertain to alpha$_1$-antitrypsin deficiency *except*:
a. Heterozygotes have no increased risk of developing emphysema if they don't smoke.
b. FEV$_1$ declines more rapidly in MZ smokers than in MM smokers.
c. The MZ phenotype is 2–5 times more common in emphysematous patients.
d. Serum levels less than 35% normal are associated with severe centrilobular emphysema.
e. Cigarette smoke oxidizes Met 358 amino acid residue in the alpha$_1$-protease inhibitor molecule.

A-17. The following statements pertain to treatment of alpha$_1$-antitrypsin deficiency:
a. Purified human alpha$_1$-protease inhibitor is prepared from pooled human plasma.
b. 140 mg/kg of active inhibitor is given every other day to homozygous patients.

c. Administration of active inhibitor weekly results in protective levels in serum and alveoli.

d. Augmentation therapy is beneficial in symptomatic ex-smokers with PiMZ phenotype.

e. Leukocytosis can develop with purified human alpha$_1$-protease inhibitor.

A-18. The following statements apply to the alpha$_1$-protease inhibitor:

a. Alpha$_1$-protease inhibitor is produced by mononuclear cells.

b. Alpha$_1$-protease inhibitor is responsible for most of the anti-elastase activity of the lower respiratory tract.

c. The half-life of alpha$_1$-protease inhibitor is 4–5 days.

d. The minimum, or threshold level needed in blood to prevent lung destruction by elastases is 44 μm.

e. The Z gene is uncommon among Asians.

A-19. The following statements apply to the alpha$_1$-protease inhibitor :

a. Free radicals in cigarette smoke reduce inhibition of elastase.

b. The phenotype can be inferred from the serum level.

c. Liver disease is a manifestation of null-null deficiency states.

d. Lung destruction occurs in the lower zones because there are more bloodborne PMNs there.

e. Liver disease is due to the absence of inhibitor.

A-20. The following statements apply to cystic fibrosis:

a. Nasal polyps are rare.

b. Cystic fibrosis and its sequelae can involve nearly every organ system.

c. The median survival is 10 years.

d. The normal range of sweat chloride concentrations is slightly higher in children than in adults.

e. Invasive aspergillosis of the tracheobronchial tree is common.

A-21. The following statements apply to cystic fibrosis:

a. Early in the disease, there is an obstructive defect.

b. Spontaneous pneumothorax is a rare occurrence in cystic fibrosis.

c. Rectal prolapse should lead to suspicion of the diagnosis of cystic fibrosis.

d. Pancreatic insufficiency is present only in one third of patients.

e. Puberty is often delayed.

A-22. The following statements apply to cystic fibrosis:

a. The risk of a cystic fibrosis mother and a father with no history of cystic fibrosis having a baby with cystic fibrosis is 1 out of 4.

b. There is a defect in neutrophil phagocytosis.

c. Airway hyperreactivity is rare in cystic fibrosis.

d. Inhaled antibiotics are nearly as effective as intravenous antibiotics in treating exacerbations of cystic fibrosis.

e. Pancreatic insufficiency in cystic fibrosis patients can lead to a deficiency of vitamins B and C.

A-23. The following statements pertain to hypogammaglobulinemia:

a. *H. influenzae* and *Pneumococcus* infections are unusual in bronchiectasis associated with common variable hypogammaglobulinemia (CVH).

b. The bronchiectasis associated with CVH is diffuse.

c. Patients with CVH are predisposed to noncaseating granulomas in the lungs.

d. Intramuscular immune globulin is more effective than the intravenous route in preventing infections and decreasing antibiotic use.

e. Replacement therapy promotes normal growth in young patients.

A-24. The following are lung disorders associated with welding *except*:

a. Metal fume fever.

b. Polymer fume fever.

c. Siderosis.

d. Silicosis.

e. Asthma.

A-25. The following statements apply to respiratory bronchiolitis *except*:

a. There is accumulation of pigmented macrophages in the respiratory bronchioles.

b. The roentgenogram shows a reticulonodular pattern.

c. Pulmonary function is obstructive pattern.

d. It primarily occurs in smokers.

e. There are granulation plugs with obliteration of small airways.

A-26. The following drugs can cause PIE syndrome:

a. Gold.

b. Sulfonamides.

c. Penicillin.

d. Cromolyn.

e. Azathioprine.

A-27. Which of the following statements are true?

a. Circadian fall in circulating levels of histamine is a major mechanism in nocturnal asthma.

b. Heightened parasympathetic tone at night is a major mechanism in nocturnal asthma.

c. A reduction in circulating cortisol concentrations is the major mechanism in nocturnal asthma.

d. Asthma is one of the most common causes of persistent cough.

e. Inhaled corticosteroid blocks exercise-induced bronchospasm.

A-28. The following statements apply to asthma:

a. There is normally a circadian rhythm in FEV_1.

b. Bronchiectasis is the most common cause of persistent cough.

c. Heightened parasympathetic tone at night is thought to be a major mechanism in nocturnal asthma.

d. Circulating levels of epinephrine are thought to be a major mechanism in nocturnal asthma.

e. Exercise-induced asthma is prevented by breathing cold air.

A-29. Which of these statements are true about antibiotics in cystic fibrosis?

a. Continuous oral antibiotics have been shown to decrease the frequency of respiratory exacerbations and hospitalizations.

b. When treating *Pseudomonas aeruginosa* infections with IV antibiotics, single drug therapy is as effective as multiple drugs.

c. The dosage of aminoglycoside required to achieve optimal blood levels in cystic fibrosis patients is often 1.5- to 2-fold higher than recommended.

d. Intravenous antibiotics should be used only when new infiltrates are demonstrated on a chest roentgenogram.

e. Inhaled antibiotics are nearly as effective as intravenous antibiotics in treating exacerbations.

A-30. Which of the following statements are true?

a. Churg-Strauss syndrome is the most likely diagnosis if a patient develops bronchiectasis, rhinitis, and sinusitis early in life.

b. Situs inversus may accompany the immotile cilia syndrome.

c. Central bronchiectasis is a major manifestation of allergic bronchopulmonary aspergillosis.

d. Asthma and allergic rhinitis are manifestations of the Churg-Strauss syndrome.

e. In the Churg-Strauss syndrome lesions are seen in the brain and kidneys.

A-31. The following are associated with the immotile cilia syndrome:

a. Chronic sinusitis and bronchiectasis.

b. Infertility greater in females than in males.

c. Gynecomastia.

d. Dynein arm abnormalities of the cilia.

e. Situs inversus.

A-32. The following statements pertain to the Williams-Campbell syndrome:

a. Bronchiectasis is generalized.

b. The bronchi are very noncompliant.

c. It is an acquired deficiency of bronchial cartilage.

d. Most patients have clubbing.

e. It is associated with an increased elastance.

A-33. Elevation of IgE may occur in all of the following *except*:

a. Atopic dermatitis.

b. Visceral larva migrans.

c. Eosinophilic pneumonia.

d. Allergic bronchopulmonary aspergillosis.

e. Aspergilloma.

A-34. The following are characteristic of Löffler's syndrome *except*:

a. Migratory pulmonary infiltrates.

b. Absent or mild symptoms.

c. The entire picture lasts less than one month.

d. The lung is apparently the only organ involved.

e. Increased serum IgE.

A-35. Which of the following are clinical manifestations of allergic bronchopulmonary aspergillosis?

a. Asthma.

b. Fleeting pulmonary infiltrates.

c. Peripheral bronchiectasis.

d. Fibrosis.

e. Increased IgE.

A-36. The following statements pertain to airway disease:

a. Bronchospasm from aspirin occurs only in patients with nasal polyps.

b. The most likely diagnosis in a patient who develops bronchiectasis, rhinitis, and situs inversus is common variable hypogammaglobulinemia.

c. Distal bronchiectasis is the primary diagnostic sign of allergic bronchopulmonary aspergillosis.

d. Lactic acidosis is a major factor in the pathogenesis of airway obstruction with exercise.

e. Beta agonist treatment does not down-regulate leukocyte function in asthma because beta-adrenergic function is already diminished.

A-37. The following statements pertain to bronchiolitis obliterans without organizing pneumonia:

a. It is characterized by extension of granulation tissue from the distal alveolar ducts into alveoli.

b. The chest radiograph shows linear interstitial markings.

c. It is a common pathologic finding in connective tissue disorders.

d. Toxic fume inhalation and organ transplantation are causes.

e. Cadmium oxide has been associated with this condition.

A-38. The following statements pertain to bronchiolitis obliterans without organizing pneumonia:

a. It is commonly due to the respiratory syncytial virus in adults.

b. It is commonly due to *Mycoplasma pneumoniae* in children.

c. The radiographic pattern is often interstitial, frequently with hyperinflation.

d. Physiologically the pattern may be restrictive or obstructive.

e. It accounts for death within a few hours after exposure to high concentrations of NO_2.

A-39. The following should heighten suspicion of cystic fibrosis *except*:

a. Malabsorption.

b. Intermittent small bowel obstruction.

c. Focal biliary cirrhosis.

d. Esophageal rupture.

e. Sinusitis and nasal polyposis.

A-40. Churg-Strauss syndrome is characterized by:
   a. Pulmonary necrotizing angiitis.
   b. Systemic necrotizing angiitis.
   c. Extravascular granulomas.
   d. Eosinophilia.
   e. Involvement of both the arteries and the veins.

A-41. The following statements apply to hypersensitivity pneumonitis *except*:
   a. May develop insidiously without acute episodes.
   b. Demonstrates a combined obstructive and restrictive defect.
   c. Bronchiolitis obliterans can be present.
   d. The presence of precipitins against thermophilic actinomycetes is diagnostic.
   e. There is progressive shrinkage of the upper lobes.

A-42. The following statements apply to hypersensitivity pneumonitis *except*:
   a. Abrupt onset of flu-like symptoms.
   b. Associated with antigen-antibody complexes.
   c. A noncaseating interstitial granulomatous pneumonitis.
   d. An obstructive ventilatory defect during acute episodes.
   e. Fleeting, micronodular, interstitial pattern in the lower zone.

A-43. Bronchiolitis obliterans may be associated with all of the following *except*:
   a. Measles.
   b. Inhalation of sulfur dioxide.
   c. Rheumatoid arthritis.
   d. Allergic bronchopulmonary aspergillosis.
   e. Inhalation of ammonia.

A-44. The following are characteristic of Löffler's syndrome:
   a. Migratory pulmonary infiltrates.
   b. Absent or mild symptoms.
   c. The entire picture lasts less than one month.

d. The skin rash resembles a vasculitis.
   e. Peripheral eosinophilia.

A-45. The following apply to respiratory bronchiolitis:
   a. May be a restrictive pattern.
   b. Normal D_LCO.
   c. May be an obstructive pattern.
   d. Diagnosis generally by transbronchial biopsy.
   e. Smoking cessation may be associated with complete resolution.

A-46. The major treatment of the immotile cilia syndrome consists of:
   a. Antibiotics.
   b. Chest physical therapy and coughing.
   c. Inhaled bronchodilators.
   d. Cromolyn.
   e. Acetylcysteine.

A-47. Which of the following are given as major mechanisms in nocturnal asthma?
   a. Circadian fall in circulating levels of epinephrine.
   b. Circadian variation in cortisol concentrations.
   c. Lessened parasympathetic tone at night.
   d. Airway cooling.
   e. Sleep.

A-48. Which of the following statements are correct about the use of beta-adrenergics in the treatment of asthma?
   a. Parenterally administered beta-adrenergics are more effective than inhaled beta agonists in the treatment of acute asthma.
   b. Beta agonist treatment is not associated with down-regulation of bronchodilation in asthma as beta-adrenergic function is already diminished.
   c. Inhaled beta-adrenergics are not effective in the treatment of acute asthmatics who have used beta agonists excessively.

d. Beta-adrenergics are more effective than intravenous aminophylline in the treatment of acute asthma.

e. Parenterally administered terbutaline sulfate can decrease serum potassium levels.

A-49. Which of the following statements about methylxanthines are correct?

a. Methylxanthines cause bronchodilation principally by inhibiting airway smooth muscle concentrations of phosphodiesterase.

b. Methylxanthine, but not enprophylline, blocks airway bronchoconstriction to adenosine.

c. Intravenous methylxanthine is an effective beta agonist for acute asthma if the patient has no detectable plasma levels of theophylline.

d. The H_2 antagonist cimetidine has no effect on theophylline metabolism.

e. Theophylline is a potent modulator of airway hyperreactivity.

A-50. Which of the following statements are true about the use of corticosteroids in the treatment of asthma?

a. Corticosteroids block cellular generation of arachidonic acid products.

b. An oral dose of prednisone (40 mg) increases total leukocyte count, primarily eosinophils.

c. Inhaled corticosteroids will diminish airway hyperreactivity to histamine.

d. Corticosteroids cause recovery of down-regulated beta-adrenergic receptors.

e. There is no evidence that corticosteroids will alter the pulmonary function in acute asthma within the first 24 hours of administration.

A-51. The pathologic lesions in chronic bronchitis without emphysema which are of importance in producing obstruction to air flow are:

a. Mural thickening of the lobar and sublobar bronchi.

b. Mucus secretion in the lumina of the major bronchi.

c. Edema and inflammation in wall of the membranous and respiratory bronchioles.

d. Goblet cell hyperplasia.

e. Hypertrophy of the mucus glands in the bronchial wall.

A-52. Which of the following is more diagnostic of allergic bronchopulmonary aspergillosis than the others?

a. Recurrent pulmonary infiltrates.

b. Positive sputum culture for *Aspergillus*.

c. Severe asthma.

d. Proximal bronchiectasis.

e. Sputum and blood eosinophilia.

A-53. Which of the following is not involved in the pathogenesis of airway obstruction with exercise?

a. Mediator release.

b. Airway water loss.

c. Airway cooling.

d. Development of lactic acidosis.

e. Airway rewarming.

A-54. In bronchopulmonary fungal hypersensitivity:

a. The fungus irritates the airways and produces asthma.

b. Fungal antigens are inducing the asthmatic response.

c. It is an invasive process.

d. Penicillin is the treatment of choice.

e. Corticosteroids are the treatment of choice.

A-55. Which of the following are clinical manifestations of allergic bronchopulmonary aspergillosis ?

a. Asthma.

b. Pulmonary infiltrates.

c. Central bronchiectasis.

d. Fibrosis.

e. Increased resistance to airflow.

A-56. The treatment of ABPA should consist of:
   a. Oral steroids following levels of blood eosinophilia and/or IgE.
   b. Oral steroids following clinical response.
   c. Inhaled steroids following clinical response.
   d. Beta agonists following clinical response.
   e. Theophylline following the blood level.

A-57. In the Churg-Strauss syndrome, which are the most common pathologic findings?
   a. Granulomas are seen in the liver and spleen.
   b. Granulomas are seen in the skin.
   c. Granulomas are seen in the nerves.
   d. Granulomas are seen in the kidneys.
   e. Necrotic lesions are seen in the lungs.

A-58. Which of the following statements are not true in the Churg-Strauss syndrome?
   a. Steroids are the treatment of choice.
   b. The shorter the interval between the onset of asthma and the onset of vasculitis, the worse the prognosis.
   c. Cytotoxic agents are necessary in severe cases.
   d. Five-year survival is 60–65%.
   e. The longer the interval between onset of asthma and onset of vasculitis, the worse the prognosis.

A-59. Centriacinar emphysema is found most commonly at these sites within the lungs:
   a. Uniformly distributed in all lobes.
   b. Predominantly in the upper lobes.
   c. Predominantly in the lower lobes.
   d. Predominantly in the middle zones.
   e. Predominantly in the dorsal segments of both lungs.

A-60. Panacinar emphysema is found most commonly:
   a. Uniformly distributed in all lobes.
   b. Predominantly in the upper lobes.
   c. Predominantly in the lower lobes.
   d. Predominantly in the young.

   e. Predominantly in the central segments of the lung.

A-61. In alpha$_1$-antiprotease deficiency emphysema is:
   a. Uniformly distributed in all lobes.
   b. Predominantly in the upper lobes.
   c. Predominantly in the lower lobes.
   d. Centriacinar in type.
   e. Panacinar in type.

A-62. The following statements apply to the alpha$_1$-protease inhibitor:
   a. Alpha$_1$-protease inhibitor is a glyco-protein of MW 102,000 produced by mononuclear cells.
   b. Alpha$_1$-protease inhibitor is responsible for more than 90% of the anti-elastase activity of the lower respiratory tract.
   c. The half-life of alpha$_1$-protease inhibitor is 6–8 days.
   d. The minimum, or threshold level needed in blood to prevent lung destruction by elastases is 35 μm.
   e. The Z gene is common among blacks.

A-63. The factors of greatest importance in producing functional impairment in emphysema are:
   a. The type of emphysema present.
   b. The extent of emphysema.
   c. The severity of the emphysema.
   d. Associated chronic bronchitis.
   e. Associated pulmonary vascular disease.

A-64. Focal emphysema:
   a. Is centriacinar emphysema localized within one lung segment.
   b. Is emphysema localized to the lung apical and subpleural regions.
   c. Is emphysema adjacent to any small scar.
   d. Is emphysema adjacent to the coal macule in simple coal worker's pneumoconiosis.
   e. Is emphysema associated with cystic fibrosis.

A-65. In bronchiolitis obliterans with organizing pneumonia (BOOP):
    a. There are granulation tissue plugs within the small airways.
    b. There is presence of peripheral honeycombing.
    c. There is extension of young connective tissue into the alveoli.
    d. There is alveolar wall edema and fibrosis.
    e. There are alveolar accumulations of neutrophils.

A-66. The pathologic changes of BOOP can be seen:
    a. In an idiopathic form.
    b. Secondary to connective tissue diseases.
    c. In cocaine abuse.
    d. In HIV infection.
    e. In radiation therapy.

A-67. Clinical features of BOOP include:
    a. Mean duration of symptoms at presentation of 12 months.
    b. End inspiratory crackles.
    c. Chest radiograph usually shows bilateral patchy infiltrates which are often fleeting.
    d. Reduced vital capacity and $D_L CO$.
    e. BAL lymphocytosis.

A-68. The differential diagnosis of BOOP includes:
    a. Eosinophilic pneumonia.
    b. Hypersensitivity pneumonitis.
    c. Eosinophilic granuloma.
    d. Usual interstitial pneumonia (UIP).
    e. Organizing infection.

A-69. A cystic fibrosis patient develops bacterial infection because of which of the following reasons?
    a. There is absent mucociliary clearance, and inhaled pathogens cannot be cleared from the tracheobronchial tree.
    b. There is a deficiency in compliment factor C3.
    c. There is a defect in neutrophil phagocytosis.

    d. There is a relative hypogammaglobulinemia, and sufficient antibodies cannot be raised to respiratory pathogens.
    e. None of the above.

A-70. Accepted criteria for the diagnosis of cystic fibrosis include:
    a. A sweat chloride greater than 60 mEq/L.
    b. Chronic obstructive pulmonary disease.
    c. Exocrine pancreatic insufficiency.
    d. A positive family history.
    e. Meconium ileus.

A-71. Sweat chloride levels may be elevated in:
    a. Untreated adrenal insufficiency.
    b. Hypothyroidism.
    c. Hypoparathyroidism.
    d. Malnutrition.
    e. Pancreatitis.

A-72. Which of the following clinical manifestations can be found in cystic fibrosis?
    a. Clubbing.
    b. Cirrhosis.
    c. Hemoptysis.
    d. Nasal polyps.
    e. Glycosuria.

A-73. Which of these statements are true regarding the inheritance of cystic fibrosis?
    a. Cystic fibrosis is the most common fatal inherited disease of Caucasians.
    b. One out of every 20 Caucasian individuals is a carrier of the disease.
    c. Cystic fibrosis is transmitted as an autosomal recessive trait.
    d. Cystic fibrosis is transmitted as an autosomal dominant trait with variable penetrance.
    e. Cystic fibrosis is transmitted as a sex-linked recessive trait.

A-74. Which of the following statements are true?
    a. The cystic fibrosis gene locus has been located on the long arm of chromosome 7.

b. The cystic fibrosis gene has been sequenced and the gene product described.

c. Using DNA linkage probes, it is possible, in certain circumstances, to detect the cystic fibrosis carrier status in at-risk families and disease status in utero.

d. The clinical presentation of cystic fibrosis is uniform in age of onset, organ system involvement, and rapidity of progression.

e. Cystic fibrosis and its sequelae can involve nearly every organ system.

A-75. Which of the following statements are true of cystic fibrosis?

a. Life expectancy of a cystic fibrosis patient has not improved substantially over the last 40 years.

b. The median survival of cystic fibrosis patients is 7 years.

c. The median survival is 14 years.

d. The median survival is 20 years.

e. 20% of cystic fibrosis patients who reach age 18 have been diagnosed after age 15.

A-76. Which of the following statements are true about sweat chloride (SC) determinations?

a. SC determination of >60 mEq/L is considered diagnostic of cystic fibrosis in children.

b. SC determination of <60 mEq/L excludes the diagnosis of cystic fibrosis.

c. 1 to 2% of individuals with clinical evidence of cystic fibrosis will have normal SC determinations.

d. The normal range of SC concentrations is slightly higher in adults than in children.

e. In individuals with COPD, the SC determination is unreliable.

A-77. Which of the following cystic fibrosis bacteriology statements are true?

a. *Pseudomonas aeruginosa* is the most frequent infectious organism in young children.

b. With advancing age, *Staphylococcus aureus* becomes the predominant pathogen.

c. The presence of *P. aeruginosa* in the tracheobronchial tree in any child strongly suggests the diagnosis.

d. Aggressive treatment with intravenous antibiotics can usually eradicate bacteria in the sputum.

e. Fungal colonization of the tracheobronchial tree is rare.

A-78. Which of the following statements regarding chest radiographs and pulmonary function tests in cystic fibrosis are true?

a. 2% of adults will have a normal chest roentgenogram.

b. Most patients will have cystic bronchiectatic changes demonstrated on chest film, predominately in the lower lung fields.

c. 10–15% of adults will have normal spirometry.

d. With severe pulmonary deterioration, pulmonary function tests reveal a mixed restrictive-obstructive ventilatory defect.

e. A progressively compromised FEV_1 is strongly correlated with a poor prognosis.

A-79. Which of the following statements are true regarding the pulmonary manifestations of cystic fibrosis?

a. Spontaneous pneumothorax is a rare occurrence in cystic fibrosis.

b. Spontaneous pneumothorax occurs most often in adolescence and in young adults who have moderately severe or severe pulmonary involvement (FEV_1 is less than 50% of predicted).

c. Hemoptysis is usually associated with worsening bronchial infection and commonly resolves with conservative treatment.

d. Cor pulmonale occurs only as a terminal event.

e. Various manifestations of rhinosinusitis are found in almost all adults with cystic fibrosis.

A-80. Which of the following clinical findings often lead to the diagnosis of cystic fibrosis?
   a. Rectal prolapse.
   b. Intestinal obstruction.
   c. Biliary cirrhosis.
   d. Idiopathic acute pancreatitis.
   e. Obstructive azoospermia.

A-81. Approximately 5–15% of cystic fibrosis patients have no clinical symptoms suggestive of malabsorption. This subgroup of cystic fibrosis patients:
   a. Has no pathologic or biochemical evidence of pancreatic disease.
   b. Will never require pancreatic enzyme replacement.
   c. Statistically have lower sweat chloride determinations and a slower progression of their pulmonary disease.
   d. May experience episodes of recurrent acute pancreatitis.
   e. Do not develop intestinal obstruction.

A-82. Which of the following statements are true regarding reproduction in cystic fibrosis?
   a. Men are nearly always infertile because of maldevelopment of the sperm.
   b. Men with cystic fibrosis mature sexually at the same rate as unaffected men.
   c. Women have normal fertility.

   d. The risk of a cystic fibrosis mother having a baby with cystic fibrosis is 1 out of 4.
   e. Pregnancy in cystic fibrosis has an increased risk of clinical deterioration during and after the pregnancy as well as increased fetal complications.

A-83. Cystic fibrosis can be misdiagnosed as which of the following diseases?
   a. Tuberculosis.
   b. Eosinophilic granuloma.
   c. Sarcoidosis.
   d. Immotile cilia syndrome.
   e. Immunoglobulin deficiency.

A-84. Which of these statements regarding cystic fibrosis treatment are true?
   a. Mucus evacuation by percussion and/or vibration with gravity drainage improves functional status better than gravity drainage alone.
   b. Mucomyst (N-acetylcysteine) is highly efficacious in promoting mucus evacuation.
   c. Airway hyperreactivity is rare in cystic fibrosis and inhaled beta agonists are of no benefit.
   d. If exercise is used to aid mucus evacuation, then exercise desaturation studies should be done prior to beginning the exercise program.
   e. In children, chronic low-dose alternate-day corticosteroids reduce hospital admissions and improve functional status.

1-3 Tumors

T-1. The following statements apply to lymphangitic carcinomatosis:
a. There is often a restrictive pattern with an increased D_LCO.
b. Pleural effusion may be seen.
c. The chest roentgenogram may be normal.
d. Hilar and mediastinal adenopathy is diagnostic.
e. Nodular or beaded thickening of bronchovascular bundles is a characteristic CT pattern.

T-2. The following statements apply to lymphangitic carcinomatosis:
a. The interstitial widening seen on roentgenogram is due to lymphatic invasion.
b. Overflow of tumor cells in lymphatics gives rise to pleural effusion.
c. The most common symptom is cough.
d. The tumor is likely to reach the intrapulmonary lymphatics by hematogenous spread of tumor emboli.
e. The most common primary is the colon.

T-3. The following statements apply to lung cancer *except*:
a. Oncogenes are cancer-causing genes that are pirated from host DNA by retroviruses.
b. Proto-oncogenes are cellular counterparts of viral oncogenes.
c. Oncogenes regulate cell growth in normal tissue.
d. Oncogenes become active in lung cancer.
e. C-myc oncogene is associated with a poor prognosis.

T-4. The following statements apply to lung cancer:
a. Lung cancer cells secrete growth factors.

b. Bombesin is produced in abundance by small cell lung cancer cells.
c. Bombesin is an autocrine growth factor.
d. Small cell lung cancers become insensitive to antineoplastic therapy even if they respond initially.
e. Small cell lung cancer cells have increased expression of the class I major histocompatibility antigens.

T-5. The following statements pertain to lung cancer:
a. Smoking cessation results in near normalization of risk for lung cancer over 10 to 15 years.
b. Smoking cessation results in a rapid decrease in the formation of new lung neoplasms.
c. The relative risk for an asbestos worker who smokes cigarettes is 25.
d. Squamous carcinoma, adenocarcinoma, and small cell lung cancer arise from squamous epithelium.
e. Screening with frequent sputum cytologies in addition to chest roentgenograms decreases overall death rate from lung cancer.

T-6. The following statements apply to lung cancer:
a. Small cell lung cancer cells demonstrate loss of chromosomal material.
b. Loss of chromosomal material is seen in the patient's normal cells.
c. Chromosome 3 abnormality is present in leukemia.
d. Chromosome 3 abnormality is present in renal cell carcinoma.
e. Cigarette smoke induces chromosome damage.

T-7. The roentgenographic features of alveolar filling disease are:

a. Acinar rosettes.

b. Diffuse consolidation.

c. Pneumothorax.

d. Kerley's B lines.

e. Obliteration of the diaphragm and heart borders.

T-8. The following statements pertain to carcinoma of the lung:

a. Screening with frequent sputum cytologies in addition to chest roentgenograms reduces the death rate in lung cancer.

b. Superior vena caval syndrome represents a true medical emergency.

c. The Eaton-Lambert syndrome in a patient with small cell lung cancer is confirmed by assessment of repeated stimulation on EMG.

d. Addison's disease is the most common endocrine syndrome in small cell lung cancer.

e. Hypercalcemia is suggestive of a non-small cell lung cancer.

T-9. The following statements apply to small cell bronchogenic carcinoma:

a. It originates in the major bronchi.

b. It narrows the bronchial lumen by infiltrating the wall of the bronchus.

c. It rarely metastasizes to hilar lymph nodes.

d. It invades blood vessels and metastasizes to distant organs.

e. It is common in uranium miners.

T-10. The following statements pertain to neurogenic mediastinal masses:

a. Neurogenic mediastinal tumors are generally in the anterosuperior mediastinum.

b. Neurilemomas arise from the axonal nerve sheath.

c. Most neurogenic tumors are benign in adults.

d. Pain is a common symptom in neurogenic mediastinal masses.

e. Elaboration of vanillylmandelic acid is associated with diarrhea and flushing.

T-11. The following statements pertain to neurogenic mediastinal masses:

a. In cases of anterior mediastinal masses, preoperative supine and erect expiratory flow volume loops should be performed.

b. Hormonally active chromaffin tumors are called pheochromocytomas.

c. Schwannoma is the most common neurogenic mediastinal mass.

d. Neurilemoma is usually detected in the sixth decade of life.

e. Posterior mediastinal masses in von Recklinghausen's disease are usually chemodectomas.

T-12. Pancoast's tumors:

a. Lie in the groove made by the subclavian artery in the apices of the upper lobes of the lungs.

b. Cause pain in the distribution of C6 through T1-T4.

c. Are largely associated with adenocarcinoma.

d. Can be caused by an aspergilloma.

e. Are less curable than other presentations of lung cancer.

T-13. The following statements apply to Pancoast's tumors:

a. Fine-needle aspirate provides the best diagnostic yield.

b. All Pancoast's tumors are T2 lesions.

c. Preoperative radiation is the standard of care.

d. Cerebral metastases are rare.

e. Involvement of the subclavian artery precludes long-term survival.

T-14. Favorable prognostic features in Pancoast's syndrome include all of the following *except*:

a. Adenocarcinoma.

b. Absence of mediastinal nodes.

c. Preoperative radiation.

d. Completeness of resection.

e. Ipsilateral Horner's syndrome.

T-15. The following lesion is not found in the trachea:
a. Carcinoma.
b. Carcinoid.
c. Cylindroma.
d. Mucoepidermoid lesion.
e. Polyps.

T-16. The following statements apply to pulmonary tumors:
a. With development of liver metastases, patients with carcinoid tumors rarely live more than two years.
b. Valvular replacement in patients with endocardial fibrosis can lead to prolonged survival even in the face of liver metastases.
c. Solitary pulmonary nodules are more common with small cell carcinomas than with non-small cell carcinomas.
d. Survival is worse following resection in patients with malignant solitary pulmonary nodules than in those with other presentations of lung cancer.
e. Lung lesions with calcification are benign.

T-17. Cardiac involvement in carcinoid entails the following except:
a. The deposition of endocardial fibrous tissue.
b. Pericardial effusion.
c. Left side of the heart involvement.
d. Tricuspid regurgitation.
e. Diffuse restrictive cardiomyopathy.

T-18. Carcinoids can be associated with all of the following except:
a. Deposition of smooth muscle cells in the endocardium.
b. Pulmonic stenosis.
c. Bronchoconstriction.
d. Flushing.
e. Mitral regurgitation.

T-19. The carcinoid syndrome may have the following features except:
a. Cutaneous flushing.
b. Tachycardia.
c. Hypotension.
d. Telangiectasias.
e. Malabsorption.

T-20. The following statements apply to bronchial carcinoids except:
a. They derive from the Kulchitsky's cells of the respiratory epithelium.
b. The carcinoid syndrome is common in bronchial carcinoid.
c. They may arise from the thyroid.
d. The treatment of choice is surgical excision.
e. They derive from the same cells as small cell carcinoma.

T-21. Bronchioloalveolar cell carcinoma presents with any of the following except:
a. Solitary nodule.
b. Multiple nodules.
c. Consolidation.
d. Atelectasis.
e. Pleural effusion.

T-22. The following apply to carcinoid tumor of the thymus:
a. It arises from a population of cells of neural crest origin.
b. Excess of serotonin is universal.
c. Carcinoid syndrome is common.
d. It is associated with elevated aromatic amino acid decarboxylase.
e. It is associated with Cushing's syndrome.

T-23. The following statements apply to carcinoids:
a. Atypical carcinoids have a lower incidence of lymph node metastases than the typical carcinoids.
b. Endocrine effects are associated with large bowel carcinoids.
c. Midgut carcinoids metastasize to bone.
d. Bronchial carcinoids never metastasize.
e. Some appear histologically as oat cell carcinomas.

T-24. The following apply to bronchiolo-alveolar cell carcinoma:
   a. Up to one third of cases presenting with a solitary nodule have multicentric disease.
   b. There is a lower lobe predominance.
   c. Cytologic yield from pleural effusions is high.
   d. The incidence of hilar adenopathy is less than for other lung tumors.
   e. Bone metastases are usually blastic.

T-25. The following statements apply to asbestos-related bronchogenic carcinoma:
   a. Incidence in smokers with asbestos exposure is 90 times that of nonsmokers without exposure.
   b. 20–35% of cigarette smokers with asbestosis will develop lung cancer.
   c. Nonsmokers with asbestos exposure develop a scar adenocarcinoma or bronchoalveolar carcinoma.
   d. The presence of a ferruginous body or pleural plaques indicates asbestosis.
   e. Asbestosis usually begins in the upper lobes.

T-26. The following statements apply to asbestos-related bronchogenic carcinoma:
   a. Bronchogenic carcinoma incidence peaks about 15 years after asbestos exposure.
   b. Asbestos-related carcinoma is predominantly in the upper lobe.
   c. There is an increased prevalence of adenocarcinoma.
   d. There is an increased frequency of multicentric and bilateral carcinomas.
   e. The frequency of bronchogenic carcinoma correlates with the severity of fibrosis.

T-27. Autologous bone marrow transplant may be beneficial in patients with:
   a. Non-Hodgkin's lymphoma.
   b. Ovarian carcinoma.
   c. Small cell carcinoma of the lung.
   d. Malignant melanoma.
   e. Nonseminomatous germ cell tumors.

T-28. The following apply to bronchoalveolar carcinoma *except*:
   a. It is a well-differentiated form of adenocarcinoma.
   b. It arises from alveolar type 2 cells.
   c. Tobacco use is important in its pathogenesis.
   d. It often appears in areas of previously scarred lung.
   e. It may develop in scleroderma lung.

T-29. The following statements are true *except*:
   a. The chest radiograph of alveolar cell carcinoma may demonstrate a diffuse consolidative pattern.
   b. Rheumatoid factor and/or antinuclear antibody are positive in 40% of patients with IPF.
   c. In alveolar cell carcinoma there may be bronchorrhea, and a salty taste to the sputum.
   d. Metastatic adenocarcinoma may produce an alveolar filling pattern on chest roentgenogram.
   e. The diagnosis of BOOP can only be made with an open lung biopsy.

T-30. Smoking cessation has the following effect on risk for lung cancer:
   a. Immediate normalization.
   b. Normalization over one year.
   c. Normalization over 3 to 5 years.
   d. Near normalization over 10 to 15 years.
   e. No effect.

T-31. Which of the following is not a respiratory carcinogen?
   a. Asbestos.
   b. Chromium.
   c. Nickel.
   d. Vitamin A.
   e. Mustard gas.

T-32. The relative risk of lung cancer for cigarette smokers is approximately 20; that for a nonsmoking asbestos worker is about 5. What is the relative risk for an asbestos worker who smokes cigarettes?
   a. 5.
   b. 20.

c. 25.
d. 100.
e. 500.

T-33. Bronchogenic carcinomas of either squamous, adenocarcinoma, or small cell lung cancer histologic types are believed to arise from:
a. Alveolar macrophages.
b. Goblet cells.
c. A variety of pulmonary cells.
d. Reserve basal cells of the bronchial mucosa.
e. Squamous epithelium.

T-34. For the majority of the natural history of a bronchogenic carcinoma, what is the major symptom?
a. None.
b. Cough.
c. Hemoptysis.
d. Malaise.
e. Weight loss.

T-35. Which of the following regarding screening for lung cancer is not true?
a. The studies performed to date are not ideal.
b. Screening with frequent sputum cytologies in addition to chest roentgenograms definitely decreases overall death rate from lung cancer.
c. Intensive screening efforts increase survival time in lung cancer.
d. 5% of those who have had a curative resection of a lung cancer develop a second primary.
e. It is more frequent in smokers.

T-36. Which is the most helpful in excluding malignancy of an asymptomatic coin lesion?
a. Size below 2.0 cm.
b. Stable size over 6 months.
c. Chest CT showing lack of mediastinal adenopathy.
d. Dense concentric calcification.
e. Patient under 35 years of age.

T-37. When confronted with a patient with a suspicious lesion which has enlarged on serial chest films, the first step should be:
a. Perform pulmonary function tests to determine ability to withstand a resection.
b. Perform metastatic work-up to determine curability by resection.
c. Establish the diagnosis and cell type of tumor.
d. Perform staging mediastinoscopy.
e. Obtain a chest CT, including images of liver and adrenals.

T-38. The major advances in surgical therapy of bronchogenic carcinoma over the past 20 years include all of the following *except*:
a. Improved postoperative and anesthetic care.
b. A decrease in the discovery of inoperable disease at the time of thoracotomy.
c. An improvement in the overall long-term survival from bronchogenic carcinoma.
d. Decreased operative mortality.
e. Introduction of lung-sparing procedures, such as wedge resection, segmentectomy, and sleeve resection.

T-39. Which of the following does not represent a true medical emergency?
a. Superior vena cava syndrome.
b. Tracheal obstruction due to tumor.
c. Cord compression due to extradural metastasis.
d. Hypercalcemia with coma.
e. Hyponatremia with seizures.

T-40. The most common site of relapse after successful chemotherapy for small cell lung cancer is:
a. Bone marrow.
b. Central nervous system.
c. Liver.
d. Site of primary lung lesion.
e. Adrenal glands.

T-41. A patient with small cell lung cancer presents with severe diffuse weakness.

Tensilon test is equivocal. In order to make a diagnosis of Eaton-Lambert syndrome, you should:
a. Obtain EMG.
b. Perform muscle biopsy.
c. Order antiacetylcholine receptor antibodies.
d. Perform nerve biopsy.
e. Order myelogram.

T-42. In small cell lung cancer, what is the most common endocrine syndrome?
a. Cushing's syndrome.
b. Addison's disease.
c. Diabetes mellitus.
d. Syndrome of inappropriate antidiuretic hormone.
e. Hypercalcemia due to parathyroid-like hormone.

T-43. The most common cause of hemoptysis is:
a. Bronchogenic carcinoma.
b. Bronchiectasis, with or without aspergilloma.
c. Tuberculosis (usually from cavitating sources).
d. Pulmonary infarction.
e. Chronic bronchitis.

T-44. Hilar adenopathy is common in the following conditions *except*:
a. Histoplasmosis.
b. Coccidioidomycosis.
c. Varicella zoster infection.
d. Blastomycosis.
e. Tropical eosinophilia.

T-45. The most important finding that distinguishes a benign from a malignant solitary pulmonary nodule is:
a. Size.
b. Regularity of borders.
c. Presence of cavitation or satellite lesions.
d. Growth over 2 years.
e. Homogeneity of the lesion.

T-46. The following statements apply to small cell carcinoma of the lung:

a. It is rarely found in smokers.
b. It classically presents as a hilar mass.
c. It can be diagnosed from a fine-needle aspirate.
d. Peripheral lesions are less likely to metastasize.
e. Thoracotomy is necessary for accurate diagnosis.

T-47. The following apply to the mediastinum:
a. The aortic arch and its branches are in the anterior mediastinum.
b. The thymus gland is in the superior mediastinum.
c. The phrenic nerve is in the middle mediastinum.
d. The vagus nerve is in the posterior mediastinum.
e. The sympathetic nervous chain is within the posterior mediastinum.

T-48. The following apply to mediastinal masses:
a. Germ cell tumors are the most common mediastinal masses.
b. Mediastinal masses occur most frequently in the posterior mediastinum.
c. In the anterior-superior mediastinum thymoma occurs most frequently .
d. Posterior mediastinal lesions are usually neurogenic tumors.
e. Bronchial cysts constitute most middle mediastinal lesions.

T-49. The following apply to mediastinal masses:
a. Pericardial cysts are usually seen in the left cardiophrenic angle.
b. Enteric cysts arise from the posterior division of the primitive foregut.
c. Inclusion cysts are usually located in the posterior mediastinum.
d. Enteric cysts usually communicate with the esophageal lumen.
e. Posterior mediastinal masses are most likely to be malignant.

T-50. The following apply to mediastinal masses:
a. The greatest proportion of malignant

mediastinal neoplasms occur in patients between 60 and 75 years of age.

b. The majority of neurogenic tumors in adults are malignant.

c. Neurogenic tumors occur most often in the middle mediastinum.

d. Intrathoracic fat protruding through the foramen of Morgagni will appear as a mediastinal mass.

e. CT yields a correct preoperative diagnosis in over 90% of patients.

T-51. The following apply to carmustine (BCNU) lung toxicity:

a. Incidence about 10% in acute exposures.

b. COPD increases risk.

c. Preexisting pneumoconiosis increases risk.

d. Tobacco exposure increases risk.

e. Focal angiitis may occur.

T-52. In BCNU pulmonary toxicity there is:

a. Alveolar epithelial metaplasia.

b. Loss of type I pneumocytes.

c. Dysplasia of type II pneumocytes.

d. A proteinaceous alveolar exudate.

e. Active inflammation.

T-53. The following apply to bronchial carcinoids:

a. They have the same neuroectodermal stem cell as small cell carcinoma.

b. A male predominance.

c. 70–80% arise centrally.

d. Central carcinoids often have a spindle-cell configuration.

e. They occur most often in the RUL/RML and lingula.

T-54. The following apply to "atypical" carcinoids:

a. They account for about 10% of all carcinoids.

b. Lymph node metastasis occurs in few cases.

c. They have areas of increased cellularity.

d. 5-year disease-free survival is greater than in typical carcinoid.

e. The vast majority exhibit the carcinoid syndrome.

T-55. The following apply to hamartoma:

a. It is composed of tissues that normally constitute the organ in which it occurs.

b. The tissue elements are immature.

c. True hamartoma grows inexorably and compresses the surrounding tissue.

d. Mesenchymomas contain a fibromyxomatous matrix and adipose tissue.

e. The male:female ratio is 1:2 or 1:3.

T-56. The following apply to hamartomas:

a. 90% are endobronchial and present centrally.

b. The peak incidence is in the third decade.

c. The risk of developing malignant degeneration is high.

d. Calcification is common.

e. The endobronchial variant has mostly adipose tissue.

T-57. The following statements apply to papillary thyroid carcinoma:

a. It is the most common type of thyroid carcinoma.

b. It arises from the thyroid follicular cell.

c. It is most often seen in young black males.

d. It is usually encapsulated.

e. It tends to spread to regional lymph nodes.

T-58. The following statements apply to papillary thyroid carcinoma:

a. Lungs are the dominant site for metastatic disease.

b. Localized pulmonary infiltration and hilar enlargement constitute the primary presentation of intrathoracic metastasis.

c. Chest roentgenogram can be clear in up to 40% of patients.

d. Therapy includes exogenous L-thyroxine.

e. Recurrence can occur as late as 25 years from presentation.

T-59. The following statements are correct:
a. A reduced thyroglobulin level in a patient with prior ablation is a good marker of recurrent thyroid carcinoma.
b. The ^{131}I total body scan is highly sensitive and specific for presence of disease.
c. False negative ^{131}I total body scan can occur if patients failed to discontinue exogenous thyroid supplementation prior to scan.
d. An elevated thyroglobulin is highly sensitive and specific for presence of disease.
e. False-positive total body scan has been reported in bronchiectasis.

T-60. The most common diagnosis of an anterior mediastinal mass is:
a. Thymoma.
b. Lymphoma.
c. Germ cell tumor.
d. Thyroid carcinoma.
e. Bronchogenic cysts.

T-61. The following statements apply to thymoma:
a. It is primarily a tumor of the 2nd to 3rd decades.
b. There is a predilection for males.
c. Myasthenia gravis occurs in approximately 35% of patients with thymomas.
d. About 15% of patients with myasthenia have thymomas.
e. Hypogammaglobulinemia is common.

T-62. The following statements about thymoma are true *except*:
a. Up to 50% of thymomas are undetectable on the PA chest roentgenogram.
b. In stage III there is invasion of neighboring structures.
c. Hematologic derangement is associated with spindle cell thymomas.
d. Treatment is extensive resection followed by radiation.
e. The epithelial subtype is associated with the best prognosis.

T-63. The following statements apply to thymoma:
a. The spindle cell type is benign.
b. The spindle cell subtype of epithelial tumor is associated with Good's syndrome.
c. Thymoma and hypogammaglobulinemia may be associated with T cell deficiency.
d. Thymectomy frequently results in remission of hypogammaglobulinemia.
e. Calcification distinguishes benign from malignant disease.

T-64. The following statements apply to thymoma *except*:
a. The thymus derives from endoderm of the third pharyngeal pouches.
b. The inferior horns of the third pharyngeal pouches become the parathyroid glands.
c. The gland regresses in size after adolescence and is replaced by fat.
d. Thymomas are slow-growing tumors.
e. Myasthenia gravis is a poor prognostic indicator.

T-65. The following apply to malignant non-Hodgkin's lymphoma:
a. It is one of the most common neoplastic complications of HIV infection.
b. It occurs predominantly in IV drug users with AIDS.
c. Most are T cell lymphomas.
d. Extranodal involvement is rare.
e. The lung is an uncommon site.

T-66. The following apply to HIV-associated pulmonary lymphoma:
a. Chest film findings are similar to those seen in non-AIDS patients.
b. Lymphadenopathy is uncommon in non-Hodgkin's lymphoma.
c. Coexistent opportunistic infections are uncommon in pulmonary non-Hodgkin's lymphoma.
d. There is an increased incidence of bacterial infections.

e. Sensitivity of fiberoptic bronchoscopy and transbronchial biopsy is greater than 75% in non-AIDS non-Hodgkin's lymphoma.

T-67. The following apply to patients with HIV:
a. Suppressed cell-mediated immunity is the hallmark of HIV infection.

b. Kaposi's sarcoma is seen predominantly in drug users.
c. Burkitt's lymphoma is associated with AIDS.
d. Nonspecific lymphocytic alveolitis is common.
e. Kaposi's sarcoma lesions in lung are more cellular than cutaneous ones.

1-4 Interstitial Disease

F-1. Pulmonary eosinophilic syndromes include:
a. Löffler's pneumonia.
b. Tropical eosinophilia.
c. Allergic bronchopulmonary aspergillosis (ABPA).
d. Churg-Strauss syndrome.
e. Eosinophilia with asthma.

F-2. Which of the following statements are true?
a. Churg-Strauss syndrome is the most likely diagnosis if a patient develops bronchiectasis, rhinitis, and sinusitis early in life.
b. Situs inversus may accompany the immotile cilia syndrome.
c. Central bronchiectasis is a major manifestation of allergic bronchopulmonary aspergillosis.
d. Asthma and allergic rhinitis are manifestations of the Churg-Strauss syndrome.
e. In the Churg-Strauss syndrome lesions are seen in the brain and kidneys.

F-3. In Löffler's syndrome there is:
a. Cough, malaise, low-grade temperature.
b. "Fleeting" peripheral pulmonary infiltrates on the chest film.
c. Hypoxemia usually.

d. A mild obstructive pattern.
e. Decreased $D_L CO$.

F-4. In Löffler's syndrome there can be:
a. Infiltration of eosinophils and macrophages into the interstitium.
b. Interstitial edema.
c. Collagen disruption.
d. Disruption of basement membranes.
e. Positive immunofluorescence.

F-5. In chronic eosinophilic pneumonia:
a. There can be drenching night sweats.
b. There can be hemoptysis.
c. There can be fluffy infiltrates in the apices and axillary regions on the chest film.
d. Circulating eosinophil count is always increased.
e. Biopsy shows giant cell infiltration.

F-6. In eosinophilic pneumonia there can be:
a. Spontaneous remission in 2–4 weeks.
b. Primary respiratory failure.
c. Eosinophilia in bronchoalveolar lavage (BAL) fluid.
d. Increased major basic protein.
e. Correlation with mycobacterial diseases.

F-7. The following apply to nervous system involvement in sarcoidosis:

a. It may occur at any stage of sarcoidosis.
b. Neurologic manifestations may occur prior to other signs.
c. Facial nerve paralysis can be bilateral.
d. Facial nerve paralysis is due to compression by an enlarged parotid gland.
e. The optic nerve is the most commonly involved cranial nerve.

F-8. The following apply to nervous system involvement in sarcoidosis:
a. Hearing loss may result from auditory nerve involvement.
b. Anosmia may occur from nasal mucosal disease.
c. Localized granulomatous mass lesions are predominantly infratentorial.
d. CT may uncover granulomas missed on MRI.
e. Treatment consists of steroids.

F-9. The following can be seen in sarcoidosis:
a. Diabetes insipidus.
b. Hyperprolactinemia.
c. Galactorrhea-amenorrhea syndrome.
d. Psychiatric manifestations.
e. Parkinsonism.

F-10. The following apply to nervous system involvement in sarcoidosis:
a. The prognosis for myopathy is better than that for cranial neuropathy.
b. Acute myopathy is more common in men.
c. CSF has neutrophil predominance in sarcoid meningitis.
d. CSF has decreased glucose in sarcoid meningitis.
e. Neuropathy most commonly involves peroneal nerves.

F-11. The following apply to respiratory bronchiolitis:
a. It is a disorder of nonsmokers.
b. It involves third- and fourth-generation respiratory bronchioles.
c. It is characterized by pigmented macrophages in respiratory bronchioles.

d. There is an associated thickening and fibrosis of alveolar septa.
e. Particles in macrophage cytoplasm stain with Prussian blue.

F-12. The following apply to respiratory bronchiolitis:
a. It is associated with interstitial lung disease (ILD).
b. There is an upper lung zone predominance.
c. It is characterized by flu-like onset.
d. Patchy reticulonodular infiltrates appear on chest roentgenogram.
e. It may look like desquamative interstitial pneumonitis.

F-13. In Goodpasture's syndrome:
a. There is a systemic vasculitis.
b. There is antibody directed against basement membrane.
c. Diffuse alveolar hemorrhage can occur without obvious renal disease.
d. Diffuse alveolar hemorrhage occurs predominantly in nonsmokers with Goodpasture's syndrome.
e. Exposure to volatile hydrocarbons and URIs are associated with exacerbation.

F-14. The following apply to systemic lupus erythematosus (SLE):
a. Male/female ratio is 10:1.
b. Subepithelial deposition of DNA on immunopathologic staining.
c. It is more common in African-American females.
d. Sulfonamides can precipitate a flair.
e. Leukocytoclastic vasculitis.

F-15. Pulmonary manifestations of systemic lupus erythematosus include:
a. Pleural effusion.
b. Pulmonary hypertension.
c. Pulmonary emboli.
d. Eosinophilic pneumonia.
e. Diaphragmatic weakness.

F-16. The following apply to acute lupus pneumonitis:
a. It may present as diffuse alveolar damage.

b. Bilateral pulmonary involvement is common.

c. It presents as an alveolar infiltrate with upper lobe predominance.

d. It can be the initial manifestation of the disease.

e. It can lead to progressive interstitial fibrosis.

F-17. Lymphangioleiomyomatosis (LAM):

a. Occurs primarily in women of reproductive age.

b. Can occur in postmenopausal women receiving estrogen supplementation.

c. Spontaneous pneumothorax occurs in approximately 50% of patients.

d. Chylous pleural effusions are common.

e. Chest roentgenogram can be normal.

F-18. The following apply to lymphangioleiomyomatosis:

a. Hallmark is abnormal proliferation of immature lung smooth muscle cells.

b. Smooth muscle has decreased glycogen stores.

c. Lymphatic obstruction can lead to ascites.

d. Obstruction of vessels can result in hemosiderosis/hemoptysis.

e. Restrictive process.

F-19. The following applies to lymphangioleiomyomatosis:

a. Airflow limitation is due to development of emphysema.

b. Symptoms are reduced with oral contraceptives.

c. Estrogen and progesterone receptors are decreased in lung tissue.

d. Patients with chylous ascites benefit from progesterone.

e. There is a correlation between estrogen receptor/progesterone receptor status and clinical response to hormonal interventions.

F-20. The following apply to acute beryllium disease:

a. It is dose related.

b. It presents with bronchospasm.

c. Treatment is with steroids.

d. It persists after the exposure is removed.

e. Long-term sequelae include bronchiectasis.

F-21. The following apply to chronic beryllium disease:

a. It affects only the lungs.

b. Renal stones are a manifestation.

c. Absence of hilar adenopathy differentiates it from sarcoidosis.

d. Absence of hypercalcemia differentiates it from sarcoidosis.

e. Pleural disease is a manifestation.

F-22. The following apply to chronic beryllium disease:

a. It can develop at variable times after exposure.

b. Lower zones are typically most affected.

c. Peripheral blood neutrophil response to beryllium is diagnostic.

d. Patch test may induce sensitization in unsensitized individuals.

e. Treatment is with lifelong steroids.

F-23. The following apply to polymyositis:

a. The presence of pulmonary fibrosis carries a high mortality rate.

b. Respiratory complaints may be the first major symptoms.

c. Pleuritic chest pain is rare.

d. Fatigue may obscure symptoms of muscle weakness.

e. Pulmonary fibrosis occurs late in polymyositis.

F-24. The following apply to polymyositis:

a. Muscle biopsy confirms the diagnosis in all cases.

b. Muscle involvement may be spotty.

c. Cryptogenic organizing pneumonia may be seen.

d. Anti-Jo1 antibodies signify a high ILD "risk."

e. Anti-Jo1 antibodies are a sensitive marker of ILD in polymyositis.

F-25. In diffuse alveolar hemorrhage with capillaritis there is:
   a. Lymphocytic invasion of the interstitium with fibrinoid necrosis and capillary thrombosis.
   b. Loss of integrity of the alveolar capillary membrane with leakage of RBCs into the alveolar space.
   c. Hemosiderin accumulation in the alveolar macrophages and the lung parenchyma.
   d. Organization of the alveolar hemorrhage.
   e. Type II cell hyperplasia.

F-26. The following apply to diffuse alveolar hemorrhage:
   a. Hemoptysis can be delayed.
   b. It can be caused by crack cocaine inhalation.
   c. It can be caused by penicillamine usage.
   d. It develops with renal disease on exposure to trimellitic anhydride.
   e. Presence of Kerley's B lines implies underlying mitral regurgitation.

F-27. The following apply to pulmonary vasculitis:
   a. $D_L CO$ is initially high and serial measurements increase.
   b. There are circulating immune IgA complexes in Henoch-Schönlein purpura.
   c. Only 20% of patients with Goodpasture's syndrome are nonsmokers.
   d. There is evidence of systemic vasculitis in Goodpasture's syndrome.
   e. Antiglomerular basement membrane antibodies are specific for Wegener's granulomatosis.

F-28. In Goodpasture's syndrome:
   a. Lung and renal disease appear simultaneously in most cases.
   b. The highest incidence is in females between 30 and 40 years of age.
   c. In older age groups, the disease is more likely to be renal limited.

   d. There is a high incidence of histocompatibility antigen HLA-DRw2.
   e. There is no relationship between severity of the renal disease and outcome.

F-29. In Wegener's granulomatosis (WG):
   a. Pulmonary capillaritis with diffuse alveolar hemorrhage can be present without typical pathologic changes or clinical presentation.
   b. A focal segmental necrotizing glomerulonephritis is uncommon.
   c. Typical histology consists of medium vessel involvement, tissue necrosis, and granulomatous inflammation.
   d. There is always a cutaneous leukocytoclastic vasculitis.
   e. Can only be differentiated from systemic necrotizing vasculitis by histology.

F-30. Systemic necrotizing vasculitis (microscopic polyarteritis):
   a. Has a predilection for the abdominal viscera.
   b. Characterized by extravascular granulomatous inflammation.
   c. Preceded by a protracted course of asthma and eosinophilia prior to the development of the systemic vasculitis.
   d. Focal segmental necrotizing glomerulonephritis is a consistent finding.
   e. Peripheral neuropathy is a feature.

F-31. The following apply to connective tissue disease:
   a. Diffuse alveolar hemorrhage is most common in scleroderma.
   b. Diffuse alveolar hemorrhage occurs without pulmonary capillaritis.
   c. Diffuse alveolar hemorrhage in SLE is immune complex–mediated.
   d. Anti-DNA antibody has been demonstrated in the lung.
   e. The underlying pathology of acute lupus pneumonitis is diffuse alveolar damage.

F-32. The following apply to Behçet's syndrome:

a. It is a chronic relapsing illness characterized by oral and genital ulceration.
b. Circulating immune complexes have been identified.
c. The lung is involved in virtually all cases.
d. There is a focal segmental necrotizing glomerulonephritis.
e. Bronchial and large pulmonary arterial involvement leads to aneurysms.

F-33. The following statements are true:
a. Henoch-Schönlein purpura presents with the purpuric rash and glomerulonephritis.
b. Henoch-Schönlein purpura is an immune complex–mediated disease.
c. In Henoch-Schönlein purpura, circulating antibody directed against IgG is found.
d. Pauci-immune glomerulonephritis is a renal-limited vasculitis.
e. Diffuse alveolar hemorrhage is common in immune complex–related glomerulonephritis.

F-34. Churg-Strauss syndrome is characterized by:
a. Pulmonary necrotizing angiitis.
b. Systemic necrotizing angiitis.
c. Extravascular granulomas.
d. Occurring almost exclusively in asthma patients or those with an allergic history.
e. Involvement of arteries but not veins.

F-35. The following apply to vasculitis:
a. Polyarteritis nodosa is characterized by necrotizing vasculitis of large arteries.
b. Cavitation and hilar adenopathy are features of necrotizing sarcoid granulomatosis.
c. Pulmonary involvement in Behçet's syndrome consists of thromboangiitis.
d. The vasculitis in Wegener's granulomatosis involves pulmonary veins.
e. Non-necrotizing granulomas involve larger vessels in Wegener's granulomatosis.

F-36. The following statements apply to idiopathic pulmonary hemosiderosis (IPH):
a. Diagnosis is one of exclusion.
b. It is predominantly a disease of children and young adults.
c. It has a male predominance.
d. It shows widespread alveolar-filling opacities on chest roentgenogram.
e. Clubbing can result.

F-37. The following statements apply to idiopathic pulmonary hemosiderosis:
a. There are reduced lung volumes and diffusing capacity.
b. Alveoli are flooded with hemosiderin-laden macrophages.
c. Vasculitis is prominent.
d. Immunofluorescent stains are positive.
e. There is degeneration of type I pneumocytes.

F-38. The following statements apply to idiopathic pulmonary hemosiderosis:
a. It is characterized by recurrent diffuse alveolar hemorrhage without other organ involvement.
b. There is evidence of marked inflammation and hemosiderin accumulation.
c. Separation, splits, and ruptures of the alveolar-capillary basement membrane are noted on electron microscopy.
d. IgA immune complexes are present in the lung.
e. Female:male ratio is 2:1.

F-39. The following are true:
a. C-ANCA is an antibody causing cytoplasmic staining and directed against proteinase 3.
b. P-ANCA is an antibody causing perinuclear staining and directed against myeloperoxidase.
c. C-ANCA is more likely to be elevated in vasculitides primarily involving kidney.
d. P-ANCA is more likely to be elevated if the upper respiratory tract is involved.

e. Circulating immune complexes are found in Henoch-Schönlein purpura.

F-40. Which of the following is true of amyloidosis?
   a. It is characterized by extracellular accumulation of an A-pleated fibrillar protein.
   b. Light-chain amyloid is associated with secondary amyloidosis.
   c. Amyloid A is found with primary amyloidosis.
   d. Primary amyloid deposition occurs without an associated disease.
   e. Diffuse parenchymal infiltrates involving the alveolar septa and the walls of small blood vessels is common in secondary amyloidosis.

F-41. Radiographic features of amyloidosis may include all of the following *except*:
   a. Atelectasis.
   b. Interstitial infiltrates.
   c. Hilar lymphadenopathy.
   d. Multiple parenchymal nodules.
   e. Pleural effusion.

F-42. Which of the following is true of acute hypersensitivity pneumonitis?
   a. It is associated with exposure to finely dispersed organic dusts.
   b. Dyspnea occurs within an hour following exposure.
   c. Fever, chills, cough, and chest tightness occur 2 hours after antigen exposure.
   d. It resolves immediately after removal from exposure.
   e. BAL CD 4+ T lymphocytes are increased.

F-43. All of the following are present in BOOP or cryptogenic organizing pneumonia *except*:
   a. Granulation tissue plugs within, and complete obstruction of, small airways.
   b. Extension of the granulation tissue into the alveoli.
   c. Intraluminal polyps comprised of connective tissue.

d. Alveolar accumulations of macrophages.
e. Fibrosis of alveolar walls.

F-44. Similar histologic findings can be seen in:
   a. Idiopathic BOOP.
   b. Connective tissue diseases.
   c. Cocaine abuse.
   d. Drug reactions.
   e. Myelodysplastic syndrome.

F-45. Clinical features of BOOP are:
   a. History of a flu-like illness in 85% of cases.
   b. Mild dyspnea.
   c. Cough with dyspnea.
   d. Hemoptysis.
   e. End inspiratory crackles.

F-46. The following apply to BOOP *except*:
   a. Mean duration of symptoms at presentation of 24 months.
   b. Bilateral patchy infiltrates which are often fleeting.
   c. Bilateral airspace consolidation and nodular opacities on chest CT.
   d. Airway obstruction.
   e. An increase in BAL lymphocytes.

F-47. The following may apply to pulmonary alveolar proteinosis:
   a. Pleuritic chest pain.
   b. Digital clubbing.
   c. Elevated lactate dehydrogenase.
   d. Unilateral nodular pattern on chest radiograph.
   e. Bilateral symmetric peripheral alveolar infiltrates.

F-48. The following apply to pulmonary alveolar proteinosis *except*:
   a. It can occur in infants.
   b. It has greater prevalence in females.
   c. It can be seen in *Pneumocystis carinii* pneumonia (PCP) infection.
   d. It is seen in patients exposed to fiberglass.
   e. It is seen in individuals exposed to volcanic ash.

F-49. In alveolar proteinosis, deposition of intra-alveolar phospholipids is due to:
   a. Excessive proliferation and desquamation of type II pneumocytes.
   b. Unproven cause.
   c. Overproduction of alveolar phospholipids.
   d. Increased secretion of lamellar bodies into the alveoli.
   e. Prolonged retention of alveolar lipoproteins.

F-50. The following apply to pulmonary alveolar proteinosis:
   a. Excessive alveolar macrophages in BAL fluid.
   b. Large acellular eosinophilic bodies.
   c. Periodic acid-Schiff staining of proteinaceous material.
   d. Elevated LDH.
   e. Increased shunt fraction.

F-51. The following apply to pulmonary alveolar proteinosis:
   a. Excessive intra-alveolar proteins.
   b. Tubular myelin in the extracellular alveolar lining layer.
   c. Irregular myelin structures in the alveolar substance.
   d. Increased alveolar phospholipids.
   e. Decreased dipalmitoyl lecithin.

F-52. The following are characteristic of Löffler's syndrome:
   a. Migratory pulmonary infiltrates.
   b. Absent or mild symptoms.
   c. The entire picture lasts less than 1 month.
   d. The lung is apparently the only organ involved.
   e. Increased serum IgE.

F-53. In bronchiolitis obliterans with organizing pneumonia:
   a. There is a febrile onset, followed by progressive dyspnea and cough.
   b. There are Masson bodies on histology.
   c. There are buds of organizing granulation tissue.

   d. The involved bronchioles are usually the terminal bronchioles.
   e. Physiology is typically obstructive in nature.

F-54. The following statements pertain to bronchiolitis obliterans with organizing pneumonia:
   a. Lymphocytes comprise more than 50% of the cells recovered by bronchoalveolar lavage.
   b. Treatment with corticosteroids results in rapid improvement.
   c. Chest radiograph shows patchy areas of airspace consolidation.
   d. Uniform temporal maturity of lesions is characteristic.
   e. Predominantly intrabronchiolar distribution.

F-55. Match the pathology with the diagnosis (1 = BOOP; 2 = idiopathic pulmonary fibrosis [IPF]):
   a. Diffuse random distribution of lesions.
   b. Predominantly airspace location.
   c. Fibrosis is fibroblastic in nature.
   d. Lesions are of varying ages.
   e. Foamy macrophages are common.

F-56. The following statements pertain to bronchiolitis obliterans with organizing pneumonia:
   a. Corticosteroids should be administered for one month.
   b. There is epithelial necrosis and denudation of epithelial basal laminae.
   c. A diffuse patchy ground-glass appearance is common on chest film.
   d. Infiltrates may be unilateral.
   e. A pleural effusion rules out bronchiolitis obliterans with organizing pneumonia.

F-57. Bronchiolitis obliterans may be associated with all of the following *except*:
   a. Measles.
   b. Inhalation of sulfur dioxide.
   c. Rheumatoid arthritis.
   d. Allergic bronchopulmonary aspergillosis.
   e. Administration of penicillamine.

F-58. The following statements pertain to bronchiolitis obliterans without organizing pneumonia:
   a. It is characterized by extension of granulation tissue organization from the distal alveolar ducts into alveoli.
   b. The chest radiograph shows linear interstitial markings.
   c. It is a common pathologic finding in connective tissue disorders.
   d. Toxic fume inhalation and organ transplantation are causes.
   e. Cadmium oxide has been associated with this condition.

F-59. The following statements pertain to bronchiolitis obliterans without organizing pneumonia:
   a. It is commonly due to the respiratory syncytial virus in adults.
   b. In children it is commonly due to *Mycoplasma pneumoniae*.
   c. The radiographic pattern is often interstitial, frequently with hyperinflation.
   d. Physiologically the pattern may be restrictive or obstructive.
   e. It may follow noncardiogenic pulmonary edema due to exposure to high concentrations of NO_2.

F-60. A common problem in eosinophilic granuloma which may be the first indicator of pulmonary disease is:
   a. Pleural effusion.
   b. Hemoptysis.
   c. Congestive heart failure.
   d. Spontaneous pneumothorax.
   e. Atelectasis.

F-61. The most prominent cells on biopsy in a case of eosinophilic granuloma are:
   a. Eosinophils.
   b. Foamy macrophages.
   c. Neutrophils.
   d. Mast cells.
   e. Lymphocytes.

F-62. Goodpasture's syndrome (GS) is characterized by:

a. Immune alveolar hemorrhage.
   b. A crescentic glomerulonephritis with widespread necrosis of glomeruli.
   c. Antiglomerular basement membrane antibodies in serum.
   d. ESR more elevated than in the vasculitides.
   e. Occurrence predominantly in nonsmokers.

F-63. In Goodpasture's syndrome:
   a. There is a female predominance.
   b. Direct immunofluorescence reveals deposition of IgG along the glomerular basement membrane.
   c. Serum complement is elevated.
   d. Antinuclear antibody (ANA) is positive.
   e. Plasmapheresis lowers antiglomerular basement membrane antibodies.

F-64. The following statements apply to pulmonary fibrosis:
   a. Sjögren's syndrome occurs in patients with lymphocytic interstitial pneumonitis.
   b. Lymphocytic interstitial pneumonitis is more common in males than in females.
   c. Lymphocytic interstitial pneumonitis can develop in AIDS.
   d. Giant cell formation is common in desquamative interstitial pneumonitis.
   e. In bronchiolitis obliterans with organizing pneumonia there is an organizing pneumonia in alveolar ducts.

F-65. The following statements apply to idiopathic pulmonary fibrosis (IPF):
   a. Lesions in collagen vascular disease are indistinguishable from IPF.
   b. Rheumatoid factor is elevated in usual interstitial pneumonitis (UIP).
   c. Circulating immune complexes are elevated in usual interstitial pneumonitis.
   d. Immunofluorescence shows immunoglobulin and complement in the bronchiolar walls.

e. The median survival in UIP is 12 years.

F-66. The following statements apply to idiopathic pulmonary fibrosis:
a. In usual interstitial pneumonitis the bulk of interstitial cells are neutrophils.
b. Honeycombing is characterized by dilated bronchioles.
c. Usual interstitial pneumonitis is a disease of nonsmokers.
d. Drug reactions may cause a mixed round cell interstitial infiltrate.
e. Desquamative interstitial pneumonia (DIP) is characterized by large numbers of desquamated type II cells in the airspaces.

F-67. The following statements apply to interstitial lung disease:
a. Lymphocytic interstitial pneumonia is seen following nitrofurantoin therapy.
b. The prognosis of usual interstitial pneumonia is considerably better than that of desquamative interstitial pneumonia.
c. In desquamative interstitial pneumonia there is a ground-glass pattern of opacification in the costophrenic angle on chest radiographs.
d. Lymphocytic interstitial pneumonia can be characterized by an interstitial infiltrate of plasma cells.
e. Patients with lymphocytic interstitial pneumonia have a serum gammopathy.

F-68. The following are characteristic of eosinophilic pneumonia:
a. Blood eosinophilia is the rule.
b. Tissue eosinophilia is a major finding.
c. Hemoptysis is a predominant complaint.
d. Steroids are generally effective therapy.
e. Radiographic changes in the lung are central.

F-69. Correct statements in pulmonary fibrosis include the following:

a. FRC is reduced.
b. The pressure-volume curve is shifted up and to the left.
c. Flow rates are low.
d. Flow resistance is normal.
e. The only abnormality may be a fall in PaO_2 during exercise.

F-70. The following statements apply to sarcoidosis:
a. The most common form of CNS involvement is VIIth nerve palsy.
b. Aseptic meningitis is a common CNS abnormality.
c. There is usually loss of hormones from the anterior pituitary.
d. The Guillain-Barré syndrome may be seen in sarcoidosis.
e. Neurologic sarcoidosis responds well to corticosteroids.

F-71. The following are manifestations of rheumatoid arthritis:
a. Usual interstitial pneumonitis.
b. Pleural effusion.
c. Necrobiotic nodules.
d. Caplan's syndrome.
e. Pulmonary arteritis and hypertension.

F-72. In patients with rheumatoid disease:
a. Extra-articular disease occurs in patients with the least severe joint involvement.
b. The majority of patients with pleuropulmonary disease have a positive sheep cell agglutination for rheumatoid factor.
c. The D_LCO and static compliance are generally abnormal.
d. Obliterative bronchiolitis common in rheumatoid disease is treated with penicillamine.
e. Patients with rheumatoid lung nodules have a relatively good prognosis.

F-73. The following statements pertain to nitrofurantoin toxicity:
a. Pulmonary toxicity to nitrofurantoin is an acute hypersensitivity reaction.

b. Nitrofurantoin may induce local production of superoxide in the lung.

c. Patients may have taken the drug previously without difficulty.

d. The chest roentgenogram may be normal.

e. Fibrosis is a late manifestation and only occurs in patients who have received therapy for more than 5 years.

F-74. The following statements apply to extrinsic allergic alveolitis:

a. It is uncommon in nonsmokers.

b. The infiltrate is predominantly of lymphocytes mixed with plasma cells.

c. The dominant lesion is interstitial pneumonia.

d. There is inflammation of the distal respiratory bronchioles.

e. The presence of bronchiolitis obliterans rules out extrinsic allergic alveolitis.

F-75. The following apply to lymphangioleiomyomatosis:

a. It afflicts only women.

b. Perivascular and alveolar smooth muscle-like cells.

c. Chylous pleural effusions.

d. Ascites.

e. Progesterone may be helpful.

F-76. The following apply to lymphangioleiomyomatosis:

a. Hemoptysis.

b. Emphysema.

c. Recurrent pneumothorax.

d. Relentless dyspnea.

e. Angiomyolipomas of the kidney.

F-77. The following apply to tuberous sclerosis:

a. It is an autosomal dominant disease.

b. Seizures.

c. Lung pathology indistinguishable from lymphangioleiomyomatosis.

d. Adenoma sebaceum.

e. Angiomyolipomas of the kidney.

F-78. The following apply to chronic beryllium disease:

a. It tends to follow a less aggressive course than sarcoidosis.

b. Lymphocytes sensitized to beryllium undergo blastic transformation with uptake of tritiated thymidine on exposure to antigen.

c. The Kveim skin test is a sensitive test of exposure and sensitization to beryllium.

d. The lymphocyte response is more consistent and sensitive in blood than in BAL lymphocytes.

e. The lymphocyte transformation test is altered by steroid therapy.

F-79. Chronic beryllium disease is unlike sarcoid in that:

a. Isolated hilar adenopathy is rare.

b. The T4:T8 ratio is decreased peripherally.

c. There is no helper T cell accumulation in the lung.

d. Reticulonodular infiltrates are present without hilar adenopathy.

e. There is an obstructive ventilatory defect.

F-80. The following apply to chronic beryllium disease *except*:

a. It occurs in nuclear and aerospace industries.

b. Acute beryllium disease is limited to the respiratory system.

c. ACE levels are normal.

d. There are sarcoid-like clinical, radiographic, and physiologic abnormalities.

e. Serum immunoglobulins may be elevated.

F-81. The following apply to allogeneic bone marrow transplantation:

a. It is marrow harvested from a non-twin sibling.

b. Idiopathic interstitial pneumonia is less common than in autologous recipients.

c. Diffuse alveolar hemorrhage is less common than in autologous recipients.

d. Graft-versus-host disease is less common than in autologous recipients.

e. CMV pneumonitis is less common than in autologous recipients.

F-82. The following statements apply to interstitial lung disease:
a. Pulmonary involvement in connective tissue disease is easily distinguishable from idiopathic pulmonary fibrosis.
b. Interstitial pneumonitis is commonly found in patients with progressive systemic sclerosis.
c. A restrictive pattern and impaired diffusing capacity are often seen before clinical or radiographic evidence of lung disease in scleroderma.
d. Chlorambucil causes fibrosis in a dose-dependent manner.
e. Concomitant use of oxygen exerts synergistic effects in drug-induced lung disease.

F-83. The following statements apply to interstitial lung disease:
a. Lung disease results in 20–50% of patients with cumulative doses of 200–550 units of bleomycin.
b. Nitrofurantoin may cause an acute, spontaneously resolving pneumonitis and eosinophilia.
c. There is a characteristic X-body within the histiocytes obtained from lung biopsy tissue or bronchoalveolar lavage in eosinophilic granuloma of the lung.
d. Lymphangioleiomyomatosis afflicts postmenopausal women.
e. The mean survival in idiopathic pulmonary fibrosis is 12 years.

F-84. The following apply to talc pneumoconiosis except:
a. Spirometry is restrictive and D_LCO is reduced.
b. The degree of fibrosis is related to the duration and degree of dust exposure.
c. Mesothelioma is four times more common with significant talc exposure.
d. The natural history of talc pneumoconiosis is very different from other pneumoconioses.

e. Radiographic characteristics include parenchymal and pleural abnormalities.

F-85. The following apply to alveolar proteinosis except:
a. The intraalveolar material consists of glycoproteins and lipids that make up normal pulmonary surfactant.
b. Occupational exposure to silica, asbestos, or cadmium is found in 50% of cases.
c. It results from an increased production of surfactant by alveolar type 2 lining cells.
d. There is decreased function of alveolar macrophages.
e. It occurs with chronic myelocytic leukemia.

F-86. The following apply to alveolar proteinosis except:
a. Nocardiosis is a fairly common complication.
b. The diagnosis is established by demonstrating the positive periodic acid–Schiff staining of the intraalveolar material.
c. The alveolar walls may show type II cell hyperplasia.
d. Therapeutic whole lung lavage with normal saline is effective.
e. Eosinophils are predominant in the lung tissue.

F-87. The following apply to the CREST syndrome except:
a. Telangiectasia.
b. Raynaud's phenomenon.
c. Esophageal dysfunction.
d. Ataxia.
e. Sclerodactyly.

F-88. Eosinophilic pneumonia is characterized by the following except:
a. An indolent progressive form of dyspnea and cough.
b. Recurrent fever, cough, and dyspnea.
c. Asthmatic symptoms.

d. A central distribution of the alveolar infiltrates.

e. Peripheral eosinophilia.

F-89. The following apply to eosinophilic pneumonia *except*:
a. Follow helminthic infestations.
b. Associated with a drug reaction.
c. Allergic bronchopulmonary aspergillosis.
d. Idiopathic form is more common in men.
e. Associated with tropical eosinophilia.

F-90. Rheumatoid arthritis is associated with the following *except*:
a. Pleurisy with or without effusion.
b. Uremic pulmonary edema.
c. Necrobiotic nodules (nonpneumoconiotic intrapulmonary rheumatoid nodules) with or without cavities.
d. Bronchiolitis obliterans.
e. Upper airway obstruction due to arytenoid arthritis.

F-91. Match the BAL findings with the condition:
a. Sarcoidosis.
b. Eosinophilic pneumonia.
c. Alveolar proteinosis.
d. Lipoid pneumonia.
e. Diffuse alveolar hemorrhage.

1. Lipoproteinaceous bodies.
2. Hemosiderin-laden macrophages.
3. Lipid-laden macrophages.
4. Eosinophils.
5. T helper lymphocytes.

F-92. The following apply to BAL fluid lymphocytes in sarcoidosis:
a. They have decreased reaction when exposed to mitogens.
b. They spontaneously proliferate and secrete IL-l.
c. They have decreased IL-2 secretion/receptors.
d. The suppressor:helper T cell ratio is high.

e. They secrete macrophage inhibitory factor.

F-93. The following are causes of alveolar hemorrhage *except*:
a. Anti–basement membrane antibody disease.
b. Systemic lupus erythematosus.
c. Eosinophilic granuloma.
d. Idiopathic pulmonary hemosiderosis.
e. D-Penicillamine.

F-94. The following apply to lymphocytic interstitial pneumonitis:
a. It has the histologic features of pseudolymphoma.
b. Hilar adenopathy is common.
c. It involves extrapulmonary tissues.
d. It is predominant in males.
e. It can occur in chronic active hepatitis.

F-95. The following statements apply to occupational lung diseases:
a. Silicosis often occurs in association with coal worker's pneumoconiosis.
b. Simple coal worker's pneumoconiosis is represented by small opacities in the lower lung zones.
c. Opacities are ≥1 cm in diameter in progressive massive fibrosis.
d. Simple coal worker's pneumoconiosis causes significant pulmonary function abnormalities.
e. Patients with progressive massive fibrosis may expectorate large quantities of dark sputum.

F-96. The pleuropulmonary manifestations of systemic lupus erythematosus are:
a. Pleurisy with or without effusion.
b. Atelectasis.
c. Acute interstitial pneumonitis.
d. Chronic interstitial pneumonia.
e. Predominance in males.

F-97. The following apply to eosinophilic pneumonia:
a. Cough, sputum production, and fever of several months' duration.

b. Asthmatic symptoms.

c. Central distribution of the alveolar infiltrates.

d. Absence of peripheral eosinophilia rules out this diagnosis.

e. It responds to corticosteroids.

F-98. Match the feature with the condition—silicosis (S) or asbestosis (A):

a. Irregular small opacities especially in the lower lung zones.

b. Found in glass manufacturers.

c. Calcified pleural plaques.

d. Susceptible to infection by atypical mycobacteria.

e. Bronchogenic carcinoma is a recognized complication.

F-99. Match the feature with the condition—silicosis (S) or asbestosis (A).

a. Scleroderma may complicate.

b. Smoking facilitates the damaging effects.

c. Bilateral pleural thickening.

d. Multinodular rounded densities in upper lung zones.

e. Workers in textile industries.

F-100. The following statements apply to talc pneumoconiosis:

a. Talc is used in leather industries.

b. The lung clears talc dust by lymphatic drainage, thereby preventing pulmonary tissue damage.

c. Lung clearance is hindered by cigarette smoke.

d. Talc induces a macrophage-mediated inflammatory response.

e. Fibrous talc can produce tumorigenesis.

F-101. The following statements apply to talc pneumoconiosis:

a. Talc and asbestos are mineralogically related.

b. Quartz is not fibrogenic.

c. Talc mined in Vermont contains only traces of quartz and asbestiform minerals.

d. Cosmetic-grade talc contains the highest quantity of asbestos and quartz.

e. Grade of talc is the major determinant in the development of talc pneumoconiosis.

F-102. The following apply to eosinophilic granuloma:

a. It can be associated with lytic bone lesions of pelvis and diabetes insipidus.

b. Peripheral blood eosinophilia is a feature.

c. It occurs almost exclusively in cigarette smokers.

d. Pneumothorax occurs in around 25% of the patients.

e. Inspiratory crackles are usual on physical examination.

F-103. Radiographically, eosinophilic granuloma shows:

a. Diffuse, symmetric increase in interstitial parenchymal markings.

b. Predominance in the lower and mid lung zones.

c. Volume loss.

d. Cavitating nodules progressing to honeycombing.

e. Pleural effusion is common.

F-104. The following apply to eosinophilic granuloma:

a. Cutaneous involvement is associated with a worse prognosis.

b. Nodules and thin-walled cysts on high-resolution CT scan.

c. Reduced lung volume.

d. Normal D_LCO.

e. Hypoxemia.

F-105. The following apply to eosinophilic granuloma:

a. Blebs or cysts on the lung surface on gross examination.

b. Absence of granulomatous lesions in the interstitium microscopically.

c. Cells with weakly basophilic cytoplasm and irregular folded and indented nucleus.

d. Intracytoplasmic inclusion bodies called Masson bodies on electron microscopy.

e. S-100 protein immunostaining differentiates Langerhans' cells from other histiocytes.

F-106. The following apply to serum IgG antibodies against neutrophil cytoplasmic components (ANCA):

a. They are present in segmental necrotizing glomerulonephritis.

b. They are present in Wegener's granulomatosis.

c. Serum titers correlate with disease activity.

d. The basis for the nuclear binding of the C-ANCA is the artifactitious redistribution of soluble cytoplasmic antigens to the nucleus.

e. Both C-ANCA and P-ANCA produce identical diffuse granular cytoplasmic staining when formalin-fixed neutrophils are used as substrate.

F-107. The following apply to serum IgG antibodies against neutrophil cytoplasmic components (ANCA):

a. Most P-ANCA in pauci-immune necrotizing glomerulonephritis is specific for myeloperoxidase.

b. ANCA are found in patients with microscopic poyarteritis nodosa.

c. ANCA are found in patients with idiopathic crescentic glomerulonephritis.

d. The glomerular lesions in Wegener's granulomatosis are specific to that disease.

e. There is marked extracapillary crescent formation in necrotizing vasculitis.

F-108. The following apply to serum IgG antibodies against neutrophil cytoplasmic components (ANCA):

a. The type of ANCA correlates with the distribution of disease.

b. P-ANCA is most commonly seen in vasculitis involving the lung, sinus, and kidney.

c. C-ANCA is more likely to be positive in patients with renal limited disease.

d. The frequency of C-ANCA and P-ANCA is equal in patients with systemic arteritis who have necrotizing granulomas.

e. A positive ANCA distinguishes between pauci-immune necrotizing glomerulonephritis and Goodpasture's disease.

F-109. Immune complexes are implicated with:

a. Postinfectious glomerulonephritis.

b. Cryoglobulinemia.

c. Henoch-Schönlein purpura.

d. Lupus erythematosus.

e. Goodpasture's or renal-limited anti-glomerular basement membrane disease.

F-110. The following statements are true:

a. A positive ANCA in the face of rapidly progressive glomerulonephritis is adequate basis for initiating treatment without a biopsy.

b. An open biopsy differentiates between Wegener's granulomatosis and microscopic polyarteritis nodosa.

c. Treatment of microscopic polyarteritis nodosa is combined steroid and cyclophosphamide.

d. Steroids alone are treatment of choice in Wegener's granulomatosis.

e. The ANCA subtype does not change during the course of disease.

F-111. In idiopathic crescentic glomerulonephritis:

a. There is a history of a flu-like illness.

b. Pulmonary infiltrates or cavitary lesions are absent on the chest radiograph.

c. C-ANCA is positive.

d. Open lung biopsy reveals evidence of vasculitis.

e. Cyclophosphamide is the therapy of choice.

F-112. Indicate the condition, either Wegener's granulomatosis (WG) or Churg-Strauss syndrome (CSS), in which the clinical features are most characteristic:

	WG	CSS
a. Mononeuritis multiplex.	____	____
b. Anticytoplasmic antibodies.	____	____
c. Alveolar infiltrates.	____	____
d. Tissue eosinophilia.	____	____
e. Response to steroids alone.	____	____

F-113. Indicate the condition, either Wegener's granulomatosis (WG) or Churg-Strauss syndrome (CSS), in which the clinical features are most characteristic:

	WG	CSS
a. Asthma.	____	____
b. Peripheral blood eosinophilia.	____	____
c. Renal disease.	____	____
d. Cutaneous nodules.	____	____
e. Cardiac abnormalities.	____	____

F-114. The following statements apply to lymphomatoid granulomatosis:
a. An angiocentric and angiodestructive lymphoreticular proliferation.
b. Confined to the lungs.
c. Progresses to lymphoma.
d. 5-year survival rate greater than 70% with steroid therapy.
e. Morphologic and clinical similarity to polymorphic reticulosis.

F-115. The following are typical lesions of Wegener's granulomatosis *except*:
a. Necrotizing granulomas.
b. Discrete granulomas.
c. Central zone of necrosis surrounded by lymphocytes, plasma cells, and histiocytes.
d. Prominent eosinophils.
e. Necrotizing angiitis.

F-116. The following statements apply to idiopathic pulmonary hemosiderosis:
a. Clubbing may be seen.
b. It is predominantly a disease of children and young adults.

c. It has a male predominance.
d. There are widespread alveolar-filling opacities on chest roentgenogram.
e. It can result in cor pulmonale.

F-117. In Wegener's granulomatosis:
a. Pulmonary capillaritis with diffuse alveolar hemorrhage can be present.
b. Necrotizing glomerulonephritis is uncommon.
c. Medium vessel involvement, tissue necrosis, and granulomatous inflammation are present.
d. There is a cutaneous leukocytoclastic vasculitis.
e. Histology differentiates it from systemic necrotizing vasculitis.

F-118. In benign lymphocytic angiitis and granulomatosis:
a. Most patients present in their late fifties with fever, nonproductive cough, dyspnea, and chest pain.
b. There are bilateral patchy or nodular infiltrates on chest roentgenogram.
c. Cavities are common.
d. The disease is widely distributed in the body in the vast majority of cases.
e. Giant cell granulomas are noted on biopsy.

F-119. The following statements apply to autologous bone marrow transplant patients:
a. They have the same spectrum of complications as those undergoing allogeneic bone marrow transplants.
b. Diffuse alveolar hemorrhage in immunocompromised hosts occurs in association with thrombocytopenia.
c. Patients with diffuse alveolar hemorrhage most often present with hemoptysis.
d. The frequency of diffuse alveolar hemorrhage is higher in patients less than 40 years of age.
e. Diffuse alveolar hemorrhage can occur 1 to 2 years after autologous bone marrow transplant.

F-120. The following apply to vasculitis:
  a. Polyarteritis nodosa is characterized by necrotizing vasculitis of large arteries.
  b. Cavitation and hilar adenopathy are features of necrotizing sarcoid granulomatosis.
  c. Behçet's syndrome consists of pulmonary thromboangiitis and multiple aneurysms.
  d. The vasculitis in Wegener's granulomatosis involves capillaries.
  e. Sarcoid-like non-necrotizing granulomas are common in Wegener's granulomatosis.

F-121. The following statements apply to idiopathic pulmonary hemosiderosis:
  a. Diagnosis is one of exclusion.
  b. It is predominantly a disease of children and young adults.
  c. It has a male predominance.
  d. Most common presentation consists of periodic episodes of cough and hemoptysis with widespread alveolar-filling opacities on chest roentgenogram.
  e. It can result in bronchiectasis.

F-122. Treatment for systemic vasculitis consists of:
  a. Corticosteroids.
  b. Watchful expectancy.
  c. BCNU.
  d. Cyclophosphamide.
  e. A combination of corticosteroids and cyclophosphamide.

F-123. The following statements apply to granulomatosis and vasculitis:
  a. Necrotizing sarcoid granulomatosis is more common in males.
  b. The arteries and veins are both affected in necrotizing sarcoid granulomatosis.
  c. Vasculitis of the systemic vessels is common in necrotizing sarcoid granulomatosis.
  d. Lymphomatoid granulomatosis is an angiocentric T cell lymphoma.

  e. Bronchocentric granulomatosis is caused by hypersensitivity to aspergillus.

F-124. The following statements apply to granulomatosis and vasculitis:
  a. Wegener's granulomatosis is more common in women.
  b. The diagnosis can be made from a transbronchial or needle biopsy.
  c. The pulmonary lesions of Churg-Strauss syndrome may resemble chronic eosinophilic pneumonia.
  d. Churg-Strauss syndrome differs from polyarteritis in that both the arteries and the veins are involved.
  e. In Churg-Strauss syndrome the pulmonary blood vessels are affected predominantly.

F-125. The following are characterized by tissue necrosis, a granulomatous reaction, and angiitis:
  a. Wegener's granulomatosis.
  b. Limited Wegener's granulomatosis.
  c. Lymphomatoid granulomatosis.
  d. Necrotizing sarcoid angiitis and granulomatosis.
  e. Bronchocentric granulomatosis.

F-126. Match the disorder with the first line therapy:
  a. Lymphomatoid granulomatosis.
  b. Benign lymphocytic angiitis.
  c. Wegener's granulomatosis.
  d. Bronchocentric granulomatosis.
  e. Allergic granulomatosis.

  1. Cyclophosphamide and steroids.
  2. Resection of involved lobe.
  3. Chlorambucil.
  4. Cyclophosphamide.
  5. Corticosteroids.

F-127. Match the disorder with the predominant clinical findings:
  a. Lymphomatoid granulomatosis.
  b. Benign lymphocytic angiitis.
  c. Wegener's granulomatosis.

d. Bronchocentric granulomatosis.

e. Allergic granulomatosis.

1. Multiple nodular densities wax and wane.
2. Unilateral lesions of upper lobe.
3. Extrapulmonary sites are rare.
4. Severe progressive asthma.

F-128. Match the disorder with the predominant inflammatory cell:
a. Lymphomatoid granulomatosis.
b. Polyarteritis nodosa.
c. Wegener's granulomatosis.
d. Bronchocentric granulomatosis.
e. Allergic granulomatosis.

1. Polymorphonuclears.
2. Eosinophils.
3. Atypical lymphoid cells.

F-129. Radiographically, patients with Wegener's granulomatosis can have:
a. Fleeting infiltrates.
b. Cavities.
c. Nodules.
d. Pleural effusion.
e. Atelectasis.

F-130. The following apply to the limited form of Wegener's granulomatosis:
a. It occurs in approximately 15% of patients with Wegener's granulomatosis.
b. It does not involve the kidney.
c. It has a favorable response to steroids.
d. It has a longer duration of remission.
e. It has a shorter survival without the use of steroid therapy.

1-5 Vascular Disease

V-1. Progressive clinical deterioration in multiple pulmonary emboli is due to:
a. Recurrent emboli.
b. Propagation of existing clot.
c. RV dysfunction associated with hypoxemia and severe pulmonary hypertension.
d. Hypertensive changes in unobstructed areas of the pulmonary vasculature.
e. Opening of the foramen ovale.

V-2. There may be one or more segmental or larger unmatched perfusion defects on $\overset{\circ}{V}/\overset{\circ}{Q}$ (ventilation/perfusion) scan in:
a. Primary pulmonary hypertension.
b. Fibrosing mediastinitis.
c. Pulmonary artery agenesis.
d. Primary tumors of the pulmonary artery.
e. Extrinsic compression of a vessel.

V-3. The following statements apply to pulmonary hereditary hemorrhagic telangiectasia.
a. It is commonly associated with pulmonary arteriovenous malformations.
b. Pulmonary arteriovenous malformations can develop with fungus infections.
c. It is a recessive disorder.
d. The lesions are secondary to endothelial cell degeneration.
e. Pulmonary hemorrhage is the most common presenting symptom.

V-4. The following statements about pulmonary arteriovenous malformations (PAVMs) are true *except*:
a. Pulmonary symptoms may be absent in up to 50% of patients.
b. The most common symptom is dyspnea, followed by atypical chest pain,

and less frequently, hemoptysis or hemothorax.

c. Hypoxemia is relatively common and is associated with orthodeoxia in 80% of cases at presentation.

d. Chest roentgenogram abnormalities include solitary nodules, masses, or minute diffuse AVMs.

e. Pulmonary hypertension is common.

V-5. The following statements apply to management of pulmonary arteriovenous malformations (PAVMs):

a. Surgical resection is an effective modality for treatment.

b. Contrast echocardiography and radionuclide angiocardiography assist in the diagnosis in micro AVMs.

c. Embolotherapy is the preferred method of treatment.

d. Air embolism and paradoxical embolization are complications of embolotherapy.

e. Lesions with feeding arteries less than 3 mm in size should be embolized.

V-6. Factors that are associated with an increased incidence of pulmonary infarction include the following *except*:

a. Left ventricular failure.

b. The number of lobes with pulmonary emboli.

c. Lung cancer.

d. Sickle cell anemia.

e. Pulmonary fibrosis.

V-7. The following statements apply to pulmonary embolism and infarction *except*:

a. Patients with indeterminate or moderate-probability lung scans have about a 40% chance of having a pulmonary embolism, and a pulmonary angiogram should be carried out.

b. A low-probability scan rules out a pulmonary embolism.

c. Venous studies of the legs should be performed in a patient with a high clinical risk for pulmonary embolism with a moderate- or high-probability lung scan and a negative angiogram.

d. A patient with a high clinical risk and a moderate- or high-probability lung scan, a negative pulmonary angiogram, and a positive venous study should be given anticoagulant therapy.

e. Mortality rate after a pulmonary embolism is related to the size of the embolus.

V-8. The following statements apply to pulmonary embolism and infarction:

a. Hypoxemia is due to alveolar hypoventilation.

b. Cavitation following pulmonary infarction may be due to superinfection.

c. Pneumothorax may complicate pulmonary infarction and cavitation.

d. Resolution of angiographic and hemodynamic signs of pulmonary emboli takes place within 5 days.

e. The completeness of resolution depends on the age of the patient.

V-9. Pulmonary edema following pulmonary embolism in the absence of left ventricular failure is due to the following *except*:

a. Reflex edema from the CNS.

b. Transudation of fluid in unobstructed vessels secondary to increased capillary hydrostatic pressure.

c. Decreased plasma oncotic pressure due to fluid overload.

d. Alteration in microvascular permeability due to regional ischemia/hypoxia.

e. Release of vasoactive mediators after pulmonary embolism.

V-10. The following apply to Swyer-James (or Macleod's) syndrome *except*:

a. The morphologic findings are virtually indistinguishable from those of obstructive emphysema.

b. There is no bronchitis or bronchiolitis.

c. It may occur in one lobe of one lung and one lobe of the other.

d. There is often a history of adenoviral pneumonia during childhood.

e. Collaterals supply peripheral parenchyma and maintain lung expansion.

V-11. The following apply to Swyer-James (or Macleod's) syndrome *except*:
   a. Most patients are asymptomatic.
   b. Pulmonary function tests (PFTs) reveal reduction in vital capacity (VC) and in $D_L CO$.
   c. Arterial blood gases (ABGs) at rest are usually normal, but hypoxemia may occur with exercise.
   d. Cor pulmonale is common.
   e. There is mediastinal shift to contralateral side during exhalation.

V-12. The following apply to Swyer-James (or Macleod's) syndrome:
   a. Unilateral hyperlucency is due to decreased blood flow.
   b. The hilum on the affected side is absent on the chest roentgenogram.
   c. The volume of the affected lung depends on the age at the time of insult.
   d. The differential diagnosis includes proximal pulmonary artery agenesis.
   e. The findings on pulmonary $\overset{\circ}{V}/\overset{\circ}{Q}$ scan are the same as those of a pulmonary embolus.

V-13. The following conditions result in a right-to-left shunt in a patent foreman ovale *except*:
   a. Valvular pulmonic stenosis.
   b. The Müller maneuver.
   c. Right ventricular myocardial infarction.
   d. Pulmonary emboli.
   e. PEEP.

V-14. In primary pulmonary hypertension:
   a. There is thromboembolic occlusion of small muscular arteries.
   b. There is an association with cirrhotic liver disease.
   c. There is veno-occlusive disease.
   d. The male/female ratio is 1:3.
   e. The low $D_L CO$ correlates with the degree of hypertension.

V-15. The following statements apply to pulmonary hypertension *except*:

a. It may be due to pulmonary veno-occlusive disease.
   b. It may be due to pulmonary schistosomiasis.
   c. Plexogenic pulmonary lesions are seen in primary pulmonary hypertension.
   d. Thromboembolic pulmonary hypertension is characterized by thickened vessel media.
   e. Vessel muscular hypertrophy is common in thromboembolic pulmonary hypertension.

V-16. Match the condition with the treatment:
   a. Submassive pulmonary embolism and shock.
   b. Massive pulmonary embolism and no shock.
   c. Massive pulmonary embolism and shock.
   d. Massive pulmonary embolism and shock with 70% vascular occlusion.

   1. Thrombolytic therapy.
   2. Heparin, thrombolytic therapy.
   3. Pulmonary embolectomy.
   4. Heparin.

V-17. The following statements apply to treatment of pulmonary embolism *except*:
   a. Low-dose subcutaneous heparin increases survival in postoperative patients.
   b. Full-dose intravenous heparin is indicated in established pulmonary embolism.
   c. Bolus intravenous heparin causes less bleeding than does continuously infused intravenous heparin.
   d. Sufficient heparin should be administered to maintain the activated partial thromboplastin time at two times the control value.
   e. Anticoagulation should be continued with at least 6 weeks of full-dose anticoagulation in the patient with no obvious predisposition.

V-18. The following statements apply to pulmonary infarction:
a. It is more common in the setting of larger more proximal emboli than in smaller emboli obstructing distal vessels.
b. It is uncommon because the lung parenchyma has several sources of oxygen supply.
c. The most common symptom is dyspnea.
d. Hampton's hump is elevation of the ipsilateral hemidiaphragm with a wedge-shaped peripheral infiltrate.
e. The pleural fluid is usually transudative with more than 10,000 RBCs.

V-19. The following statements apply to pulmonary embolism and infarction:
a. Pleural effusion with pulmonary infarction has a lymphocyte predominance early.
b. There is a polymorphonuclear predominance in pleural effusion with pulmonary infarction later in the course.
c. More than 50% of patients suspected of having a pulmonary embolus have normal angiograms.
d. Venograms are normal in more than 50% of patients suspected of having deep venous thrombosis.
e. More than 50% of patients with pulmonary emboli have clinical evidence of deep venous thrombosis.

V-20. The following apply to pleural effusions with pulmonary infarction *except*:
a. They tend to be small.
b. They tend to appear late in the course.
c. Infected infarction after pulmonary embolus is an uncommon cause of empyema.
d. An increase after appropriate therapy may indicate empyema.
e. An increase after appropriate therapy may indicate hemothorax.

V-21. At sea level, an increased right-to-left shunt in the heart or lungs can be ruled out if:

a. The roentgenogram and hemoglobin are normal.
b. SaO_2 is greater than 100% on 100% oxygen.
c. PaO_2 is greater than 500 mm Hg on 100% oxygen.
d. Hemoglobin is more than 15 mg/ml.
e. Oxygen content rises above 16 ml/L of plasma.

V-22. In a patient with congestive heart failure during exercise:
a. Maximum oxygen consumption may be reached at a lower than expected work load.
b. There may be an early inordinate rise in respiratory quotient.
c. The systolic and diastolic blood pressure may fall.
d. There is an inordinate increase in tidal volume.
e. The dead space/tidal volume ratio falls.

V-23. The following statements apply to patent foreman ovale:
a. It is potentially a route for left-to-right shunt.
b. The Valsalva maneuver results in higher left atrial than right atrial pressure and a left-to-right shunt.
c. Right ventricular myocardial infarction can cause a right-to-left shunt.
d. Right ventricular infarction usually presents with clear lung fields and jugular venous distention.
e. Vasodilators may decrease any right-to-left shunt.

V-24. The following statements apply to fat embolism:
a. Fractures of both femur and tibia have a higher mortality than fracture of the femur alone.
b. Fracture of the tibia has a worse prognosis than isolated femur fracture.
c. Direct embolization of fat results from mechanical disruption of large fat stores and venous drainage of bone marrow.

d. Complement activation is specific for the diagnosis.

e. Frozen clot section assays for fat are specific for the diagnosis.

V-25. Pulmonary lesions in Behçet's syndrome include the following *except*:
a. Pleurisy.
b. Bronchiectasis.
c. Tuberculosis.
d. Airflow obstruction.
e. *In situ* thromboses.

V-26. The differential diagnosis of postcapillary hypertension includes:
a. Right ventricular dysfunction.
b. Tricuspid regurgitation.
c. Atrial myxoma.
d. Pulmonary veno-occlusive disease.
e. Anomalous pulmonary drainage.

V-27. In sickle cell disease there is:
a. Lymphocytosis.
b. SaO_2 is increased at a given PaO_2.
c. Cell-mediated immunity.
d. Clinical course of acute chest syndrome shorter than that of bacterial pneumonia.
e. Exchange transfusion is treatment of acute chest syndrome.

V-28. Uremia is associated with:
a. Pleural effusion.
b. Interstitial fibrosis.
c. Pulmonary calcification.
d. Decreased pulmonary capillary permeability.
e. Increased susceptibility to pulmonary tuberculosis.

V-29. The following apply to pulmonary edema secondary to airway obstruction:
a. It may develop in croup and epiglottitis.
b. It is manifested after relief of the obstruction.
c. It can develop prior to relief of the obstruction.
d. It is due to generation of a markedly negative intrapleural pressure.
e. It is due to increased afterload.

V-30. In sickle cell disease there is the following *except*:
a. Microvascular obstruction by rigid red blood cells.
b. Heightened susceptibility to pulmonary infection.
c. Recurrent pulmonary infiltrates in multiple lobes.
d. Substitution of valine for glutamic acid at position 6 of beta globulin subunit of hemoglobin.
e. Increased T4:T8 cell ratio.

V-31. Pulmonary venous hypertension causes the following *except*:
a. Distention of lower lobe vessels and narrowing of upper lobe vessels.
b. Kerley's B lines.
c. Perivascular edema.
d. Medial hypertrophy of veins and venules.
e. Alveolar hemorrhage.

V-32. The following apply to atrial tumors:
a. Atrial myxomas occur mostly in the second decade.
b. Malignant fibrous histiocytomas affect older women.
c. Myxomas have a predilection for Black people.
d. Myxomas are hypocellular, nonvascular tumors.
e. Myxomas can cause postcapillary pulmonary hypertension.

V-33. The following apply to pulmonary arteriovenous malformations:
a. They are associated with Rendu-Osler-Weber syndrome in 15% of cases.
b. They are present in 50% of patients with Rendu-Osler-Weber syndrome.
c. Congenital malformations are usually recognized in the first decade.
d. They can occur in schistosomiasis infections.
e. They have a feeding vessel from the right atrium and a draining vessel to the hilum.

V-34. The following apply to pulmonary arteriovenous malformations:
   a. They have a lower lobe predominance.
   b. The are rarely subpleural.
   c. Bronchial vessels in the afferent limb rule out this diagnosis.
   d. There is a male preponderance.
   e. 50% have epistaxis without associated Rendu-Osler-Weber syndrome.

V-35. The following apply to pulmonary arteriovenous malformations:
   a. Pulmonary hypertension due to chronic hypoxia is prevalent.
   b. They can develop systemic emboli.
   c. Digital clubbing is rare.
   d. They can manifest as a coin lesion.
   e. Sharp margins of lesions are characteristic.

1-6 Pleural Disease

PL-1. The following statements apply to pleural disease:
   a. Pleural fluid eosinophilia is common in tuberculous pleurisy.
   b. Nitrofurantoin can cause a pleural fluid eosinophilia.
   c. More than 10% basophils in pleural fluid suggests cryptococcal infection.
   d. Mesothelial cells are a predominant cell in exudative pleural effusions.
   e. More than 5% mesothelial cells virtually rules out tuberculous pleurisy.

PL-2. The following statements apply to pleural disease:
   a. A milky pleural effusion that remains opaque following centrifugation indicates a large number of leukocytes.
   b. It is likely a chylothorax if the triglyceride concentration is greater than 110 mg/dl.
   c. A triglyceride concentration less than 80 mg/dl rules out a chylothorax.
   d. The presence or absence of chylomicrons can be determined by lipoprotein electrophoresis.
   e. Chromosomal analysis is helpful in the diagnosis of mesothelioma when cytologic examination proves negative.

PL-3. The following statements apply to pleural disease:
   a. Relief of dyspnea following therapeutic thoracentesis is due to reduction in the size of the thoracic cage.
   b. Unilateral pulmonary edema most commonly occurs with a trapped lung.
   c. A grossly bloody effusion in the absence of trauma is most likely to be due to malignancy.
   d. Whitish pleural effusion indicates the presence of chyle.
   e. Anchovy-colored fluid suggests *Aspergillus* infection.

PL-4. The following statements apply to pleural disease:
   a. In effusions with elevated LDH levels the percentage of LDH-4 and LDH-5 is higher than in the corresponding serum.
   b. A titer of rheumatoid factor in pleural fluid of ≥1:120 is suggestive of rheumatoid pleurisy.
   c. Chances of finding LE cells in pleural fluid decrease if the fluid is allowed to stand at room temperature for several hours.
   d. A pleural fluid/serum antinuclear antibody (ANA) ratio of 1.0 or greater is suggestive of lupus pleuritis.

e. Total hemolytic complement and complement components are high in pleural fluid in most patients with lupus pleuritis.

PL-5. The following statements pertain to asbestos and malignant pleural mesothelioma:
a. Virtually all of cases have a history of asbestos exposure.
b. Prevalence of asbestos bodies is high in the general public.
c. The latency period after exposure to asbestos can be 45 years.
d. The risk of developing bronchogenic carcinoma is 25%.
e. The latency period from exposure to tumor development is about 10 years.

PL-6. The following statements pertain to malignant pleural mesothelioma:
a. The risk varies with the type of asbestos fiber.
b. Chrysotile fibers are worse than amosite.
c. The main determinant appears to be whether a fiber is straight or curved.
d. Amphiboles are not readily deposited and seem to dissolve over time.
e. Asbestos fibers are incompletely phagocytosed.

PL-7. The following statements pertain to malignant pleural mesothelioma:
a. Hematogenous spread to other organs is common.
b. The tumor is rarely locally invasive.
c. Histology is sarcomatous in most cases.
d. It has a characteristic pattern of staining for keratin.
e. Mean survival at one year is 50%.

PL-8. The following statements pertain to malignant pleural mesothelioma:
a. The most common symptom is dyspnea.
b. Left-sided pleural effusion is more common than right-sided.
c. Pleural plaques or interstitial fibrosis may be evident.

d. The pleural fluid is typically a transudate.
e. Cigarette smoking does not increase the risk.

PL-9. The following statements pertain to the yellow nail syndrome:
a. Pleural biopsy may reveal dilated lymphatic channels.
b. The pleural fluid is an exudate.
c. The pleural fluid has an elevated pH.
d. There is a polymorphonuclear predominance.
e. LDH is low in pleural fluid.

PL-10. The following statements pertain to the yellow nail syndrome:
a. Ascites is often present.
b. Pleural effusion is usually bilateral.
c. Chronic bronchitis can be associated with the classic triad.
d. Abnormal ciliary motility is the basis of the recurrent sinopulmonary infection.
e. There may be mixed obstructive and restrictive physiology.

PL-11. The following statements pertain to the yellow nail syndrome:
a. It includes chronic lymphedema and recurrent sinopulmonary infections.
b. The edema and effusions are due to impaired lymphatic drainage.
c. There is overproduction of pleural fluid.
d. Nail changes may precede the other signs by months or years.
e. There is a 2:1 male predominance.

PL-12. The following applies to pleural effusion in rheumatoid arthritis *except*:
a. A serous exudate that is predominantly lymphocytic.
b. Occurs almost exclusively in women.
c. May antedate signs and symptoms.
d. Glucose concentration is low.
e. More often right-sided than left-sided.

PL-13. The following statements pertain to chylothorax:
  a. Immune deficiency may develop.
  b. The majority of traumatic chylothoraces will resolve spontaneously.
  c. Pseudochylous effusions usually have an elevated cholesterol level.
  d. Chyle is an irritant of the pleural surface.
  e. A chylomicron band on lipoprotein electrophoresis is proof of a chylous effusion.

PL-14. The following statements pertain to chylothorax:
  a. Chylothorax is due primarily to obstruction of the thoracic duct.
  b. An effusion with triglyceride greater than 110 is virtually diagnostic.
  c. With a triglyceride level less than 50, there is less than 5% chance that it is a chylothorax.
  d. The fluid has a high LDH.
  e. Cells consist of more than 25% B lymphocytes.

PL-15. The following statements pertain to chylothorax:
  a. The most common cause of chylothorax is mediastinal malignancy.
  b. Milky fluid can stain negative for fat and still be chylous.
  c. Chylothorax can be bloody, turbid, or even serous.
  d. The glucose level in chyle is less than the plasma level.
  e. The cholesterol/triglyceride ratio is usually >1.0.

PL-16. The following statements pertain to chyle:
  a. The thoracic duct ascends from the abdomen into the chest along the left paravertebral gutter and then crosses over to the right paravertebral gutter until it reaches the left subclavian vein.
  b. Normally, chyle flow is between 1500 and 2500 cc/day.
  c. The volume of chyle flow depends on the level of activity of the individual.

  d. Disruption of the duct below the fifth thoracic vertebra usually leads to left-sided effusions.
  e. Disruption above the fifth thoracic vertebra commonly causes right-sided or bilateral effusion.

PL-17. The following applies to parapneumonic effusions:
  a. Primarily lymphocytes, normal glucose, and normal pH characterize the exudative stage.
  b. In the fibrinopurulent stage the fluid contains PMNs, glucose and pH decrease, and high LDH.
  c. In the organization stage fibroblasts grow and produce a "pleural peel."
  d. Empyema can develop in the absence of pneumonic infection.
  e. Decortication should be carried out as soon as possible.

PL-18. The following apply to tuberculous pleural effusions:
  a. Always a manifestation of primary TB in young patients.
  b. Develop when subpleural caseous material ruptures into the pleural space.
  c. Result from a delayed hypersensitivity reaction to tubercular proteins.
  d. Classically consist predominantly of neutrophils, <50 mg/dl glucose, and LDH >1000.
  e. Have adenosine deaminase levels that are highly sensitive and specific for tuberculosis.

PL-19. The following apply to tuberculous pleural effusions:
  a. A negative PPD rules out the diagnosis.
  b. Sputum is usually negative unless there are infiltrates.
  c. Pleural effusion has >10% eosinophils.
  d. Prednisone is effective in markedly symptomatic patients.
  e. Treatment consists of INH and rifampin for 12–18 months.

PL-20. The following statements apply to pleural disease:
   a. Black pleural fluid suggests rupture of an amebic liver abscess into the pleural space.
   b. A putrid odor is diagnostic of an anaerobic empyema.
   c. An ammonia odor suggests urinothorax.
   d. In the nephrotic syndrome pleural effusions are frequently subpulmonic and bilateral.
   e. Pleural effusions in peritoneal dialysis usually occur a week after dialysis.

PL-21. The following statements apply to pleural disease:
   a. In acute exudative effusions, there are high leukocyte counts with a predominance of mononuclear cells.
   b. In the subacute or chronic exudative effusions cell counts may be low with a predominance of polymorphonuclear leukocytes.
   c. Exudates have a pleural fluid/serum total protein ratio >0.5.
   d. Exudates have a pleural fluid/serum LDH ratio >0.6.
   e. Exudates have a pleural fluid/serum total protein ratio <0.5.

PL-22. The following statements apply to pleural disease:
   a. Pleural leukocyte counts greater than 50,000/μl suggest empyema.
   b. Chronic malignant exudates usually have more than 25,000 leukocytes/μl.
   c. Tuberculous effusions have less than 5000 leukocytes/μl.
   d. Effusion in pancreatitis has less than 10,000 leukocytes/μl.
   e. Effusion in pulmonary infarction has more than 10,000 leukocytes/μl.

PL-23. The following statements apply to pleural disease:
   a. An isolated elevation of pleural fluid LDH suggests a parapneumonic effusion.

   b. Pleural fluid/serum protein ratio >0.5 in patients with congestive heart failure.
   c. An isolated elevation of pleural fluid LDH suggests malignancy.
   d. In tuberculous pleural effusions protein concentrations <3.0 gm/dl.
   e. Malignant pleural effusions are always exudates.

PL-24. The following statements apply to pleural disease:
   a. The leukocyte count may be less than anticipated in purulent pleural fluid because of lysis of polymorphonuclear leukocytes.
   b. Soon after the onset of symptoms in pneumonia and effusion, there is a lymphocyte predominance.
   c. Pleural fluid increase in polymorphonuclears is highly suggestive of tuberculous pleurisy.
   d. There is more than 50% lymphocytes in carcinomatous pleural effusions.
   e. There may be greater than 10% eosinophils in pleural fluid following a pneumothorax.

PL-25. The following statements apply to pleural disease:
   a. A large number of plasma cells in pleural fluid suggests eosinophilic granuloma.
   b. The pleural fluid/serum glucose ratio is <0.5 in rheumatoid pleurisy.
   c. In lupus pleuritis, the glucose concentration is generally normal.
   d. Pleural fluid acidosis occurs in an esophageal rupture.
   e. Chest tube drainage is indicated in an empyema if the pleural fluid pH is <7.10, glucose <40 mg/dl, and LDH >1000 U/L.

PL-26. The following statements apply to pleural disease:
   a. A pH greater than 7.40 predicts a short survival time in a malignant pleural effusion.

b. Pleural fluid/serum amylase ratio is greater than 1.0 in malignancy.

c. Pleural effusion in patients with acute pancreatitis resolves over several days to weeks.

d. Pleural fluid amylase levels are elevated in esophageal rupture.

e. LDH levels are less than 1000 U/L in a rheumatoid pleurisy.

PL-27. The following apply to hepatic pleural effusions:

a. They are most likely to be due to a <2 cm defect in the tendinous diaphragm.

b. Diagnosis is established by intrapleural injection of technetium colloid.

c. Diagnosis is established by creating a pneumoperitoneum.

d. Diagnosis can be established by thoracoscopy.

e. Treatment should include chemical pleurodesis.

PL-28. Treatment of pleural effusions associated with ascites involves:

a. Sodium restriction.

b. Diuretics.

c. Thoracentesis.

d. CT thoracostomy.

e. Pleurodesis.

PL-29. The following apply to hepatic pleural effusions:

a. They occur in 5–10% of cirrhotic patients.

b. They occur only in cirrhotic patients with ascites.

c. They are always transudates.

d. Majority are right-sided.

e. They are usually small.

PL-30. All of the statements concerning pleural effusions associated with benign asbestos pleural effusion (BAPE) are true *except*:

a. The diagnosis is based on asbestos exposure, exclusion of other causes, and observation.

b. Most present with chest pain, and a minority have fever, cough, or dyspnea or are asymptomatic.

c. BAPE is the most common pleuropulmonary manifestation in the 20 years after the first exposure but may occur 1 to 58 years after exposure.

d. The effusion is a small, unilateral hemorrhagic exudate, commonly with eosinophilia, that resolves over several months.

e. Following BAPE, there may be recurrence, diffuse pleural thickening with or without progression, blunting of costophrenic angle, or no residual.

PL-31. The following applies to pleural effusion in tuberculosis *except*:

a. A serous exudate that is predominantly lymphocytic.

b. Skin test may be negative in early cases.

c. Subsequent active pulmonary disease is likely to occur if untreated.

d. It is more common in children than in adults.

e. It is frequently unilateral.

PL-32. The following disorders are associated with a pleural effusion *except*:

a. Staphylococcal pneumonia.

b. *Streptococcus pyogenese* infection.

c. Actinomycosis.

d. Eosinophilic pneumonia.

e. *Haemophilus influenzae* pneumonia.

PL-33. Subacute or chronic effusion associated with pancreatitis:

a. Can occur weeks to months after an episode of pancreatitis.

b. Can be associated with pancreatic carcinoma.

c. Is usually small.

d. More than 25% have associated ascites.

e. Is a transudate.

PL-34. Elevated pancreatic amylase in pleural effusions are seen in the following *except*:

a. Acute pancreatitis.
b. Chronic pancreatitis with pseudocysts.
c. Pancreatic abscess.
d. Diabetes.
e. Esophageal rupture.

PL-35. The following apply to pleural effusions in acute pancreatitis:
a. They occur at the time of acute pancreatitis.
b. Majority are right-sided.
c. They are usually asymptomatic.
d. Effusion is usually large.
e. Mononuclear cells are predominant.

PL-36. Subacute or chronic pleural effusion after pancreatitis resolves with:
a. Bowel rest.
b. Hyperalimentation.
c. Repeated thoracentesis.
d. Chest tube drainage.
e. Pancreatic surgery.

PL-37. The following apply to pleural effusions associated with Kaposi's sarcoma:
a. Closed-needle pleural biopsy is typically diagnostic.
b. There is lymphatic obstruction of mediastinal lymph nodes.
c. There is relative sparing of the visceral pleura.
d. Radiation therapy is effective in cutaneous lesions.
e. Treatment of pleural effusion is tube thoracostomy with tetracycline sclerosis.

PL-38. The following apply to pleural effusions in Kaposi's sarcoma:
a. Typically there is a serosanguineous exudate.
b. There is a polymorphonuclear cell predominance.
c. Glucose is usually elevated.
d. They have low pH values.
e. They may be chylous.

PL-39. In Kaposi's sarcoma:
a. Visceral involvement precedes cutaneous lesions.

b. It is more common in IV drug users than in homosexuals.
c. Radiograph shows mediastinal adenopathy.
d. Radiograph demonstrates diffuse interstitial infiltrates.
e. Radiograph demonstrates pleural effusions.

PL-40. In Kaposi's sarcoma:
a. The cell of origin is the pluripotential angioblast.
b. Cytomegalovirus stimulates a sarcomatous change.
c. Non–AIDS-related Kaposi's sarcoma disseminates commonly.
d. AIDS-related Kaposi's sarcoma metastasizes to visceral organs in only a few cases.
e. Raised, violaceous nodules can be seen in the tracheobronchial tree.

PL-41. In pleural effusions secondary to ascites:
a. The pleural fluid is an exudate.
b. Pleural fluid is usually more transudative than the ascites.
c. Peritoneal fluid passes into the pleural space but not vice versa.
d. Pleural exudates occur in the presence of transudative ascites.
e. Bloody pleural effusions may be present with clear ascites.

PL-42. Pleural effusions secondary to ascites primarily result from:
a. Azygos vein hypertension.
b. Increases in lymphatic flow and pressure.
c. Hypoalbuminemia.
d. Congenital diaphragmatic defects.
e. Pleural arteriovenous malformations.

PL-43. Pleural effusions secondary to ascites:
a. Occur in 5–10% of patients with cirrhotic ascites.
b. Often present as massive effusions.
c. Are typically left-sided.
d. Only occur with tense ascites.
e. May be indicative of Meigs' syndrome.

PL-44. Spontaneous pneumothorax may be associated with:
   a. Chronic obstructive pulmonary disease.
   b. Tuberous sclerosis.
   c. Marfan syndrome.
   d. Hydatid disease.
   e. Lymphangioleiomyomatosis.

PL-45. Which of the following are true?
   a. Chyle is composed largely of proteins.
   b. Chylomicrons from the jejunal mucosa comprise most of thoracic duct lymph.
   c. A triglyceride level less than 50 virtually rules out a chylothorax.
   d. The glucose level in chyle is not different from the plasma level.
   e. The T4:T8 ratio in chyle is about 4.0.

PL-46. Which of the following are true?
   a. Normally, chyle flow is between 1500 and 2500 cc/day.
   b. The pattern and volume of chyle flow depend on the level of activity.
   c. The most common cause of chylothorax is mediastinal malignancy.
   d. Chylothorax is alkaline.
   e. Milky fluid can stain negative for fat and still be chylous.

PL-47. Which of the following statements concerning CHF and pleural effusion are true?
   a. Generally there is a unilateral left pleural effusion.
   b. There is a serous, lymphocytic transudate with a pH <7.40.
   c. Pleural effusions are associated with pulmonary venous but not systemic venous hypertension.
   d. An isolated left pleural effusion does not exclude CHF as the etiology.
   e. Acute diuretic therapy may convert pleural fluid from a transudate to an exudate.

PL-48. All of the following statements concerning cirrhosis and pleural effusions are true *except*:

   a. 5% of patients with cirrhosis and clinical ascites have pleural effusions.
   b. Effusions are right-sided in 70% of cases.
   c. Pleural fluid and ascitic fluid proteins are equivalent.
   d. A massive pleural effusion is associated with a diaphragmatic defect.
   e. In a diaphragm defect, radioactivity is not detected over the thorax until 12–20 hours after intraperitoneal injection.

PL-49. Which of the following statements concerning nephrotic syndrome and pleural effusions are true?
   a. About 25% of patients develop pulmonary embolism.
   b. There is an associated increase of clotting inhibitors.
   c. There is a predilection for a subpulmonic location.
   d. Pleural fluid is a transudate.
   e. Bilateral effusions of disparate size should heighten suspicion of thromboembolism.

PL-50. All of the following statements concerning parapneumonic effusion are true *except*:
   a. It occurs in almost half of all patients with pneumonia.
   b. Clinical presentation distinguishes between a complicated and uncomplicated effusion.
   c. Patients with purulent fluid and a pH <7.10 need chest tube drainage.
   d. Pneumonia with pleural effusion requires increased antibiotics.
   e. A complicated effusion has a pH <7.30 and LDH >1000 U/L.

PL-51. All of the following statements concerning malignancy and pleural effusions are true *except*:
   a. A pH <7.30 usually predicts a survival of less than 5 months.
   b. Pleural fluid cytology has greater sensitivity than closed pleural biopsy in diagnosing a malignant effusion.

c. Pleural effusion in lung cancer is ipsilateral.

d. Malignant effusions have a predominance of mononuclear cells.

e. A pleural effusion in lung cancer excludes curative resection.

PL-52. All of the following concerning mesothelioma are true *except*:

a. Virtually all patients with malignant mesothelioma are symptomatic at presentation.

b. Patients with benign fibrous mesothelioma have an asbestos exposure.

c. Pleural effusion occurs early in the course of mesothelioma.

d. Effusions in malignant mesothelioma have a predominantly low pH and a low glucose.

e. An apparent large effusion and an ipsilateral mediastinal shift suggest a malignant mesothelioma.

PL-53. All of the following statements concerning pulmonary embolism and pleural effusion are true *except*:

a. Pleural effusions occur in approximately 50% of patients with pulmonary embolism.

b. Effusions are present within 24 hours of admission in almost all patients.

c. Effusions are usually unilateral.

d. Most effusions are transudates.

e. Hemorrhagic, PMN-predominant exudate is found in one third of patients.

PL-54. All of the following statements concerning postcardiac injury syndrome are true *except*:

a. Pleural effusions can occur in 80% of patients.

b. Typical presentation is pleuritic chest pain and fever 3 weeks following cardiac surgery.

c. PMN-predominant exudate with fluid glucose is equal to that in serum.

d. Effusions are usually right-sided.

e. It is associated with high levels of serum antimyocardial antibodies.

PL-55. Which of the following statements concerning rheumatoid pleurisy are true:

a. The male:female incidence is 1:4.

b. Rheumatoid pleurisy can precede articular manifestations.

c. Characteristically, pH 7.00, glucose >60 mg/dl.

d. Characteristically, fluid LDH is <1000 U/L.

e. It may result in an effusion high in cholesterol.

PL-56. All of the following statements concerning lupus pleuritis are true *except*:

a. It is the most common pleuropulmonary manifestation of SLE.

b. It is almost always symptomatic.

c. Finding LE cells in pleural fluid is diagnostic.

d. Native and drug-induced lupus neuritis can be distinguished by pleural fluid analysis.

e. It is a bilateral small to moderate effusion.

PL-57. All of the following statements concerning chylothorax are true *except*:

a. Lymphoma is the most common cause of chylothorax in adults.

b. 75% of patients with LAM will develop a chylothorax.

c. A pleural fluid cholesterol level of less than 75 mg/dl virtually excludes a chylothorax.

d. A chylothorax may be milky, serous, turbid, or bloody.

e. A major problem with prolonged tube thoracostomy treatment of chylothorax is immune compromise.

PL-58. All of the following statements concerning spontaneous esophageal rupture (Boerhaave's) are true *except*:

a. It can follow a severe bout of vomiting or retching.

b. The most common site of rupture is the lower third of the esophagus.

c. The low pleural fluid pH results from gastric acid reflux.

d. Pleural fluid may be transudate with normal pH.

e. Diagnosis and surgical treatment within 24 hours result in excellent survival.

PL-59. All of the following statements concerning pleural effusions associated with diseases below the diaphragm are true *except*:

a. In urinothorax, there is a transudate with pH 7.30, pleural fluid/serum creatinine of 1.0.

b. In a splenic infarction, fluid is a serous, PMN-predominant exudate.

c. In a subphrenic abscess, fluid has pH 7.10, glucose <40 mg/dl.

d. In pancreatitis, fluid is serous, pleural fluid/serum amylase >1.0.

e. In amebic liver abscess, fluid is a turbid, PMN-predominant exudate.

PL-60. All of the following statements concerning pleural effusions associated with diseases of the lymphatics are true *except*:

a. Involvement of the respiratory tract in the yellow nail syndrome may be manifested by sinusitis.

b. Pleural effusion and yellow nails without lymphedema is rare in the yellow nail syndrome.

c. Noonan's syndrome is a Turner's phenotype with a normal karyotype.

d. Noonan's syndrome may be associated with chylothorax due to pulmonary lymphangiectasia.

e. Lipoprotein electrophoresis is necessary to diagnose chylothorax even with triglyceride concentrations >150 mg/dl.

PL-61. Pleural effusion after endoscopic variceal sclerotherapy for esophageal varices:

a. Is an exudate.

b. Has normal pH.

c. Has low glucose.

d. Has high amylase.

e. Occurs unilaterally.

1-7 Infection

I-1. Which of the following are true of herpes simplex virus?

a. Smokers and burn patients are predisposed to herpes infection.

b. A defect in humoral immunity predisposes to infection.

c. Diagnosis is made by a positive HSV culture in sputum.

d. A lack of rise in antibody titer is an ominous sign in HSV infection.

e. Penicillin is the treatment of choice.

I-2. Histologic findings in herpes simplex infection include all of the following *except*:

a. Tissue necrosis.

b. Degeneration of cells.

c. Multi-nucleated giant cells.

d. Hypertrophied type 2 cells.

e. Eosinophilic intranuclear inclusions.

I-3. The following statements pertain to infection :

a. Ciprofloxacin would constitute appropriate therapy for aspiration pneumonia in a non-immunosuppressed patient admitted from the community.

b. Abnormalities in serum complement play a role in the pathogenesis of pulmonary disease associated with HIV.

c. *Pseudomonas aeruginosa* is one of the most common pulmonary pathogens in patients with AIDS.

d. Intrathoracic adenopathy is seen on chest roentgenogram with *Pneumocystis carinii* pneumonia.

e. Giemsa stain can be used to identify *P. carinii*.

I-4. The following statements about chronic pulmonary histoplasmosis are true *except*:

a. A positive histoplasmin skin test has little or no diagnostic value in endemic areas.

b. An elevated complement fixation is specific and diagnostic of histoplasmosis.

c. Sputum cultures are often negative.

d. Wright's stains of sputum are positive when cultures of the sputum are positive.

e. Urinary cultures are useful in the diagnosis of histoplasmosis.

I-5. The following statements apply to histoplasmosis:

a. Hilar lymphadenopathy is common in primary disease.

b. Pleural effusion is common.

c. Cavitation may be present in post-primary disease.

d. Hilar adenopathy is common in post-primary disease.

e. A calcified focus is common in post-primary disease.

I-6. The following statements apply to *Legionella* infection:

a. The serogroup 2 is the most prevalent of 12 serogroups of *Legionella pneumophila*.

b. A rising serum titer can be seen in other bacterial infections.

c. The direct fluorescent antibody (DFA) is only effective for serogroups 7–12.

d. Latex agglutination tests are only specific for *L. pneumophila* serogroup 1.

e. *Legionella* takes 2–3 weeks to grow on culture medium containing buffered

charcoal yeast extract medium, supplemented with alpha-ketoglutarate.

I-7. The following statements pertain to *Legionella* infection:

a. Nosocomial legionellosis accounts for 75% of the nosocomial pneumonias in some hospitals.

b. Superheating water and hyperchlorination helps prevent *Legionella* infections.

c. Age and cigarette smoking are risk factors for legionellosis.

d. The organism breeds in hot water tanks at temperatures greater than 180°F.

e. Up to 50% of cases of *Legionella* pneumonia occur in surgical patients, particularly after transplantation.

I-8. The following statements pertain to *Legionella* infection *except*:

a. Prophylactic erythromycin may prevent *Legionella* infection.

b. Erythromycin increases serum cyclosporine levels by competing with the same hepatic enzyme system for its metabolism.

c. 50% of patients have bilateral effusions.

d. *Legionella* pneumonia may lead to interstitial fibrosis that is indistinguishable from many other fibrotic pulmonary disorders.

e. Clinical response to treatment with erythromycin usually occurs within 72 hours.

I-9. The following statements apply to *Legionella* infection:

a. The clinical features in *Legionella bozemanii* infection are similar to those seen in *L. pneumophila* infection.

b. Rifampin may be beneficial in cases unresponsive to erythromycin.

c. A two-fold increase in titer in indirect immunofluorescent assay to ≥64 is diagnostic.

d. Seroconversion can be detected in many patients within the first week of the illness.

e. Most cultures will be positive in 1–2 days.

I-10. Which of the following are true of nocardiosis?
a. *Nocardia* is soil-borne.
b. Consolidation is always confined to lobes or segments.
c. Concomitant corticosteroid therapy or antineoplastic agents are associated with high mortality.
d. Sulfonamides are effective therapy.
e. Serum complement is positive in active infection.

I-11. In nocardiosis:
a. Two thirds of patients are female.
b. *N. asteroides* causes Madura foot.
c. Sputum culture is rapidly positive.
d. The pleura is commonly involved.
e. Most pulmonary disease is due to *N. brasiliensis*.

I-12. All of the following are correct *except*:
a. Pneumococcal pneumonia is most common in patients with poor defense functions of the respiratory tract.
b. *Streptococcus pneumoniae* initially produces hyperemia and edema and neutrophils in the alveoli.
c. Resolution results in incomplete healing and tissue necrosis.
d. Serotype 3 causes the most severe disease.
e. The *Pneumococcus* elaborates neuraminidase.

I-13. The following increase the likelihood of tuberculosis infection *except*:
a. The concentration of organisms in ambient air.
b. The duration of exposure.
c. Previous infection with tuberculosis.
d. Laboratory handling of infected sputum.
e. End-stage renal disease.

I-14. The following statements apply to tuberculosis:

a. 30% of individuals who are close contacts of patients with infectious tuberculosis become infected.
b. INH prophylaxis reduces the possibility of TB infection in HIV-positive patients.
c. Obesity is a risk factor for tuberculosis.
d. Previous BCG vaccination reduces the severity of extrapulmonary TB.
e. In 90% of individuals who are close contacts of patients with infectious tuberculosis, the TB is contained and active infection does not ever develop.

I-15. The following are risk factors for TB *except*:
a. Intravenous drug abuse.
b. Radiographic "old TB."
c. Immunosuppression.
d. Smoking.
e. End-stage renal disease.

I-16. The following statements apply to the tuberculin skin test:
a. A positive test indicates active infection.
b. It is positive in about 20% of asymptomatic HIV-positive patients with TB.
c. It is positive in about 80% of HIV-positive patients with TB.
d. A positive test requires intact cell-mediated immunity.
e. IL-3 and IL-5 are involved in a positive response.

I-17. The following should receive prophylactic INH *except*:
a. A 54-year-old with a 16-mm PPD that was 3 mm 3 months ago.
b. A 32-year-old who is HIV-positive with a 12-mm PPD.
c. A 42-year-old suffering from sarcoidosis.
d. A 36-year-old with a negative PPD who has been in contact with a new case.
e. A 62-year-old from China with upper lobe scarring, a positive PPD, but negative smear and culture.

I-18. Erythema nodosum is occasionally seen in the following chronic pulmonary diseases *except*:
a. Tuberculosis.
b. Histoplasmosis.
c. Coccidioidomycosis.
d. Blastomycosis.
e. Invasive pulmonary aspergillosis.

I-19. The following statements apply to aspergilloma:
a. It is unusual in sarcoidosis.
b. It may resolve spontaneously.
c. It may be the cause of recurrent hemoptysis.
d. Amphotericin is effective therapy.
e. Prednisone therapy can result in dissemination.

I-20. Signs suggestive of endobronchial tuberculosis include all of the following *except*:
a. Lung collapse.
b. Air trapping.
c. Consolidation.
d. Intrathoracic adenopathy.
e. Pleural effusion.

I-21. All of the following apply to endobronchial tuberculosis:
a. It can be manifest in a "cobblestone" mucosa usually with sterile granuloma.
b. It can be manifest in an obstructing mass containing caseous material.
c. In early lesions, caseating granulomas are usually acid-fast bacillus-free.
d. In late lesions, there may be fibrosis without granulomas and acid-fast bacilli.
e. PPD is positive in 45% of patients.

I-22. In adult patients with pulmonary candidiasis the most common mode of transmission is:
a. Aerosolization of spores that are ubiquitous in the environment.
b. Aspiration of *Candida* that has colonized the oral pharynx.

c. Hematogenous seeding from gastric contents in patients who have gastrointestinal candidiasis.
d. Injection of *Candida* spores into the lung during respiratory tract maneuvers such as mechanical respiratory ventilation and aerosol nebulization.
e. Needles and syringes.

I-23. The following statements apply to varicella pneumonia in adults:
a. It has the same morbidity and mortality as in children.
b. The chest radiograph typically displays a patchy or diffuse bilateral nodular infiltrate.
c. Tobacco use is a risk factor.
d. Pneumonia occurs 1–6 days after the onset of the rash.
e. Intravenous acyclovir should be administered to normal hosts with clinically evident pneumonia.

I-24. The following statements apply to therapy in AIDS:
a. Intrathoracic adenopathy or diffuse infiltration on the chest roentgenogram in patients with HIV infection should trigger suspicion of tuberculosis.
b. Neutropenia is associated with pentamidine therapy in patients with AIDS.
c. Toxic delirium may occur with administration of pentamidine in patients with AIDS.
d. Hyperglycemia may occur with administration of pentamidine in patients with AIDS.
e. Hypoglycemia has been reported with administration of pentamidine in patients with AIDS.

I-25. The following statements apply to the acquired immunodeficiency syndrome:
a. Primary pulmonary hypertension in HIV-positive patients develops primarily in hemophiliacs.
b. HIV-positive patients may have pulmonary hypertension.

c. Pulmonary hypertension in intra-venous drug abusers is granulomatous.

d. The anticardiolipin antibody in AIDS is associated with an increased risk of deep venous thrombosis/pulmonary emboli.

e. The CD 4 depletion is on a retroviral cytopathic basis.

I-26. The following statements are true:

a. Diffuse hypergammaglobulinemia and two or more monoclonal "spikes" are found in Sjögren's syndrome.

b. T cells are infected with the Epstein-Barr virus during the course of mono-nucleosis.

c. Cellular immunity is frequently de-pressed during the acute phase of mononucleosis.

d. Rheumatoid factor can be positive in Epstein-Barr virus infections.

e. Anticardiolipin antibodies can be positive in patients with acute Epstein-Barr virus infections.

I-27. The following statements pertain to the anticardiolipin antibodies:

a. Patients with SLE have clinically sig-nificant anticardiolipin antibodies.

b. Anticardiolipin antibody is in the same family as the false-positive VDRL.

c. Antiphospholipid antibody has been associated with pulmonary hyperten-sion.

d. Phospholipid antibodies may alter platelet membranes leading to decreased platelet adhesion.

e. Phospholipid antibodies may affect endothelial membranes and increase prostacyclin release.

I-28. The following statements apply to the lupus anticoagulant *except*:

a. It is an IgG antibody.

b. It is present in AIDS.

c. It inhibits the prothrombin time.

d. It inhibits coagulation at the level of the prothrombin activator complex.

e. It causes hemorrhagic events.

I-29. The following statements apply to the lupus anticoagulant:

a. It results in thrombotic events.

b. It may be associated with immune-mediated thrombocytopenia.

c. There is no relationship between ele-vated PTT and lupus anticoagulant in the plasma.

d. There is no relationship between opportunistic infections and the lupus anticoagulant.

e. The presence of lupus anticoagulant increases the risk of thromboembolic disease in patients who are HIV-positive.

I-30. The following statements apply to roentgenograms of the chest:

a. Pleural effusion is common in *Enta-moeba histolytica* infection.

b. Cavitation is uncommon in actinomy-cosis.

c. Pleural effusion is common in actino-mycosis.

d. Chest wall involvement is common in actinomycosis.

e. Cavitation is uncommon in coccid-ioidomycosis.

I-31. The following disorders are usually asso-ciated with cavitation *except*:

a. *Klebsiella* pneumonia.

b. Löffler's syndrome.

c. Actinomycosis.

d. Ankylosing spondylitis.

e. Wegener's granulomatosis.

I-32. Which of the following are true of *Cryptococcus neoformans*?

a. Infection is by inhalation.

b. Infection presents most commonly as subacute meningitis.

c. It is the leading cause of opportunistic infection in AIDS.

d. Chest film findings include cavitary lesions.

e. Diagnosis is made by mucicarmine staining.

I-33. The following apply to lung development:
   a. Lobar bronchi appear at the third week of gestation.
   b. The bronchial tree is fully developed by the sixteenth week of intrauterine life.
   c. Respiratory bronchioles appear before the tenth week.
   d. The acini develop between the sixteenth week and birth.
   e. The adult complement of alveoli are attained within 12 months after birth.

I-34. The following apply to bronchopulmonary dysplasia:
   a. It occurs in premature infants who require mechanical ventilation.
   b. It occurs in infants requiring high oxygen concentrations at birth.
   c. Necrotizing bronchiolitis is present.
   d. There are arterial changes characteristic of pulmonary hypertension.
   e. Patients who survive demonstrate reactive airway disease.

I-35. The following apply to bronchopulmonary infection in children:
   a. Type 7 adenovirus causes significant bronchiolitis in infants.
   b. Bronchiolar obliteration in infancy can cause unilateral radiolucency of the lung.
   c. Alveolar development is not affected in Macleod's syndrome.
   d. Expiratory films show little change in lung volume in affected area in Swyer-James syndrome.
   e. Patients are usually asymptomatic in Macleod's syndrome.

I-36. The radiographic findings with *Pneumocystis carinii* infection in AIDS are:
   a. Bilateral or diffuse radiographic densities of alveolar filling.
   b. Upper lobe predominance if patient is receiving prophylactic inhaled pentamidine.
   c. Negative chest films despite impressive clinical pneumonia.

   d. Pleural effusion.
   e. Pneumothorax.

I-37. *Pneumocystis carinii* pneumonia in AIDS differs from that in other immune deficiencies in that:
   a. The incidence is greater.
   b. Recurrence is frequent.
   c. The clinical onset is more rapid.
   d. Organisms are less often detected on sputum examination.
   e. Incidence of adverse reactions to drug therapy is increased.

I-38. In the tuberculosis of advanced HIV infection:
   a. Pulmonary infiltrates favor an apical location.
   b. Sputum is commonly positive on smear or culture.
   c. Extrapulmonary tuberculosis is common.
   d. Mediastinal lymphadenopathy is rare.
   e. It responds promptly to antituberculous drug therapy.

I-39. In HIV infection:
   a. Mediastinal and hilar adenopathy is common.
   b. Kaposi's sarcoma can cause mediastinal and hilar adenopathy.
   c. Cytomegalovirus is the most frequent agent found post mortem in AIDS.
   d. Evidence of Cytomegalovirus increases as blood helper T cell count drops below 200/mm^3.
   e. Fungal pneumonia is common in AIDS patients.

I-40. In HIV infection:
   a. The incidence of disseminated histoplasmosis and coccidioidomycosis depends on the prevalence of endemic disease in the region.
   b. Nonspecific diffuse bilateral reticulonodular or nodular infiltrates are most characteristic of cryptococcosis.
   c. *Streptococcus* pneumonia is common in the AIDS population.

d. *Legionella* and *Nocardia* pneumonias are rare.

e. Lymphoid interstitial pneumonia (LIP) is seen predominantly in adults.

I-41. The disease process in tuberculosis is caused by:

a. Toxins secreted by *Mycobacterium tuberculosis*.

b. The physical load caused by growth of *Mycobacterium tuberculosis*.

c. Delayed-type hypersensitivity responses to *Mycobacterium tuberculosis*.

d. Cytotoxic T cells reacting against *Mycobacterium tuberculosis*.

e. *Mycobacterium tuberculosis* endotoxin.

I-42. Hepatitis associated with isoniazid may be characterized as follows:

a. It is age-related and is highest in patients over the age of 50.

b. It is more common among rapid acetylators of INH.

c. It always occurs in the first month.

d. It is more common among postpartum women.

e. Most often it is followed by chronic hepatic dysfunction.

I-43. The following apply to HIV-positive patients:

a. They are susceptible to opportunistic infections because of defects in macrophage function.

b. Pyogenic bacteria are the cause of a substantial number of respiratory infections.

c. They are approximately seven times more likely to develop pneumococcal pneumonia than are HIV-negative patents.

d. B cells undergo spontaneous activation, producing a nonspecific, polyclonal hypergammaglobulinemia.

e. Of all the states of HIV infection, only those with AIDS are affected by pneumonia.

I-44. The following apply to HIV infection:

a. B cell differentiation and proliferation in response to specific antigens is markedly reduced in patients with AIDS.

b. B cell differentiation and proliferation in response to specific antigens is normal in patients with other stages of HIV infection.

c. HIV-infected patients with pneumococcal pneumonia produce type-specific antibodies following disease.

d. Neutrophil chemotaxis is decreased in advanced HIV infection.

e. In HIV infection, B cells undergo spontaneous activation, producing histamine.

I-45. The following apply to pneumococcal pneumonia in HIV-positive patients:

a. The clinical manifestations are indistinguishable from those in HIV-negative patients.

b. The duration of symptoms is always less than 1 week.

c. Only a small proportion of cases have positive blood cultures.

d. Response to therapy is slow.

e. There is a high rate of recurrence of pneumococcal pneumonia.

I-46. The following apply to TB in HIV-positive patients:

a. The clinical presentation when CD 4 counts are >300 may be indistinguishable from classic reactivation.

b. Impaired cell-mediated immunity hinders formation of granulomas.

c. Most are primary infections.

d. The diagnosis of TB often precedes the diagnosis of AIDS.

e. Extrapulmonary disease is rare.

I-47. The following apply to tuberculosis in HIV-infected individuals:

a. Infiltrates are predominantly in the lower lobes.

b. Early in HIV infection acid-fast smears are frequently positive.

c. Patients with advanced disease are often anergic.

d. INH should be given to any patient with 5 mm or more induration regardless of age or prior skin testing results.

e. INH, rifampin, and pyrazinamide (PZA) should be given for drug-susceptible infection.

I-48. The following apply to tuberculosis in HIV-infected individuals:

a. INH, rifampin, PZA, and ethambutol hydrochloride are recommended in disseminated TB with CNS involvement.

b. If the organisms are drug-resistant, treatment should be continued for at least 12 months after cultures become negative.

c. Antifungals can result in subtherapeutic levels of rifampin.

d. Ketoconazole can result in subtherapeutic levels of rifampin.

e. TB occurs later in the course of HIV infection than other "opportunistic" infections.

I-49. Diffuse hypergammaglobulinemia and two or more monoclonal "spikes" are found in:

a. EBV.

b. CMV.

c. Multiple myeloma.

d. Polyclonal B cell lymphomas.

e. Sjögren's syndrome.

I-50. The following applies to EBV infection and acute mononucleosis:

a. Infected B cells cause polyclonal immunoglobulin secretion.

b. Activated infected B cells in mononucleosis decrease by week 2–3.

c. Cellular immunity is depressed during the acute phase.

d. B suppressor cell function gradually returns to normal in 4–8 weeks.

e. T cell activation can exist for 6–12 months.

I-51. The following are true of EBV infection:

a. Patients with infectious mononucleosis have heterophile antibodies.

b. Rheumatoid factor can be positive.

c. The ANA is usually at low titer with a speckled pattern.

d. Anticardiolipin antibodies are low titer IgG.

e. Anticardiolipin antibodies are in same family as false-positive VDRL and lupus anticoagulant.

I-52. The antiphospholipid antibody is associated with:

a. Arterial thrombosis.

b. Polycythemia.

c. Recurrent spontaneous abortions.

d. Pulmonary hypertension.

e. Erythema multiforme.

I-53. Appropriate statements about therapy for patients with anticardiolipin Ab include:

a. Continue anticoagulation as long as the Ab is present in patients with a documented thrombotic event and an ACA.

b. No therapy is required in patients who have not had a disorder attributable to the Ab.

c. Steroids and/or immunosuppressives should be considered in patients with repeated episodes despite adequate anticoagulation.

d. Corticosteroids decrease the titer of ACA.

e. Corticosteroids decrease the incidence of thrombosis in the absence of anticoagulation therapy.

I-54. The following apply to tuberculosis in chronic renal failure:

a. There is an increased incidence in patients with chronic renal failure.

b. 10% of all deaths in patients on chronic hemodialysis are due to TB.

c. Proclivity toward TB is mediated by impaired humoral immunity.

d. Blood lymphocytes from uremic patients have increased responsiveness to mitogenic stimuli.

e. Serum from uremic patients suppresses the mitogenic response of normal polymorphonuclears.

I-55. The following apply to treatment in tuberculosis *except*:
a. Rifampin is hepatically metabolized.
b. Isoniazid is acetylated in the liver.
c. Metabolites of isoniazid are excreted in the stool.
d. Isoniazid is not dialyzable.
e. Ethambutol hydrochloride is dependent on renal function for excretion.

I-56. The following apply to tuberculosis:
a. There is an increased incidence of miliary tuberculosis in pregnancy.
b. Right middle lobe atelectasis is most commonly due to tuberculosis.
c. The thoracolumbar spine is the most common site of spinal tuberculosis.
d. INH, streptomycin, and PAS are recommended therapy in bone lesions.
e. Chemotherapy for extrapulmonary TB should be given for at least 18 months.

I-57. The following are true:
a. Trauma is a leading cause of paralysis of the larynx.
b. Supraclavicular nodes are rare in tuberculous lymphadenitis.
c. Tuberculous meningitis is usually due to the rupture of a tubercle into the subarachnoid space.
d. Tuberculous meningitis is always associated with other evidence of extracranial TB.
e. Corticosteroids and usual treatment of pulmonary TB are recommended in tuberculous pericarditis.

I-58. The following apply to nocardiosis:
a. Two thirds of patients are male.
b. The majority of cases occur in old age.
c. Pulmonary disease alone occurs in more than 75% of cases.

d. The pleura is not involved.
e. It may complicate lupus erythematosus.

I-59. The following apply to nocardiosis:
a. In the majority of cases, infection occurs through the skin.
b. *N. brasiliensis* usually produces 80% of pulmonary disease.
c. *N. asteroides* causes the classic Madura foot.
d. It causes suppurative necrosis and nonencapsulated abscess formation.
e. It disseminates hematogenously.

I-60. Radiographic findings in nocardial pulmonary infections include:
a. A solitary irregular mass.
b. Diffuse tiny nodules.
c. An interstitial reticular pattern.
d. A normal chest roentgenogram.
e. Hilar and mediastinal lymphadenopathy.

I-61. The following apply to *Aspergillus* infection:
a. The mainstay of therapy of aspergilloma is systemic amphotericin B.
b. Invasive aspergillosis can affect the eyes.
c. Invasive aspergillosis can affect the heart.
d. Disseminated aspergillosis can involve the kidney.
e. There is synergy between amphotericin B and INH.

I-62. The following apply to invasive aspergillosis:
a. Isolation of *Aspergillus* from specimens of the lower respiratory tract (sputum or BAL) is diagnostic.
b. A positive culture alone is proof of tissue invasion.
c. Fungal hyphae in tissues is diagnostic.
d. Serum precipitins are negative in 70–80% of patients.
e. There is an association between invasive pulmonary aspergillosis (IPA) and influenza A infection.

I-63. The following apply to invasive aspergillosis:
  a. In 70% of cases the lung is the only site of invasive aspergillosis.
  b. *Aspergillus flavus* accounts for almost 75% of clinical disease.
  c. Patients with hematopoietic or lymphoreticular malignancies account for over 80% of all cases.
  d. Approximately 40% of patients have hemoptysis.
  e. Oral itraconazole may be more efficacious than amphotericin B.

I-64. The following apply to blastomycosis *except*:
  a. It is endemic in the southeastern and southwestern United States.
  b. It presents as a flu-like illness.
  c. It can involve prostate.
  d. There is meningeal involvement in HIV patients.
  e. Nearly all disseminated cases have pulmonary involvement.

I-65. The following apply to blastomycosis:
  a. The organism takes 2–4 weeks to culture.
  b. Positive serology is highly suggestive of the diagnosis.
  c. Amphotericin B is the treatment of choice.
  d. Ketoconazole or itraconazole provides chronic suppression.
  e. HIV patients have a rash about 80% of the time.

I-66. The following apply to acute epiglottitis:
  a. It can involve the lingular tonsils.
  b. Classically, it is suppurative.
  c. Drooling is common.
  d. Bacteremia is uncommon.
  e. Hoarseness is a common symptom.

I-67. The following apply to acute epiglottitis:
  a. *Haemophilus influenzae* is the major cause of adult epiglottitis.
  b. Lateral neck radiography is critical.

  c. Pulmonary edema can follow relief of obstruction.
  d. Treatment includes Unasyn.
  e. Rifampin is useful for prophylaxis.

I-68. The following apply to patients with HIV:
  a. There is suppressed cell-mediated immunity.
  b. Kaposi's sarcoma is seen in up to 40% of cases.
  c. Burkitt's lymphoma is associated with AIDS.
  d. Nonspecific lymphocytic alveolitis is common.
  e. Kaposi's sarcoma lesions in the lung are more cellular than cutaneous ones.

I-69. The following statements apply to lung abscess:
  a. Hospital-acquired lung abscess is often colonized with *Legionella*.
  b. Bronchoscopy should be performed to rule out carcinoma.
  c. Penicillin V-K is the first choice in therapy.
  d. Clindamycin is an effective therapy.
  e. Mortality is the same with prolonged medical and surgical management.

I-70. Complications of a lung abscess include:
  a. Brain abscess.
  b. Massive hemoptysis.
  c. Pyopneumothorax.
  d. Bronchopulmonary fistula.
  e. Amyloidosis.

I-71. The following statements apply to bronchial secretions:
  a. The majority of lymphocytes in normal bronchoalveolar lavage are B cells.
  b. Most alveolar macrophages display surface membrane HLA-DR.
  c. IgG and IgE are present in bronchial secretions.
  d. IgG exceeds IgA in the bronchial secretions.
  e. The concentration of IgA exceeds that of IgG in lavage fluid.

I-72. The following apply to development of acid-fast infection in renal failure *except*:
   a. It is particularly common in Whites.
   b. Extrapulmonary disease predominates.
   c. Rifampin frequently causes nephrotoxicity.
   d. Frequency of infection with atypical mycobacteria is increased.
   e. Ethambutal hydrochloride therapy can cause ophthalmic damage.

I-73. Lung conditions associated with anaerobic bacterial infection include the following *except*:
   a. Pulmonary infarction.
   b. Bronchogenic carcinoma.
   c. Bronchiectasis.
   d. Sjögren's syndrome.
   e. Bronchial adenoma.

I-74. Anaerobic bacterial infection is most common in:
   a. Hypogammaglobulinemia.
   b. Complement deficiency.
   c. Altered mucocutaneous barrier.
   d. Neutropenia.
   e. Defective cell-mediated immunity.

I-75. Anaerobic bacterial infection is prevalent in:
   a. Pulmonary abscess.
   b. Aspiration pneumonia.
   c. Empyema.
   d. Community-acquired pneumonia.
   e. Hospital-acquired pneumonia.

I-76. The following apply to histoplasmosis in AIDS:
   a. It is virtually always disseminated.
   b. IV drug users are more susceptible to histoplasmosis than homosexuals.
   c. Skin lesions are present almost uniformly.
   d. Most cases show some CNS involvement.
   e. Complement fixation assay is limited by cross-reaction with *Cryptococcus*.

I-77. Diffuse alveolar filling on radiograph and symptoms of short duration suggest the following *except*:
   a. Mycoplasmal pneumonia.
   b. *Legionella* pneumonia.
   c. Viral pneumonia.
   d. *Pneumocystis carinii* infection.
   e. Coccidioidomycosis.

I-78. The following apply to histoplasmosis:
   a. The histoplasma polysaccharide antigen is the most sensitive test.
   b. This test is more sensitive in CSF than in urine.
   c. Response to amphotericin is good.
   d. Response to ketaconazole is good.
   e. Lifelong therapy is necessary.

I-79. In legionnaires' disease the following may be present:
   a. Elevated CPK.
   b. Abnormal liver function tests.
   c. Myoglobinuria.
   d. Hyponatremia.
   e. Hyperphosphatemia.

I-80. The following apply to legionnaires' disease:
   a. *L. pneumophila* can be readily isolated from the sputum.
   b. Bronchoalveolar lavage gives a higher yield than bronchial washings.
   c. Saline and lidocaine may inhibit *Legionella* growth.
   d. Indirect immunofluorescent antibody is a fast test for identification.
   e. Urinary antigen detects *L. pneumophila* serogroup 1.

I-81. The retropharyngeal space:
   a. Is bounded anteriorly by pharyngeal constriction.
   b. Is bounded posteriorly by the prevertebral fascia.
   c. Is bounded laterally by the carotid sheaths.
   d. Extends inferior to the superior mediastinum.
   e. Prevertebral tissues >22 mm at C7 indicate a pathologic process.

I-82. A retropharyngeal abscess:
  a. Usually is due to a contiguous infection of the ears, nose, or throat.
  b. Presents initially with dysphagia.
  c. Is more common in adults.
  d. The most frequent complication is mediastinitis.
  e. Surgical drainage of the abscess is mandatory.

I-83. The following apply to blastomycosis:
  a. The skin is the most frequent site of infection.
  b. The spores convert to mycelial form in the lung.
  c. The chest film is frequently abnormal even in asymptomatic patients.
  d. Hilar and mediastinal adenopathy are common.
  e. Blastomyces is not a frequent opportunistic pathogen in the immunocompromised.

I-84. In patients with AIDS:
  a. Multiple pulmonary nodules are common in advanced disease.
  b. Nodular infiltrates are seen most frequently with infection.
  c. *Pneumocystis carinii* can present as a solitary pulmonary nodule.
  d. *Mycobacterium avium-intracellulare* causes focal lung nodules more frequently than *M. tuberculosis.*
  e. *Histoplasma capsulatum* is a cause of focal lung nodules.

I-85. The following apply to patients with AIDS:
  a. Non-Hodgkin's lymphoma presents as multiple pulmonary nodules.
  b. Pulmonary non-Hodgkin's lymphoma presents as extranodal involvement.
  c. Kaposi's sarcoma presents as well-defined pulmonary nodules.
  d. Pleural effusions are frequent in Kaposi's sarcoma.
  e. They are at higher risk to develop adenocarcinoma of the lung.

I-86. Which of the following statements about TB in the elderly are true?
  a. Most cases are due to reactivation of a remote, latent infection.
  b. Reactivation is due to diminished immunity associated with aging.
  c. Age-adjusted case rates are 2- to 5-fold higher in nursing homes.
  d. Epidemic TB with recent infection occurs in nursing homes.
  e. Isoniazid prophylactic therapy limits nursing home epidemics.

I-87. Which statements about extrapulmonary TB are true?
  a. It is usually accompanied by active pulmonary disease.
  b. It constitutes about 15% of new TB in the United States.
  c. It may be treated with usual short-course regimens.
  d. It is more prevalent among non-Whites.
  e. Disordered immunity is usually involved.

I-88. The antiphospholipid antibody causes:
  a. Thrombocytopenia.
  b. Spontaneous abortion.
  c. Increased platelet adhesion.
  d. Increased prostacyclin release.
  e. Increased BAL lymphocytes.

I-89. The following statements apply to varicella in adults:
  a. It can be associated with significant morbidity and mortality.
  b. Pneumonia is the most common complication.
  c. Pregnancy and tobacco use are risk factors.
  d. Pneumonia occurs 1–6 days after the onset of the rash.
  e. Intravenous acyclovir should be administered to normal hosts with clinically evident pneumonia.

I-90. The most common etiology of viral pneumonia is:

In children	In adults
a. Respiratory syncytial virus.	a. Respiratory syncytial virus.
b. Influenza A.	b. Influenza A.
c. Adenovirus.	c. Adenovirus.
d. Coxsackie virus B.	d. Coxsackie virus B.
e. Cytomegalo-virus.	e. Cytomegalo-virus.

I-91. Which of the following bacteria are associated with postinfluenza pneumonia (i.e., secondary bacterial pneumonia)?
   a. *Staphylococcus aureus.*
   b. *Streptococcus pneumoniae.*
   c. *Branhamella catarrhalis.*
   d. *Pseudomonas aeruginosa.*
   e. *Proteus mirabilis.*

I-92. Which of the following agents can be used as prophylaxis for influenza?
   a. Amantadine hydrochloride.
   b. Rimantadine hydrochloride.
   c. Acyclovir.
   d. Ganciclovir.
   e. AZT (azido-dideoxythymidine).

I-93. For which high risk group(s) have pneumococcal vaccine been recommended?
   a. Children older than 2 years with sickle cell disease.
   b. Elderly adults with cardiovascular disease.
   c. Asplenic patients.
   d. Children with leukemia.
   e. Individuals with cerebrospinal fluid leaks.

I-94. Bronchoscopy specimens are superior to sputum for the following pulmonary pathogens:
   a. *Streptococcus pneumoniae.*
   b. *Haemophilus influenzae.*
   c. *Legionella* species.
   d. *M. tuberculosis.*
   e. *Pneumocystis carinii.*

I-95. In toxic strep syndrome:
   a. There are thin yellow bullae on the skin.
   b. There is thrombocytopenia and hypo-prothrombinemia.
   c. There is progressive azotemia and hypocalcemia.
   d. Multi-organ failure with adult respiratory distress syndrome (ARDS) is common.
   e. The treatment of choice is penicillin G.

I-96. The following apply to toxic shock syndrome:
   a. Staphylococci can produce alpha toxin which is dermonecrotic.
   b. Gamma toxin causes acute diarrhea.
   c. Exfoliatin is responsible for systemic and cutaneous symptoms of TSS.
   d. Beta toxin degrades sphingomyelin in erythrocytes.
   e. TSST-1 is responsible for staphylococcal scalded skin syndrome.

I-97. Which of the following reservoirs has been convincingly implicated in legionnaires' disease?
   a. Air conditioners.
   b. Evaporative condensors.
   c. Cooling towers.
   d. Whirlpools.
   e. Potable water distribution systems.

I-98. Which of the following clinical signs occur more often in legionnaires' disease than in pneumonias of other etiology and therefore are useful in clinical diagnosis?
   a. Abdominal pain.
   b. Diarrhea.
   c. Relative bradycardia.
   d. Hepatic dysfunction with elevated liver function tests.
   e. Hyponatremia.

I-99. All of the following are true *except:*
   a. Pneumonia caused by *L. bozemanii* can originate in soil.
   b. The clinical features in *L. bozemanii* infection are different from those seen in *L. pneumophila.*

c. *Legionella* infections can be diagnosed by serologic techniques.

d. The pathogen can be isolated in culture.

e. Direct immunofluorescence has only a 25–50% sensitivity.

I-100. Which of the following pulmonary diseases are associated with HIV infection?

a. Pneumococcal pneumonia.

b. Eosinophilic granuloma.

c. Lymphoid interstitial pneumonia.

d. Lymphoma.

e. Tuberculosis.

I-101. Which of the antibiotic(s) below would constitute appropriate therapy for aspiration pneumonia in a non-immunosuppressed patient admitted from the community?

a. Penicillin.

b. Clindamycin.

c. Cefotaxime.

d. Ciprofloxacin.

e. Ceftazidime plus amikacin.

I-102. Which of the following are common pulmonary pathogens in patients with AIDS?

a. Oropharyngeal anaerobes.

b. *Branhamella catarrhalis*.

c. *Pseudomonas aeruginosa*.

d. *Mycobacterium avium-intracellulare*.

e. Cytomegalovirus.

I-103. Which of the following stains can be used to identify *P. carinii*?

a. Fluorescein-tagged monoclonal antibody.

b. Gram's stain.

c. Giemsa stain.

d. Methenamine silver stain.

e. Fite's stain.

I-104. In nocardiosis:

a. Two thirds of patients are female.

b. Pulmonary disease alone occurs in about one third of cases, and disseminated disease occurs in about one third.

c. Sputum culture is rapidly positive.

d. The pleura is commonly involved.

e. Most pulmonary disease is due to *N. asteroides*.

I-105. TWAR is an acronym for:

a. A new antiviral agent used for therapy of cytomegalovirus pneumonia in AIDS patients.

b. A newly discovered agent of pneumonia.

c. The selective culture media on which mycoplasma will grow.

d. A silver stain that preferentially stains *Pneumocystis carinii* in sputum.

e. The CDC code name for *Legionella pneumophila* because it was first isolated from blood in a febrile patient, Thomas Ward.

I-106. Which of the following abnormalities in host defenses may play a role in the pathogenesis of pulmonary disease associated with HIV?

a. Abnormalities in serum complement.

b. Impaired macrophage function.

c. Reduced PMN chemotaxis.

d. Abnormalities in production of immunoglobulins.

e. Reduced cell-mediated immunity.

I-107. The following radiographic findings are consistent with a diagnosis of *P. carinii* pneumonia *except*:

a. Pneumothorax.

b. Pneumatocele formation.

c. Intrathoracic adenopathy.

d. Diffuse infiltration.

e. Focal infiltration.

I-108. Which of the following studies should always be performed on BAL specimens in patients with suspected HIV-associated lung diseases?

a. Culture for anaerobic organisms.

b. Mycobacterial cultures.

c. Cell count and differential.

d. Stain for *P. carinii*.

e. Culture for *Chlamydia*.

I-109. Tuberculosis in patients with HIV infection most often causes which of the following radiographic findings?
   a. Intrathoracic adenopathy.
   b. Cavitary upper lobe lesions.
   c. Diffuse infiltration.
   d. Nodular infiltration.
   e. Pleural effusion.

I-110. The therapy of choice for pulmonary and disseminated candidiasis is:
   a. Ketoconazole.
   b. Flucytosine.
   c. Miconazole.
   d. Amphotericin B.
   e. Rifampin.

I-111. Which of the following adverse reactions may occur with administration of pentamidine in patients with AIDS?
   a. Thrombocytopenia.
   b. Toxic delirium.
   c. Hypoglycemia.
   d. Hyperglycemia.
   e. Hypotension.

I-112. Trimethoprim-sulfamethoxazole is associated with which of the following adverse reactions in patients with AIDS?
   a. Fever.
   b. Skin rash with mucositis.
   c. Hepatitis.
   d. Neutropenia.
   e. Cardiac arrhythmia.

I-113. The most common underlying disorder associated with aspergilloma (fungus ball) of the lung is:
   a. Asthma.
   b. Tuberculosis.
   c. Coccidioidomycosis.
   d. Neutropenia associated with leukemia.
   e. Organ transplantation.

I-114. Which statement concerning the utility of sputum cultures for diagnosis of invasive pulmonary aspergillosis is correct?
   a. Sputum culture is worthless because of the ubiquitousness of the organism.
   b. Sputum culture may be misleading because of the relatively high presence of the organism in air and the ready contamination in the microbiology laboratory.
   c. Sputum culture is useful only if *Aspergillus* is also isolated from another site, especially blood.
   d. A positive sputum culture in neutropenic and immunosuppressed patients is highly suggestive of invasive aspergillosis.
   e. Blood culture is highly sensitive in the diagnosis of invasive aspergillosis.

I-115. Which of the following are susceptible to coccidioidomycosis?
   a. Archaeology students digging in infected soils in endemic regions.
   b. Dark-skinned races visiting endemic areas.
   c. Residents in Central and South America and the San Joaquin Valley.
   d. Chronic alcoholics.
   e. Immunosuppressed patients who have resided in endemic areas.

I-116. The therapy of choice for disseminated histoplasmosis is:
   a. Ketoconazole.
   b. Miconazole.
   c. Amphotericin B.
   d. Amphotericin B plus flucytosine.
   e. Itraconazole plus oral rifampin.

I-117. Infection control for bronchoscopy in patients with HIV infection should include:
   a. Gloves, mask, eye wear, and gown.
   b. Air hygiene.
   c. Concern with fomites for transmitting *M. tuberculosis*.
   d. 24-hour gas sterilization of bronchoscope.
   e. Laminar flow rooms.

I-118. The most common clinical presentation of cryptococcal infection is:
   a. Urinary tract infection.

b. Fungus ball in a preexisting tuberculosis cavity.

c. Pneumonitis.

d. Cryptococcoma of the central nervous system.

e. Meningitis.

I-119. Which of the following are true?

a. Direct immunofluorescence is positive in legionnaires' disease.

b. A 4-fold increase in indirect immunofluorescence assay titer during convalescence is diagnostic.

c. A presumptive diagnosis can be made with a single titer >256.

d. Legionella grows in buffered charcoal yeast extract agar with the addition of various antibiotics.

e. Most cultures will be positive in 3–5 days.

I-120. Which of the following drugs are bactericidal for TB?

a. Isoniazid (INH).

b. Pyrazinamide (PZA).

c. Streptomycin (SM).

d. Rifampin.

e. Ethambutol hydrochloride (EMB).

I-121. Which of these TB regimens are acceptable for general use?

a. 1 month of INH and RIF daily, followed by 8 months of INH and RIF twice weekly.

b. 2 months of INH, RIF, and EMB daily, followed by 7 months of INH and RIF daily.

c. 2 months of INH, RIF, and PZA daily, followed by 4 months of INH and RIF twice weekly.

d. 6 months of INH, RIF, PZA, and SM thrice weekly.

e. 4 months of INH, RIF, PZA, and SM daily.

I-122. Which of these assertions regarding human *M. avium-intracellulare* disease are true?

a. It is common in AIDS.

b. It is invariably disseminated in AIDS.

c. Pulmonary cases are seen mainly with preexisting lung disease.

d. The disease is primarily found in the southeastern United States.

e. Most *M. avium-intracellulare* complex infections are invasive.

I-123. In *M. avium-intracellulare* infection:

a. Treatment has never been proved efficacious.

b. The usual patient should begin on INH, RIF, EMB, and SM.

c. Drug susceptibility data are useless in choosing treatment.

d. Resectional surgery may be useful in selected patients.

e. The only drug necessary is streptomycin.

I-124. Which of the following are true about *M. fortuitum-chelonei* disease?

a. It is almost as prevalent as *M. kansasii* infection.

b. It is associated with esophageal dysfunction.

c. It is a common nosocomial pathogen.

d. It is totally unresponsive to anti-TB drugs.

e. The tetracyclines may be effective.

I-125. Which of these mycobacterial sputum isolates are often pathogens?

a. *M. szulgai.*

b. *M. terrae.*

c. *M. simiae.*

d. *M. gordonae.*

e. *M. xenopi.*

I-126. Which of these statements about pulmonary disease due to *M. kansasii* are true?

a. It occurs mostly among elderly patients with underlying lung diseases such as COPD.

b. Chemotherapy alone is sufficient to cure.

c. There is frequently low-level resistance to TB drugs such as INH.

d. Patients can be successfully managed with 6 month TB regimens.

e. Clinically significant drug resistance can be acquired with an inadequate drug regimen.

I-127. Which of the following statements on the epidemiology of TB are true?

a. TB is predominantly a disease of minorities in the United States.

b. The greatest recent increase in incidence is among people aged 45 to 64 years.

c. Recent increase in incidence is due to immigrants.

d. It may be easily spread in nursing homes.

e. Prevalence of drug-resistance has fallen over the past 10 years.

I-128. The AIDS virus causes decreased resistance to infection by mycobacteria because:

a. The AIDS virus infects CD 8+ cytotoxic T cells which are required for resistance.

b. The AIDS virus infects CD 4+ helper T cells and CD 8+ cells, thus decreasing immune responses.

c. The AIDS virus infects CD 4+ helper T cells, which stimulate B cells to make antibacterial antibodies.

d. The AIDS virus infects CD 4+ helper T cells, which regulate growth of cytotoxic T cells, which control infection.

e. The AIDS virus infects CD 4+ helper T cells, which secrete lymphokines.

1-8 Critical Care

C-1. The following apply to amyotrophic lateral sclerosis:

a. It mainly affects men 25 to 35 years of age.

b. There is loss of upper and lower motor neurons in the spinal cord.

c. Anal and bladder sphincters are usually spared.

d. Atrophy and fasciculations are common.

e. Bulbar deficits are uncommon.

C-2. The following apply to amyotrophic lateral sclerosis:

a. Glottic and pharyngeal paresis can lead to pneumonia.

b. These patients are vulnerable to upper airway closure when sleeping.

c. Upper airway closure is primarily associated with non-REM sleep.

d. Upper airway closure is exacerbated by negative pressure ventilators.

e. Succinylcholine chloride is the preferred muscle relaxant for intubation.

C-3. The following apply to colchicine:

a. It interferes with microtubule assembly and function.

b. It interferes with neutrophil granule release.

c. Doses over 50 mg are usually fatal.

d. Overdose can be detected in routine toxicology screens.

e. Overdose causes mitotic figures in PMNs on peripheral blood smear.

C-4. The following are seen in colchicine overdose:

a. Nausea, vomiting, abdominal pain and diarrhea.

b. Metabolic alkalosis.

c. Seizures.

d. Ascending paralysis.

e. Thrombocytopenia.

C-5. The following apply to treatment of colchicine overdose:

a. Potassium permanganate is given as an antidote.

b. Aggressive fluid resuscitation.

c. Bicarbonate.

d. Early mechanical ventilation.

e. Most of the drug is cleared in <24 hours.

C-6. The following statements are true:

a. Pulmonary emboli occur almost solely from deep venous thrombosis.

b. Right heart thrombi form as emboli from systemic veins.

c. *In situ* emboli can occur in association with pacer wires.

d. Right ventricular clot is more common than right atrial clot.

e. Serpiginous or "worm-like" thrombi are not visible on echocardiography.

C-7. The following statements are true:

a. Sessile thrombi generally are not associated with deep venous thrombosis.

b. Serpiginous or "worm-like" thrombi occur mostly in the setting of right ventricular failure.

c. Left-sided thromboemboli can occur with a patent foramen ovale.

d. Treatment of sessile thrombi is heparin/coumadin.

e. Catheter-related thrombi are successfully treated with thrombolysis.

C-8. Segmental or larger unmatched perfusion defects on $\dot{V}/\dot{Q}$ scan occur in:

a. Primary pulmonary hypertension.

b. Fibrosing mediastinitis.

c. Pulmonary artery agenesis.

d. Primary tumors of the pulmonary artery.

e. Extrinsic compression of a vessel.

C-9. ARDS patients suffer from:

a. PaO_2/FiO_2 <250.

b. Decreased permeability to plasma proteins.

c. Increased venous admixture.

d. Acute bilateral diffuse radiographic infiltrates.

e. A pulmonary capillary wedge pressure of >40 mm Hg.

C-10. The following apply to early ARDS:

a. Elevated pulmonary artery pressure and resistance with a normal PaO_2.

b. Infusing nitroprusside reduces cardiac output.

c. Inhaled nitrous oxide decreases pulmonary vascular resistance.

d. Inhaled nitrous oxide decreases the systemic vascular resistance.

e. Inhaled nitrous oxide may increase right ventricular ejection fraction.

C-11. The following apply to ARDS:

a. Pulmonary artery thromboembolism is common at autopsy.

b. There is growth of smooth muscle into distal regions of the pulmonary artery.

c. The right ventricular ejection fraction increases as pulmonary artery pressure (PAP) increases.

d. It can be caused by anaphylactic reaction to drugs.

e. In late stage, pulmonary capillary wedge pressure may be high.

C-12. The following apply to animal models of ARDS:

a. Intravenous lipopolysaccharide increases transpulmonary flux of edema.

b. Lipopolysaccharide causes the release of thromboxane.

c. Thromboxane is a profound pulmonary vasoconstrictor.

d. Tumor necrosis factor alpha is produced by neutrophils.

e. Tumor necrosis factor alpha following endotoxin injection causes shock.

C-13. The following statements apply to auto-PEEP in COPD:

a. It is measured by occluding the expiratory port and observing the pressure.

b. The incidence is lower when minute ventilation is high.

c. The incidence rises with increasing patient age.

d. It can be reduced by decreasing inspiratory flow.

e. It rises with low compressible volume circuit.

C-14. The following statements apply to auto-PEEP in COPD:

a. It increases with smaller endotracheal tubes.

b. Static compliance is overestimated.

c. It is reduced by addition of PEEP up to a level equal to the auto-PEEP.

d. It is increased by reducing frequency and V_T.

e. The magnitude depends on the time available for expiration.

C-15. In healthy individuals at rest:

a. Inspiratory muscles overcome elastance and flow resistance of the total respiratory system.

b. Expiratory muscle activity is usually absent.

c. Part of the expiratory pressure is dissipated against the postinspiration activity of the inspiratory muscles.

d. Elastic recoil pressure stored during the preceding inspiration drives expiration.

e. There is braking early in expiration due to activity of inspiratory muscles.

C-16. In patients with chronic airflow limitation:

a. Auto-PEEP may develop because the rate of lung emptying is slow.

b. When a patient is acutely ill, tachypnea promotes dynamic hyperinflation.

c. The pressure-generating capability of the inspiratory muscles is reduced.

d. CPAP (continuous positive airway pressure) is valid in airflow limitation only if it further increases end expiratory lung volume.

e. The inspiratory muscle pressure required to initiate lung inflation should be increased by an amount approximately equal to end-expiratory elastic recoil pressure + CPAP.

C-17. Amyotrophic lateral sclerosis (ALS) can present with:

a. Focal muscle weakness.

b. Atrophy and fasciculations (90%).

c. Polycythemia.

d. Dysarthria.

e. Swallowing difficulties.

C-18. The most important aspect in treating disseminated intravascular coagulation is to:

a. Administer heparin.

b. Administer platelets.

c. Treat the underlying disease process.

d. Achieve normal levels of fibrinogen.

e. Transfuse with fresh frozen plasma and cryoprecipitate.

C-19. "Freebasing" of cocaine can result in:

a. Decreased diffusing capacity due to pulmonary vasoconstriction.

b. Pneumomediastinum secondary to alveolar rupture.

c. Noncardiogenic pulmonary edema.

d. An acute syndrome with dyspnea and hypoxemia.

e. Bronchiolitis obliterans and organizing pneumonia (BOOP).

C-20. Methemoglobin:

a. Is formed by the oxidation of deoxyhemoglobin to the ferric state.

b. Binds with oxygen so that oxyhemoglobin is reduced.

c. Causes a shift to the right of the oxygen dissociation curve.

d. Impairs oxygen delivery to tissues.

e. Is formed in small amounts under normal circumstances.

C-21. Methemoglobinemia:

a. May be hereditary.

b. Is associated with increase of NADH-dependent metHb reductase.

c. May result from exposure to well water.

d. May result from exposure to sulfa drugs and Pyridium.

e. Has as its earliest sign bluish-brown cyanosis.

C-22. In methemoglobinemia:

a. Headache may be present when metHb approaches 10% of total Hb.

b. Levels of 50–70% are associated with arrhythmias.

c. Levels >70% are frequently fatal.

d. Diagnosis is made by dark brown blood that brightens with exposure to oxygen.

e. Treatment usually consists of IV methylene blue.

C-23. In pulse oximetry:

a. Oxygen saturation is estimated by ratio of absorption of light at two wavelengths.

b. Oxyhemoglobin absorbs light primarily at a wavelength of 600.

c. Deoxyhemoglobin absorbs light mainly at a wavelength of 940.

d. It is accurate even with a variety of hemoglobins present.

e. With metHb, the ratio of the two wavelengths is less than 0.6.

C-24. In hypothyroidism or myxedema one may encounter:

a. Alveolar hypoventilation.

b. Sleep apnea.

c. Transudative pleural effusion.

d. Pulmonary edema.

e. Cardiomegaly.

C-25. In patients with myxedema *and* obesity one sees:

a. Reduced lung volumes.

b. Normal maximum breathing capacity.

c. Normal $D_L CO$.

d. Alveolar hypoventilation.

e. Reduced hypercapnic ventilatory responsiveness.

C-26. In most patients with myxedema without obesity one sees:

a. Normal lung volumes.

b. Normal gas exchange.

c. Reduced maximum breathing capacity.

d. Normal $D_L CO$.

e. Normal hypercapnic ventilatory responsiveness.

C-27. The Guillain-Barré syndrome has been associated with the following *except*:

a. *Campylobacter* infections.

b. *Mycoplasma*.

c. Trauma.

d. Epidural and general surgery.

e. Hodgkin's disease.

C-28. The clinical presentation of Guillain-Barré syndrome includes the following *except*:

a. Progressive symmetric muscle weakness which spreads proximally.

b. Hyperreflexia.

c. Paresthesias, pain, numbness.

d. Cranial nerve involvement.

e. Flushing.

C-29. The clinical presentation of Guillain-Barré syndrome includes:

a. Hypertension.

b. Very cellular CSF.

c. Normal CSF protein.

d. Increase in glucose.

e. Increased nerve conduction.

C-30. The following apply to ethylene glycol poisoning:

a. Organ toxicity is due to deposition of calcium-oxalate crystals in blood vessel walls.

b. Oxalate is capable of causing renal damage if ingested directly.

c. Hypocalcemia is common.

d. Hippuric acid crystals are found in the urine.

e. Ethylene glycol has a 100-fold greater affinity for alcohol dehydrogenase than ethanol.

C-31. Three stages of ethylene glycol poisoning have been described. Match the toxic manifestations of ethylene glycol poisoning with the stage:
a. Cranial nerve abnormalities.
b. Optic atrophy.
c. Pulmonary edema.
d. Ophthalmoplegia.
e. Acute tubular necrosis.

C-32. Treatment of ethylene glycol poisoning consists of the following *except*:
a. HCO$_3$.
b. Carbonic anhydrase inhibitors.
c. Ethanol.
d. Hemodialysis.
e. Alkaline diuresis.

C-33. Autologous bone marrow transplant may be beneficial in patients with:
a. Non-Hodgkin's lymphoma.
b. Ovarian carcinoma.
c. Small cell carcinoma of the lung.
d. Malignant melanoma.
e. Nonseminomatous germ cell tumors.

C-34. Match the following advantages and disadvantages with pressure-controlled inverse-ratio ventilation (P) and volume-controlled inverse-ratio ventilation (V):
a. Guaranteed minute ventilation.
b. Precise control of flow pattern.
c. Peak alveolar pressures can vary.
d. Deep sedation is usually necessary.
e. Tidal volume varies with changing respiratory mechanics.

C-35. The causes of an anion gap are the following *except*:
a. Salicylate intoxication.
b. Theophylline intoxication.
c. Uremia.
d. Paraldehyde toxicity.
e. Ethylene glycol toxicity.

C-36. Tracheoesophageal fistula may result from the following *except*:
a. A cervical Zenker's diverticulum.
b. *Candida* tracheal infection.
c. Blunt chest trauma.
d. Wegener's granulomatosis.
e. Gastric ulcer.

C-37. The following apply to allopurinol:
a. It reduces incidence of urate nephropathy in asymptomatic hyperuricemia.
b. Dosage must be adjusted for renal function.
c. Complications include ocular sequelae.
d. Steroids reduce side effects.
e. Toxicity is due to immune complex deposition and vasculitis.

C-38. The following statements apply to bone marrow transplant:
a. Pulmonary complications of autologous bone marrow transplant are different from those of allogeneic bone marrow transplant.
b. "Immunocompromised" hosts develop a "primary" or idiopathic form of diffuse alveolar hemorrhage.
c. Diffuse alveolar hemorrhage in autologous bone marrow transplant recipients is seen in association with invasive fungal infection.
d. The frequency of alveolar hemorrhage correlates with the type of chemotherapy.
e. Alveolar hemorrhage most commonly occurs within 40 days of transplantation.

C-39. The following statements apply to inverse-ratio ventilation:
a. It extends the expiratory time.
b. It is volume-cycled ventilation with a decelerating expiratory flow rate.
c. It leads to better outcome than conventional ventilator therapy in ARDS.
d. It is volume-cycled ventilation with an end inspiratory pause.
e. Is pressure-controlled ventilation with a long inspiratory time.

C-40. The following apply to the adult respiratory distress syndrome:
a. Tissue injury in the adult respiratory

distress syndrome is homogeneously distributed.

b. The incidence of sepsis and multiple organ failure rises with the duration of mechanical ventilation.

c. Volume-cycled ventilation with applied positive end expiratory pressure injures alveolar tissues.

d. Inverse-ratio ventilation may improve gas exchange while limiting or decreasing the peak airway pressures.

e. Even with ventilatory support, most patients with the adult respiratory distress syndrome die of respiratory insufficiency.

C-41. The following apply to the adult respiratory distress syndrome:

a. The proportion of venous admixture correlates with the proportion of non-aerated lung.

b. The surface tension of alveoli may be lower than normal at low lung volumes.

c. Aerated lung volume at functional residual capacity (FRC) is significantly less than in other patients requiring mechanical ventilation.

d. The inflation portion of the pressure-volume (P-V) curve is typically normal.

e. There is significant hysteresis of the P-V curve.

C-42. The following apply to ventilation in the adult respiratory distress syndrome:

a. Gas extravasated from alveoli during ventilatory support may cause pneumothoraces.

b. Alveolar rupture occurs when pressure gradient is low across alveoli along bronchovascular sheath.

c. Peak alveolar pressure exceeding 20 cm H_2O increases the risk of tissue rupture.

d. Ventilator-induced alveolar edema will not occur at low levels of peak airway pressure.

e. Large tidal volumes can contribute to increased lung edema.

C-43. The following apply to ventilator therapy:

a. Peak alveolar pressure exceeds peak airway pressure during volume controlled ventilation.

b. Peak airway pressure and the peak alveolar pressure equilibrate during pressure-controlled inverse-ratio ventilation.

c. With inverse-ratio ventilation, cardiac output may rise as mean airway pressure increases.

d. During volume-controlled inverse-ratio ventilation, alveolar pressures may rise dangerously if the patient is allowed to trigger the ventilator.

e. Increasing the frequency during pressure-controlled inverse-ratio ventilation increases the alveolar ventilation.

C-44. In the allopurinol hypersensitivity syndrome:

a. Aspartate aminotransferase is elevated.

b. The leukocytosis may be accompanied by eosinophilia.

c. The leukocytosis may be accompanied by a left shift.

d. Many patients have diabetes mellitus.

e. Onset of the syndrome is immediate within hours of receiving the drug.

C-45. Management of myxedema includes the following:

a. Administration of CNS depressants.

b. Administration of hypotonic fluids.

c. Meticulous search for a precipitating event or infection.

d. Passive cooling to avoid peripheral vasodilation.

e. Initial administration of corticosteroids to cover possible coexistent adrenal insufficiency.

C-46. Hypothyroidism is characterized by:

a. Central sleep apnea which is reversible.

b. Hyperglycemia, suggesting coexistent adrenal insufficiency.

c. Renal impairment with hypernatremia.

d. Inappropriate ADH secretion or inability to suppress ADH with a water load.

e. Altered renal hemodynamics with reduced delivery of water to the distal nephron.

C-47. The following statements pertain to hypothyroidism and myxedema:
a. Decompensation is usually caused by a precipitating event or illness.
b. The yellow tinge of the skin is due to deposits of carotene.
c. It may follow Hashimoto's thyroiditis.
d. Ventilatory responses to chemical stimuli are reduced.
e. Iodide and lithium carbonate cause hypothyroidism in susceptible individuals.

C-48. In toxic strep syndrome:
a. There are thin yellow bullae on the skin.
b. There is marked leukopenia.
c. There is progressive hypercalcemia.
d. Multi-organ failure with ARDS is common.
e. The treatment of choice is tetracycline.

C-49. These statements pertain to the toxic shock syndrome:
a. Staphylococcal alpha toxin can lyse cells.
b. Staphylococcal beta toxin degrades sphingomyelin in erythrocytes.
c. Staphylococcal gamma toxin increases water absorption from the bowel.
d. TSST-1 antibody in plasma is diagnostic.
e. Toxin in serum is demonstrated by a monoclonal antibody assay.

C-50. The following are major physical signs of respiratory distress *except*:
a. Arrhythmias.
b. Diaphoresis.
c. Nasal flaring.
d. Bulging out of the suprasternal/supraclavicular/intercostal spaces.
e. Tachypnea.

C-51. The following statements pertain to bacterial meningitis:

a. Cerebral edema is common in patients with bacterial meningitis.
b. Secretion of antidiuretic hormone contributes to the pathogenesis of edema.
c. The inflammatory response in CSF increases with inhibition of arachidonic acid.
d. Cyclooxygenase inhibitors along with beta-lactam antibiotics reduce inflammation.
e. Dexamethasone along with antibiotics decreases CSF tumor necrosis factor.

C-52. The following statements pertain to bacterial meningitis:
a. *Staphylococcus aureus* is a major cause of bacterial meningitis.
b. Meningitis follows colonization of the nasopharynx by an organism.
c. Host defense mechanisms are inadequate if bacteria enter the subarachnoid space.
d. Specific antibody formation and complement levels are increased in the CSF.
e. Tumor necrosis factor in CSF may be specific for bacterial meningitis.

C-53. The following apply to diabetic ketoacidosis:
a. Phospholipase A is involved in mediating increased permeability in ARDS.
b. Acute pancreatitis is common during diabetic ketoacidosis.
c. ARDS in diabetic ketoacidosis is always bilateral.
d. An elevated serum amylase is related to the severity of diabetic ketoacidosis.
e. Fulminant ARDS occurs primarily with hemorrhagic pancreatitis.

C-54. With pressure-support ventilation, the following apply *except*:
a. It delivers a breath until the patient's inspiratory flow decreases to a minimal level.
b. Every breath must be triggered by the patient.
c. The delivered tidal volume decreases if effort decreases.

d. Low minute-ventilation alarm may fail if utilizing in-line continuous nebulizers.

e. Respiratory work is reduced if respiratory drive is heightened.

C-55. The following apply to ventilator therapy:

a. Prolonged mechanical ventilation predisposes to respiratory muscle fatigue.

b. Insufficient support may produce weakness of the respiratory muscles.

c. Spontaneous gas exchange may improve after negative-pressure ventilation in some patients with COPD.

d. Work of breathing increases during intermittent mandatory ventilation.

e. Work of breathing is performed entirely by the ventilator during a machine breath.

C-56. The following apply to gastric distension *except*:

a. It may follow a decrease in mouth pressure during the delivery of manual ventilation.

b. It may cause deterioration in ventilation-perfusion relationships.

c. It is induced by elevated airway pressure above lower esophageal sphincter pressure, during mechanical ventilation.

d. It may result from a prolonged or difficult attempt at intubation.

e. If massive, it can result in gastric rupture.

C-57. The following apply to critically ill patients *except*:

a. An increased respiratory drive may result from severe respiratory alkalosis.

b. Lying on one side can cause hypoxemia in patients with unilateral lung disease.

c. Agitation or seizures may result from use of theophylline.

d. Aminoglycoside antibiotics can produce respiratory embarrassment.

e. Hypoxemia may result following use of bronchodilators.

C-58. In a patient who is "fighting the ventilator," one should first carry out the following *except*:

a. Adjust the trigger sensitivity.

b. Adjust the inspiratory flow.

c. Adjust the delivered tidal volume.

d. Alter the mode of mechanical ventilation.

e. Administer diazepam, 2–5 mg IV every 5 minutes to a maximum of 20–30 mg.

C-59. The following statements apply to management of head injuries:

a. Hypercapnia lowers an elevated intracranial pressure.

b. Mean intrathoracic pressure is increased with mechanical ventilation.

c. Rapid ventilator rates may raise the intracranial pressure.

d. High-frequency jet ventilation is associated with high peak airway pressures.

e. High-frequency jet ventilation reduces intracranial pressure when elevated by intermittent positive-pressure ventilation (IPPV).

C-60. The following statements apply to ventilator therapy in head injuries *except*:

a. IPPV in excess of 12 breaths per minute may result in an increase in intracranial pressure.

b. Hypercarbia reduces the intracranial pressure.

c. Peak airway pressure is low in high-frequency jet ventilation.

d. High-frequency jet ventilation reduces the elevations of intracranial pressure.

e. Addition of continuous positive airway pressure (CPAP) and intermittent mandatory ventilation (IMV) to high-frequency jet ventilation produces good oxygenation.

C-61. The following statements apply to auto-PEEP in a ventilator patient:

a. Auto-PEEP or intrinsic PEEP develops because of insufficient inspiratory time.

b. The complications are different from those of applied or extrinsic PEEP.

c. Intrathoracic vascular pressure measurements can be inaccurate.

d. Auto-PEEP can result in an increased intracranial pressure.

e. Patients with a small-diameter endotracheal tube are at risk of auto-PEEP.

C-62. Which of the following are true of auto-PEEP in ventilator patients?

a. Patients with airflow limitation are at greater risk of auto-PEEP.

b. High respiratory rates increase the risk of auto-PEEP.

c. Institution of a high minute ventilation reduces the risk of auto-PEEP.

d. It can be eliminated by decreasing expiratory time.

e. It is measured by occlusion of the inspiratory port at end expiration.

C-63. Treatment of auto-PEEP on a ventilator consists of:

a. Use of a smaller endotracheal tube.

b. Shortening expiratory time.

c. Use of a circuit with low compressible volume.

d. Decreasing the respiratory frequency and or minute ventilation.

e. Addition of positive end expiratory pressure.

C-64. The following statements apply to auto-PEEP in a patient on a ventilator:

a. The level can be read continuously on the ventilator pressure manometer.

b. It predisposes to barotrauma and hemodynamic embarrassment.

c. It reduces the work of breathing.

d. It increases the efficiency of force generation of the respiratory muscles.

e. A negative pressure in addition to the minimum circuit pressure drop must be generated to initiate an assisted breath.

C-65. The following apply to the end expiratory lung volume:

a. It approximates the relaxation volume of the respiratory system in normal subjects.

b. It is below predicted FRC because of dynamic airway collapse in critically ill patients.

c. It is above the predicted FRC in some critically ill patients.

d. Relaxation pressure of the respiratory system is zero at end expiration in normals.

e. It falls with expiratory obstruction.

C-66. The following statements apply to the anticholinergic syndrome:

a. Cardiac muscle is affected most by anticholinergic agents.

b. It may be potentiated by antihistamines.

c. Tricyclic antidepressants may be useful in mild conditions.

d. Phenothiazines are beneficial in severe CNS toxicity.

e. Physostigmine can cause excessive salivation.

C-67. The following apply to the patient who is failing a weaning trial *except*:

a. Rapid respiratory rate.

b. Increased ventilation.

c. Reduced tidal volume.

d. Reduced alveolar ventilation.

e. Reduced V_D / V_T ratio.

C-68. Endoscopic intravariceal sclerotherapy (EVS):

a. Is the treatment of choice for esophageal varices prophylactically.

b. Results in a pleural effusion in up to 50% of patients.

c. The effusion is transudate with normal pH, glucose, and amylase.

d. There is a retrocardiac density emulating RLL infiltrate.

e. Causes esophageal perforation.

C-69. Hydrocarbon poisoning:

a. It can cause an acute alveolitis.

b. The alveolitis disappears in 10 days.

c. It can cause a chronic proliferative process.

d. The chronic proliferative process resolves over several weeks.

e. There is necrosis of bronchial, bronchiolar, and alveolar tissues.

C-70. The following applies to hydrocarbon ingestion and pneumonitis:
a. Pulmonary lesions are caused by gastrointestinal absorption.
b. Vomiting should be induced.
c. Corticosteroids are beneficial.
d. Antibiotics are indicated.
e. Bronchodilators are useful.

C-71. Hypophosphatemia is particularly associated with:
a. Hyperparathyroidism.
b. Alcohol withdrawal.
c. Diabetic ketoacidosis.
d. Sepsis.
e. Malnutrition.

C-72. Phosphate deficiency may result from:
a. Malabsorption.
b. Diuretics.
c. Respiratory acidosis.
d. Insulin administration.
e. Aggressive nutrition.

C-73. The following apply to hypophosphatemia:
a. Phosphate deficiency may occur with a normal serum phosphate level.
b. Clinical symptoms rarely occur in the absence of markedly reduced levels.
c. Significant problems generally do not occur until levels are <1 mg/dl.
d. A reduction in red cell 2,3 DPG and ATP leads to a right shift in the oxyhemoglobin dissociation curve.
e. A Guillain-Barré-like ascending paralysis may develop.

C-74. The following apply to hypophosphatemia:
a. Levels <2 mg/dl in diabetes require intravenous supplementation.

b. Levels of 1–2.5 mg/dl can be treated with skim milk.
c. Potassium and magnesium may be reduced.
d. Precipitation of calcium phosphate crystals potentially complicates IV phosphate therapy.
e. Hypercalcemia can develop if phosphate is administered too quickly.

C-75. The following apply to Reye's syndrome:
a. There is a genetic susceptibility.
b. It is associated with aspirin use.
c. It does not occur in adults.
d. It often follows a URI/influenza illness.
e. It is an infectious phase followed by an encephalitic phase.

C-76. The following apply to Reye's syndrome:
a. There is increased activity of mitochondrial enzymes in encephalitic phase.
b. There is increased activity of mitochondrial enzymes involved in oxidative phosphorylation.
c. Activity of cytosolic enzyme is increased.
d. Biochemical differences parallel mitochondrial degeneration in brain.
e. Clinical severity parallels mitochondrial distortion.

C-77. When the oxygen delivery fails to meet cellular energy needs:
a. Lactate production increases.
b. ATP is generated anaerobically.
c. Glucose metabolism shifts to pyruvate production.
d. Hydrogen ion concentration falls.
e. Oxygen debt develops.

C-78. In septic patients:
a. Vo_2 is independent of 0_2 delivery below 350 ml/min/m².
b. Vo_2 is dependent on 0_2 delivery above 350 ml/min/m².
c. Systemic alkalosis is characteristic.
d. Lactic acidosis indicates ongoing tissue hypoxia.

e. Elevated lactate levels indicate a bad outcome.

C-79. In the allopurinol hypersensitivity syndrome:
a. About 40% of patients develop some reaction to allopurinol.
b. There is diffuse maculopapular rash.
c. There is exfoliative dermatitis.
d. There is worsening renal function.
e. There is eosinophilia.

C-80. The following apply to the allopurinol hypersensitivity syndrome:
a. Male/female incidence is 2:1.
b. There is elevated aspartate aminotransferase in majority of cases.
c. Renal failure develops in few cases.
d. Corticosteroids are effective treatment.
e. Reduction of asymptomatic high serum urate levels reduces urate nephropathy incidence.

C-81. The following apply to the allopurinol hypersensitivity syndrome:
a. It is believed to be a hypersensitivity reaction to oxypurinol.
b. It involves immune-complex deposition.
c. Vasculitis is present.
d. Oxypurinol accumulation is directly related to renal function.
e. Mortality is most likely with acute or acute-on-chronic renal failure.

C-82. The following are complications of nitrofurantoin:
a. Fevers and chills.
b. Eosinophilia.
c. Bibasilar interstitial infiltrate on radiograph.
d. Hives.
e. Chronic interstitial pneumonitis is most common.

C-83. The following apply to nitrofurantoin toxicity:

a. Acute reaction is due to direct effect of oxygen radicals.
b. Circulatory collapse can occur.
c. Resolution occurs quickly after the drug is discontinued.
d. Symptoms recur on re-exposure.
e. Chronic pulmonary toxicity can occur years after seemingly uncomplicated therapy.

C-84. The following applies to nitrofurantoin toxicity:
a. Men comprise 80% of cases.
b. Pleural effusions are frequent.
c. Eosinophilia and leukocytosis are common in patients with chronic pneumonitis.
d. Lung biopsy shows an interstitial pneumonitis that can be distinguished from other causes of interstitial pneumonitis.
e. It can cause a desquamative interstitial pneumonia.

C-85. The following apply to nitric oxide:
a. It is the same as endothelium-derived relaxing factor (EDRF).
b. It is the etiologic agent responsible for silo filler's disease.
c. A decrease in intracellular calcium stimulates the production of nitric oxide.
d. It directly inhibits cyclic guanosine monophosphate (GMP) in vascular smooth muscle causing relaxation.
e. Production is stimulated by hypoxia.

C-86. Inhaled nitric oxide (NO):
a. Avidly binds to hemoglobin.
b. Activates the cytochrome system required for electron transport.
c. Causes marked systemic vasodilatation.
d. Causes selective vasodilatation of poorly ventilated areas.
e. Decreases pulmonary vascular resistance (PVR) in patients with primary pulmonary hypertension.

C-87. The following apply to prolonged neuromuscular blockade in the ICU:

a. Atracurium besylate accumulates in patients with renal failure.

b. Pancuronium bromide accumulates in patients with liver failure.

c. It can be associated with metabolic alkalosis.

d. It can be associated with male sex.

e. It can be associated with hypomagnesemia.

C-88. The following apply to prolonged neuromuscular blockade in the ICU:

a. High-dose corticosteroids and neuromuscular blocking agents increase risk.

b. The myopathy is similar to chronic corticosteroid myopathy.

c. CPK frequently is elevated.

d. The deficits are typically reversible.

e. Specific treatment consists of nonsteroidal anti-inflammatory agents.

C-89. Critical illness polyneuropathy syndrome is characterized by:

a. Lower extremity paralysis.

b. Increased deep tendon reflexes.

c. Variable sensory deficits.

d. Axonal degeneration involving both motor and sensory fibers.

e. Occurrence in patients with the multiple organ dysfunction syndrome.

C-90. The following apply to salicylates:

a. Therapeutic levels for anti-inflammatory effects range from 5–10 mg/dl.

b. Toxic effects occur with levels greater than 30 mg/dl.

c. Acute intoxication has a poorer outcome than chronic intoxication.

d. Hepatocellular necrosis occurs only when levels exceed 75 mg/dl.

e. IV sodium bicarbonate indicated if salicylate greater than 35 mg/dl.

C-91. The pathophysiologic effects of salicylate intoxication include:

a. Noncardiogenic pulmonary edema.

b. Stimulation of Krebs cycle.

c. Interference with the synthesis of factor VIII.

d. Decrease in renal excretion of bicarbonate.

e. Initial hypoglycemia.

C-92. Treatment of salicylate intoxication consists of:

a. Gastric lavage.

b. Activated charcoal.

c. Hydration.

d. Intubation and mechanical ventilation.

e. Maintaining a urinary pH less than 7.0.

C-93. Specific indications for hemodialysis in cases of salicylate intoxication include:

a. Levels greater than 50 mg/dl in acute ingestion.

b. Levels greater than 30 mg/dl in chronic toxicity.

c. Rising blood levels.

d. CNS abnormalities.

e. Urinary pH less than 7.0.

C-94. The following apply to burns:

a. There is inhalation injury in about 33% of major burns.

b. Death is the result of carbon monoxide poisoning.

c. Inhalation of air at 150°C results in burns of lung parenchyma.

d. The patient is symptomatic when levels of CO reach 5%.

e. Death occurs when levels of CO reach 25%.

C-95. The following apply to carbon monoxide:

a. The half-life in the body is 4 hours.

b. The half-life is reduced to 45–60 minutes with 100% FiO_2.

c. It shifts the oxyhemoglobin desaturation curve to the right.

d. It binds to myoglobin causing decreased O_2 transport to cardiac muscle.

e. It interferes with the cytochrome oxidase system of cellular respiration.

C-96. The following apply to amyotrophic lateral sclerosis (ALS):

a. Mean survival is 10 years.

b. Survival tends to be decreased with progressive bulbar palsy.

c. Survival is shorter for females.

d. PFTs reveal reduced residual volume (RV) and total lung capacity (TLC).

e. Maximum ventilation possible (MVV) is the most abnormal pulmonary function test.

C-97. Critical factors needed to cause lung injury in aspiration are:

a. pH of gastric aspirate <2.5.

b. Bacterial content.

c. Particulate matter/content.

d. pH of gastric aspirate >2.5.

e. Volume of the aspirate.

C-98. A ventilator-supported patient develops sudden severe respiratory distress. You would first:

a. Increase tidal volume.

b. Disconnect the patient from the ventilator and manually ventilate with 100% oxygen using an anesthesia bag.

c. Check the ventilator for leaks.

d. Increase the inspired oxygen concentration.

e. Change the ventilator.

C-99. The following is true of *Clostridium botulinum*:

a. A neurotoxin is produced by the organism.

b. It is a gram-negative, rod-shaped, spore-forming, anaerobic genus of bacteria.

c. It is widely distributed in the soil and water.

d. Spores are killed by 100°C in 3 hours.

e. Formed toxin is denatured at 80°C.

C-100. The following is true of botulism:

a. Most cases of human disease are the result of toxin types C and D.

b. Type A disease is found east of the Mississippi river.

c. Type B disease is found west of the Mississippi river.

d. Type E is associated with marine products.

e. Type A has the shortest latency between ingestion and symptoms.

C-101. The botulism toxin:

a. Targets the presynaptic terminal of neuromotor end plates in peripheral nerves.

b. Prevents acetylcholine release from the nerve terminal.

c. Can have effects that last for months.

d. Is absorbed from its source (GI or wound) into the blood stream and lymphatics.

e. Causes sore throat by interruption of the cholinergic autonomic system.

C-102. The following tests are most likely to be positive in the patient with botulism:

a. Tensilon test.

b. Lumbar puncture.

c. EMG.

d. Serum *Clostridium botulinum* assay.

e. Culture of stool.

C-103. The following are true of botulism:

a. Clinical manifestations begin within 12–36 hours of toxin ingestion.

b. Nausea and vomiting are more common in type B toxin.

c. Early symptoms include weakness, lassitude, and dizziness.

d. Most cases are due to improper home canning of fruits and vegetables.

e. Autonomic dysfunction can lead to an ileus, constipation, and urinary retention.

C-104. The following are true of botulism:

a. Diplopia, blurred vision, photophobia, dysphonia, dysarthria, and dysphagia occur.

b. Symmetric ascending weakness of the extremities occurs.

c. Sensation is classically not affected.

d. Ventilatory support may be necessary for months.

e. Symptoms can persist for up to a year.

C-105. The following apply to botulism:

a. Clindamycin is effective therapy.

b. Antitoxin shortens the course of the disease.

c. Antitoxin has a significantly greater effect if given within 24 hours.

d. Amoxicillin is effective therapy.

e. Guanidine is effective therapy.

C-106. The following apply to botulism:

    a. Paralysis is due to binding of the toxin to calcium channels at the motor neuron end plate.

    b. Acetylcholine release is inhibited.

    c. Symptoms begin within 12–36 hours of ingestion.

    d. Distal muscles are more involved than proximal.

    e. Sensory function is markedly disturbed.

C-107. The following apply to high-altitude pulmonary edema:

    a. It is a noncardiogenic pulmonary edema.

    b. It develops in people who ascend to over 8000–9000 feet of elevation.

    c. Symptoms usually occur within 24–96 hours.

    d. Fever would rule out high-altitude pulmonary edema.

    e. Leukopenia is found in the majority of patients.

C-108. Hemodialysis may result in the following *except*:

    a. A fall in PaO_2.

    b. Increased $P(A-a)O_2$.

    c. Reduced $D_L CO$.

    d. Complement activation.

    e. Bicarbonate dialysate increases the incidence of pulmonary complications.

C-109. In sickle cell disease:

    a. Hemoglobin O_2 saturation curve is shifted to the left.

    b. 2–3 DPG is decreased.

    c. Pulmonary capillary blood volume is decreased.

    d. PaO_2 at 50% Hb saturation (P50) is decreased.

    e. Reducing the percentage of Hb S cells increases the oxygen-carrying capacity.

C-110. The following statements apply to gastroesophageal function *except*:

    a. Lower esophageal sphincter pressure is decreased by theophilline.

    b. Lower esophageal sphincter pressure is increased by beta agonists.

    c. Lower esophageal sphincter pressure is decreased by smoking.

    d. The forced vital capacity (FVC) and forced expiratory volume (FEV_1) are reduced with gastric but not duodenal ulcer.

    e. Theophylline increases gastric acid secretion.

C-111. Injuries causing ARDS include:

    a. Bacteremia.

    b. Aspiration of gastrointestinal contents.

    c. Hydrocarbon ingestion.

    d. Acute vasculitis.

    e. Anaphylactic reaction to drugs and blood.

C-112. The following apply to ventilator therapy:

    a. During volume-controlled ventilation, the peak alveolar pressure always exceeds the peak airway pressure.

    b. During pressure-controlled inverse-ratio ventilation, the peak airway pressure and the peak alveolar pressure equilibrate.

    c. With inverse-ratio ventilation, cardiac output may rise as mean airway pressure increases.

    d. During positive-pressure ventilation, mean airway pressure over the entire respiratory cycle reflects the average pressure applied by the ventilator.

    e. Increasing the frequency during pressure-controlled inverse-ratio ventilation will increase the alveolar ventilation.

C-113. ARDS is characterized by which of the following:

    a. Diffuse roentgenographic infiltrates.

    b. Refractory hypoxemia.

    c. Normal left ventricular filling pressures.

    d. Carbon dioxide retention.

    e. Respiratory acidosis.

C-114. A sample of blood has a hemoglobin concentration of 15 gm/dl and a pO_2 of 40 mm Hg. This sample of blood:
   a. Has a hemoglobin saturation with oxygen of less than 50%.
   b. Contains about 20 ml of O_2 per 100 ml.
   c. Is likely to be a mixed venous sample from a patient with severe congestive heart failure.
   d. Is likely to have been drawn from the right atrium of a normal person.
   e. Is likely to be an arterial blood sample from a normal person residing at 10,000 ft. altitude.

C-115. In primary pulmonary hypertension, the most common presentation for a patient with plexogenic pulmonary arteriopathy is:
   a. A male teenager with dyspnea and increased bronchovascular markings on chest roentgenogram.
   b. A middle-aged female with normal-appearing lung fields on chest film and normal distribution of radionuclide on pulmonary perfusion lung scan.
   c. An elderly female with increased bronchovascular markings on chest film and subsegmental perfusion defects on perfusion lung scan.
   d. A middle-aged female with a normal chest film, but patchy distribution of radionuclide on lung scan.
   e. An elderly male with normal chest film and lung scan, but a pulmonary arteriogram that shows widespread segmental and subsegmental filling defects and occlusions.

C-116. Which of the following is correct about vasodilator therapy and pulmonary hypertension?
   a. Vasodilator drugs are usually effective treatment for pulmonary veno-occlusive disease.
   b. Pulmonary arterial blood pressure may rise in response to vasodilator therapy.
   c. When total pulmonary resistance falls with vasodilator drug therapy it is because of a direct vasodilator effect of the drug.
   d. Generally, with vasodilator therapy, the fall in pulmonary vascular resistance is proportional to the fall in systemic vascular resistance.
   e. Morphologic abnormalities in the pulmonary resistance vessels correlate well with increases in pulmonary arterial blood pressure.

C-117. The clinical condition most often associated with ARDS is:
   a. Hypotension.
   b. Multiple transfusions.
   c. Sepsis.
   d. Trauma.
   e. Drug overdosage.

C-118. The pathology of ARDS is characterized by:
   a. Interstitial and alveolar edema.
   b. Neutrophil and platelet aggregation.
   c. *In situ* thrombosis.
   d. Hyaline membranes.
   e. All of the above.

C-119. Pathogenic factors *not* implicated in ARDS include:
   a. Inflammation.
   b. Vascular obstruction.
   c. Atelectasis.
   d. Fibrosis.
   e. Immune deficiency.

C-120. All of the following pulmonary function abnormalities occur in ARDS *except*:
   a. Increased airflow obstruction.
   b. Decreased lung volumes.
   c. Hypoxemia.
   d. Decreased diffusion capacity.
   e. Hypocapnia.

C-121. Which of the following are correct?
   a. In head injury hypocapnia is effective in lowering elevated intracranial pressure.
   b. IPPV in excess of 12 breaths per minute may result in an increase in

intrathoracic pressure and a rise in intracranial pressure.

c. High-frequency jet ventilation is characterized by low tidal volumes, high respiratory rates, and low peak airway pressures, and helps to reduce the elevations of intracranial pressure.

d. An elevated serum amylase is common in diabetic ketoacidosis.

e. Fulminant ARDS can be seen with hemorrhagic pancreatitis or ongoing pancreatic inflammation.

C-122. ARDS is best diagnosed by:
a. Greater than 15,000 white blood cells/mm³.
b. Increased intrapulmonary shunt.
c. Clinical picture.
d. Increased dead space.
e. Circulating immune complexes.

C-123. Therapies of proven value in preventing or ameliorating ARDS include:
a. Prophylactic heparin.
b. Prophylactic antibiotics.
c. Prophylactic corticosteroids.
d. Prophylactic positive end expiratory pressure (PEEP).
e. None of the above.

C-124. Other therapies of proven value in treating ARDS include:
a. Heparin.
b. Antibiotics.
c. Corticosteroids.
d. PEEP.
e. Acetylcysteine.

C-125. PEEP is beneficial because of all of the following *except*:
a. Redistributing extravascular lung water.
b. Decreasing extravascular lung water.
c. Preventing atelectasis.
d. Opening airways.
e. Increasing lung volume.

C-126. The ventilation-perfusion lung scan pattern most likely to be associated with a pulmonary embolism is:

a. Subsegmental perfusion defects associated with a normal ventilation scan.

b. Segmental perfusion defects associated with matched ventilation defects with a normal chest roentgenogram.

c. Segmental and lobar perfusion defects associated with a normal ventilation scan.

d. Subsegmental defects associated with matched ventilation defects and infiltrates in the corresponding positions on chest roentgenogram.

e. A single lobar perfusion defect associated with a matched ventilation defect and corresponding evidence on the chest film for lobar atelectasis.

C-127. Patients with ARDS are best monitored by:
a. Systemic arterial oxygen tension.
b. Wedge pressure.
c. Cardiac output.
d. Systemic oxygen transport.
e. Tissue oxygen extraction.

C-128. Which of the following statements is true of oxygen consumption in patients with ARDS?
a. It determines tissue oxygen delivery.
b. It is dependent on tissue oxygen delivery.
c. It bears no relationship to tissue oxygen delivery.
d. It cannot be increased by expanding intravascular volume.
e. It cannot be increased by giving vasoactive drugs.

C-129. The cardiovascular effects of mechanical ventilation and PEEP are most likely to be related to:
a. Decreased venous return to the right ventricle.
b. Decreased left ventricular filling.
c. Increased left ventricular afterload.
d. Increased venous return to right ventricle.
e. High wedge pressure.

C-130. Which of the following are true?
   a. Phospholipase A and the complement cascade are thought to be involved in mediating increased permeability.
   b. Diabetic ketoacidosis can cause ARDS.
   c. ARDS can be unilateral.
   d. Controlling intracranial pressure is beneficial in neurologic recovery of patients with a head injury.
   e. Mechanical ventilation inducing hypocapnia is effective in acutely and chronically lowering elevated intracranial pressure.

C-131. Mortality in ARDS is usually due to:
   a. Respiratory failure.
   b. Pulmonary embolism.
   c. Viral infection.
   d. Disseminated intravascular coagulation.
   e. Multiple organ system failure.

C-132. Most survivors of ARDS should have:
   a. Few pulmonary function abnormalities.
   b. Decreased life expectancy.
   c. Persistent airflow obstruction.
   d. Hypoxemia on exercise.
   e. Decreased diffusion capacity.

C-133. For long-term treatment of deep venous thrombosis with warfarin, which of the following statements about the prothrombin time is correct?
   a. A prothrombin time prolongation between 1.5 and 2.0 times control is necessary to significantly lower recurrent thromboembolism.
   b. A prothrombin time prolongation between 1.3 and 1.5 times control results in fewer severe bleeding complications than does a prolongation between 1.5 and 2.0 times control.
   c. A prothrombin time prolongation between 2.0 and 2.5 times control is necessary to significantly reduce recurrent thromboembolism.
   d. Bleeding is not related to prolongation of prothrombin time but rather to the dose of warfarin.
   e. One mg of warfarin daily is adequate therapy in most patients.

C-134. The best prophylactic regimen for venous thromboembolism in a 60-year-old patient undergoing craniotomy for removal of an astrocytoma is:
   a. Subcutaneous heparin at 5000 units every 12 hours.
   b. Intravenous dextran for 3 days.
   c. Warfarin in a dose to prolong the prothrombin time to 1.2 times control.
   d. TED stockings and early ambulation.
   e. Pneumatic leg compression.

C-135. In the initial treatment of proximal deep venous thrombosis heparin should be given:
   a. Intravenously at a dose to prolong the activated partial thromboplastin time to 2 to 2.5 times control.
   b. Intravenously at a dose based on body weight without laboratory monitoring.
   c. Subcutaneously at a dose to prolong the activated partial thromboplastin time to 1.2 to 1.5 times control.
   d. Subcutaneously at a dose of 5000 units every 3 hours.
   e. Intravenously at a dose to prolong the activated partial thromboplastin time to 1.5 to 2.0 times control.

C-136. For treatment of deep venous thrombosis, which of the following is correct about the overlap period during which heparin and warfarin anticoagulant therapy should be given concurrently?
   a. All four vitamin K-dependent coagulation factors (II, VII, IX, X) generally reach therapeutic levels within 2 days of initiation of warfarin therapy; thus a 2-day overlap of therapy is adequate.
   b. Protein C is dependent on vitamin K and has a plasma half-life similar to that of factor VII.
   c. A large loading dose of warfarin (30 mg) will achieve the desired effect of therapeutic plasma levels of K-depen-

dent factors much more quickly and allow earlier discontinuation of heparin.

d. Heparin causes marked prolongation of the prothrombin time and must be stopped prior to initiation of warfarin therapy.

e. Excessive blood levels of protein C have been associated with hemorrhagic necrosis of the skin.

C-137. Following application of the ABCs of basic resuscitation (A=establish an airway, B=ensure that the patient is breathing properly, and C=ensure adequacy of circulation), immediate intervention is indicated in all of the following life-threatening emergencies *except*:

a. Open pneumothorax.

b. Airway obstruction.

c. Tension pneumothorax.

d. Bronchial disruption.

e. Cardiac tamponade.

C-138. In a patient with chest trauma, a high suspicion for an associated abdominal injury should be considered in all of the following situations *except*:

a. A flail chest in an unconscious patient.

b. A patient with a steering wheel injury.

c. A knife wound in the right 5th intercostal space, midaxillary line.

d. A gunshot wound to the right anterior chest in the second interspace with no exit wound.

e. A left parascapular stab wound with a left hemopneumothorax.

C-139. The clinical distinction between a tension pneumothorax and a massive hemothorax may be difficult. All of the following statements are true *except*:

a. Both conditions result in a prominent hemithorax with diminished breath sounds.

b. Both result in a shift of the trachea to the opposite side.

c. Both are likely to produce prominent neck veins and airway compression.

d. Percussion will be hyperresonant in tension pneumothorax but dull in hemothorax.

e. Hemothorax is more likely to occur than tension pneumothorax if the patient sustained a blunt injury.

C-140. A suspected tension pneumothorax that is life threatening requires:

a. Obtaining a STAT chest film.

b. Insertion of an anterior chest tube in the 2nd intercostal space midclavicular line.

c. Insertion of a lateral chest tube in the 6th intercostal space midaxillary line.

d. Insertion of an open-ended needle percutaneously into the pleural space.

e. Endotracheal intubation and positive pressure ventilation.

C-141. In chest trauma, subcutaneous emphysema may be associated with all of the following *except*:

a. Complete obstruction of a main stem bronchus by a foreign body.

b. A ruptured bronchus.

c. A ruptured esophagus.

d. A pneumothorax with a tear in the mediastinal pleura.

e. A lung laceration in an area of pleural symphysis.

C-142. Thoracentesis can successfully diagnose and treat many traumatic hemothoraces. However, chest tube insertion is indicated in all of the following situations *except*:

a. The patient is in shock on admission to the Emergency Department.

b. It is a means of monitoring blood loss from a suspected torn thoracic aorta.

c. Chest film reveals a hemopneumothorax.

d. The patient has associated abdominal injuries requiring exploratory laparotomy under general anesthesia.

e. Blood rapidly accumulates in the pleural space after thoracentesis.

C-143. The most clinically useful method for diagnosing rib fractures is:

a. PA and lateral chest films.

b. Anteroposterior compression of the thorax.

c. Detailed rib radiographs.

d. Chest wall tomography.

e. Direct palpation of individual ribs.

C-144. In a patient with suspected rib fractures, PA and lateral chest roentgenograms are obtained to:

a. Delineate and document the fracture sites.

b. Ascertain the extent of the soft tissue injury.

c. Rule out an associated pneumo- or hemopneumothorax.

d. Diagnose a possible flail segment.

e. Evaluate the lung for possible pulmonary contusion.

C-145. Respiratory failure in a patient with a flail chest is mainly related to all of the following *except*:

a. Pendelluft.

b. Pain.

c. Loss of the chest cage bellows function.

d. Retained secretions.

e. An underlying pulmonary contusion.

C-146. Flail chest of 5 or less rib segments is best treated by:

a. External traction using towel clips and a weighted pulley system.

b. Continuous positive pressure ventilation.

c. Internal fixation with surgically implanted Kirschner wires.

d. Supplemental oxygen, vigorous pulmonary therapy, analgesics, and local anesthetics.

e. A Velcro rib binder.

C-147. All of the following are common sites for esophageal perforation secondary to a foreign body *except*:

a. The cricopharyngeus.

b. The level of the aortic arch.

c. The level of the carina.

d. The lower esophageal sphincter.

e. An area of previous stricture formation.

C-148. Post-traumatic myocardial contusion is best diagnosed by:

a. Serial electrocardiograms.

b. CPK.

c. A thallium scan.

d. Chest pain.

e. None of the above.

C-149. In a patient with chest trauma presenting in shock, the diagnosis of pericardial tamponade is best substantiated by:

a. A pulsus paradoxus greater than 15 mm Hg.

b. The presence of Beck's triad.

c. Chest radiographic evidence of cardiomegaly.

d. Direct monitoring of the central venous pressure.

e. EKG evidence of myocardial ischemia.

C-150. The most sensitive sign of disruption of the thoracic aorta as a result of blunt chest trauma is:

a. Widened mediastinum on chest roentgenogram.

b. Fractured 1st or 2nd rib.

c. Upper extremity hypertension.

d. Left hemothorax.

e. Chest film evidence of left main stem bronchial deviation.

C-151. Traumatic rupture of the thoracic aorta occurs:

a. Almost exclusively in the arch.

b. Only at the isthmus (just distal to the left subclavian artery).

c. Anywhere in the thoracic aorta.

d. Commonly at the isthmus but also at the aortic valve and at the diaphragmatic hiatus.

e. In the ascending aorta just before the arch.

C-152. The allopurinol hypersensitivity syndrome consists of:

a. Fever.

b. Diffuse maculopapular rash.

c. Exfoliative dermatitis.

d. Worsening lung function.

e. Leukopenia.

1-9 Case Problems

P-1. In a patient breathing 21% O_2, in New York (barometric pressure 747 mm Hg), the respiratory quotient was 0.7, tidal volume was 600 ml, expired CO_2 was 5 %, PaO_2 was 35 mm Hg, $PaCO_2$ was 70 mm Hg, and pH was 7.33. The $P(A-a)O_2$ was roughly:
a. 12 mm Hg.
b. 37 mm Hg.
c. 55 mm Hg.
d. 32 mm Hg.
e. 67 mm Hg.

P-2. In this patient, the respiratory rate was 30/min. The alveolar ventilation was:
a. 18.0 L/min.
b. 6.0 L/min
c. 12.0 L/min.
d. 9.0 L/min.
e. 15.0 L/min.

P-3. In a patient at sea level the following blood gas values were obtained:

	On Room Air	On O_2
PaO_2	55 mm Hg	525 mm Hg
PAO_2	72 mm Hg	687 mm Hg
P(pulm-end cap) O_2	71 mm Hg	685 mm Hg
$PaCO_2$	56 mm Hg	62 mm Hg

The low PaO_2 on room air is primarily due to:
a. Diffusion defect.
b. Ventilation/perfusion mismatch.
c. True venous admixture.
d. Alveolar hypoventilation.
e. Dead space-like ventilation.

P-4. Examine Figure 1, which is the graphic report of exercise testing in a patient. This represents:
a. Abnormal gas exchange.
b. Cardiovascular limitation.
c. Ventilatory limitation.
d. Lack of effort.
e. Pulmonary vascular abnormality.

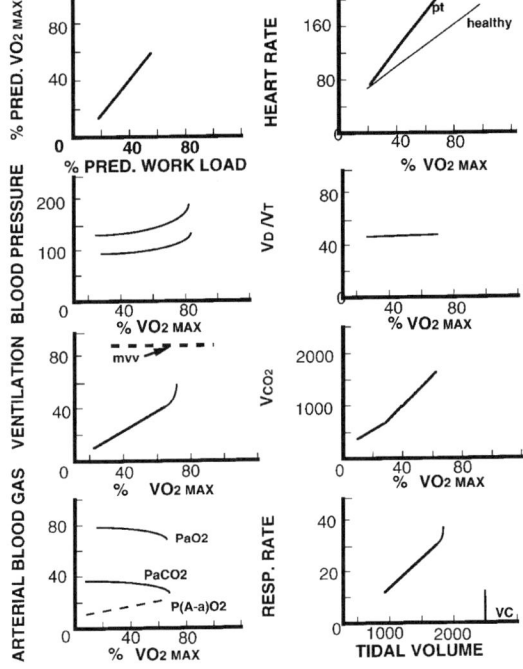

Figure 1

P-5. In a patient who has taken an overdose of sedative and is brought to the emergency room at midnight in New York (barometric pressure 747 mm Hg), the PaO_2 was 40 mm Hg and $PaCO_2$ was 80 mm Hg while breathing room air. He was transferred to the ICU, placed on a ventilator without supplemental oxygen. One hour later the PaO_2 is 70 mm Hg and $PaCO_2$ is 40 mm Hg. The nurse in the unit phones you to tell you:
a. The patient is improving.
b. The patient is deteriorating.
c. The patient needs supplemental oxygen.
d. There is a diffusion defect.
e. Alveolar hypoventilation has developed.

P-6. For the following blood gas measurements match correct diagnosis:

	pCO_2	pH	pO_2	Diagnosis
a.	30	7.43	60	1. Acute exacerbation in COPD.
b.	30	7.52	110	2. Asthma.
c.	30	7.41	110	3. Acute anxiety.
d.	48	7.33	55	4. Chronic hyperventilation.

P-7. You are called to the emergency ward to see a 25-year-old man with known asthma. He normally uses oral theophylline and an inhaled beta agonist. For the past 24 hours he has been using his inhaler every 20 minutes with decreasing relief of symptoms. What would be your approach?

    a. Do not give beta agonists; he has developed tachyphylaxis to these agents.

    b. Repeat inhaled beta agonists by the nebulized route.

    c. Give large doses of intravenous aminophylline.

    d. Give large doses of oral corticosteroids.

    e. Give inhaled anticholinergics.

P-8. These are his test results. The following were found:

Parameter	Pred	Obs	% Pred	Post-BD
FVC	5.0	3.3	66	3.4
FEV_1	4.0	1.1	27	1.2
V_{max25}	4.0	3.3	55	3.5
V_{max50}	2.0	2.0	50	2.1
FRC	3.0	5.9	190	5.0
TLC	6.0	7.5	125	6.5

The data indicate:

    a. Airflow limitation.

    b. Restriction.

    c. Normal function.

    d. Mixed disorder.

    e. Poor effort or muscle disease.

P-9. You would:

    a. Prescribe a beta agonist.

    b. Bronchoscope the patient.

    c. Ask a surgeon to perform a lung biopsy.

    d. Prescribe an antibiotic.

    e. Institute mechanical ventilation.

P-10. A 55-year-old woman presents with a bilateral destructive sinusitis and ocular inflammation, which progressed to bilateral severe corneal melting, scleritis, and conjunctivitis. The patient denies a history of asthma, drug use, cardiovascular disease, skin lesions, or joint ailments. CT scans of the nasopharynx reveal bilateral mucoperiosteal thickening of maxillary and ethmoid sinuses with destruction of the posterolateral and medial walls of the right maxillary sinus. The chest roentgenogram shows bilateral noncavitating nodules. Peripheral blood eosinophilia and rheumatoid factor were absent, and antinuclear antibody tests and cultures were negative. You would next carry out:

    a. An open lung biopsy.

    b. Bronchoscopy and lavage.

    c. Needle aspiration of one of the lesions.

    d. Transbronchial lung biopsy.

    e. A therapeutic trial of corticosteroid therapy.

P-11. A 65-year-old man with progressively increasing dyspnea on exertion has an open lung biopsy, which is depicted in Figure 2. This is:

    a. Cryptogenic organizing pneumonia.

    b. Desquamative interstitial pneumonitis.

    c. Sarcoidosis.

    d. Alveolar proteinosis.

    e. Lymphangioleiomyomatosis.

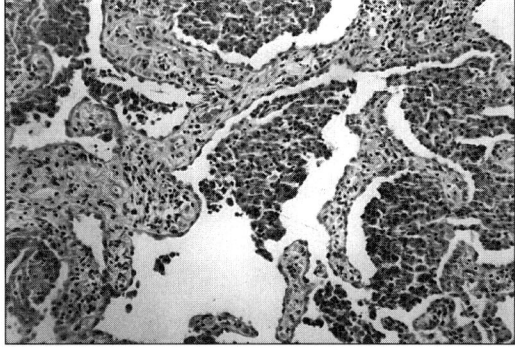

Figure 2

P-12. Examine Figure 3, which is the graphic report of exercise testing in a patient. This represents:

a. Abnormal gas exchange.

b. Cardiovascular limitation.

c. Ventilatory limitation.

d. Lack of effort.

e. Pulmonary vascular abnormality.

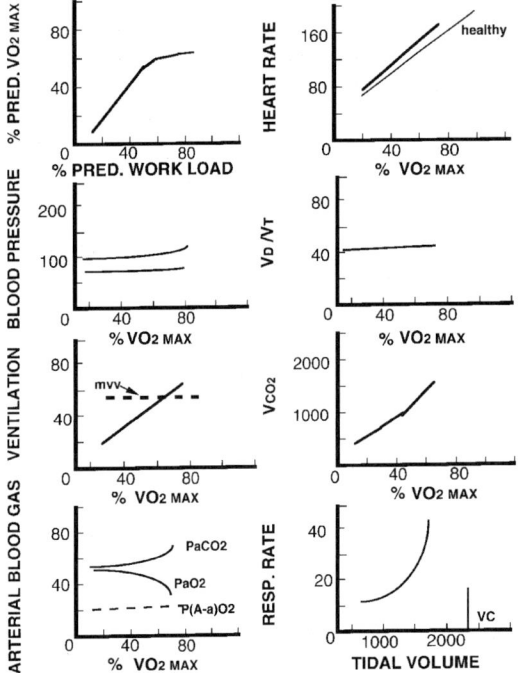

Figure 3

P-13. You have just completed treatment of a patient with acute asthma. The patient's FEV_1 has gone from 25% predicted to 60% predicted; 125 mg of methylprednisolone is given.

a. The patient is less likely to require hospitalization.

b. There will be no effect on the course of asthma therapy.

c. High-dose corticosteroids will precipitate severe hyperglycemia.

d. In acute asthma, corticosteroids principally promote recovery of beta-adrenergic function.

e. Pulmonary function effect will be noted within 15 minutes.

P-14. A patient is seen in the emergency room who has had severe asthma for 2 days. On examination, there is intercostal retraction, peripheral cyanosis, and apparent fatigue. FEV_1 is 32% of predicted. There is no response to inhaled beta agonists. Which of the following arterial blood values would you expect?

a. $pO_2 = 60$ mm Hg; $pCO_2 = 25$ mm Hg; pH = 7.55.

b. $pO_2 = 50$ mm Hg; $pCO_2 = 30$ mm Hg; pH = 7.40.

c. $pO_2 = 75$ mm Hg; $pCO_2 = 37$ mm Hg; pH = 7.42.

d. $pO_2 = 40$ mm Hg; $pCO_2 = 60$ mm Hg; pH = 7.25.

e. $pO_2 = 70$ mm Hg; $pCO_2 = 60$ mm Hg; pH = 7.43.

P-15. A 79-year-old man with a 50 pack/year history of smoking comes to the ER with a history of excessive cough and expectoration of sputum for 5 months and weight loss of 30 pounds in one year. There has been no exposure to TB or travel from his home state. On physical examination the trachea is shifted to the right and there is dullness to percussion and diminished breath sounds on the right side. This is:

a. Atelectasis on the right.

b. Left pleural effusion.

c. Left pneumothorax.

d. Right pleural effusion.

e. Atelectasis on the left.

P-16. A 30-year-old man presents with a history of having had allergic rhinitis 15 years ago, and the development of asthma 10 years ago. Five years ago he was told that his blood eosinophil count was high, and that there were some infiltrates on the chest film. He now presents with abdominal pain, skin rash, and mononeuritis multiplex. The most likely diagnosis is:

a. Wegener's granulomatosis.

b. Systemic lupus erythematosus.

c. Churg-Strauss syndrome.

d. Scleroderma.

e. Lymphangioleiomyomatosis.

P-17. Examine Figure 4, which is the graphic report of exercise testing in a patient. This represents:
   a. Abnormal gas exchange.
   b. Cardiovascular limitation.
   c. Ventilatory limitation.
   d. Lack of effort.
   e. Pulmonary vascular abnormality.

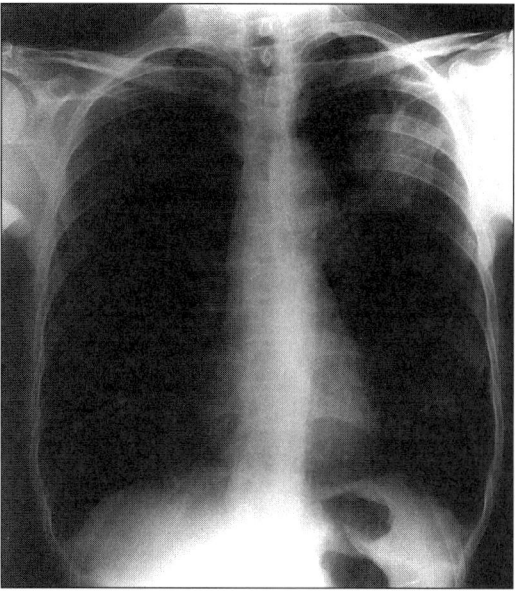

Figure 5a

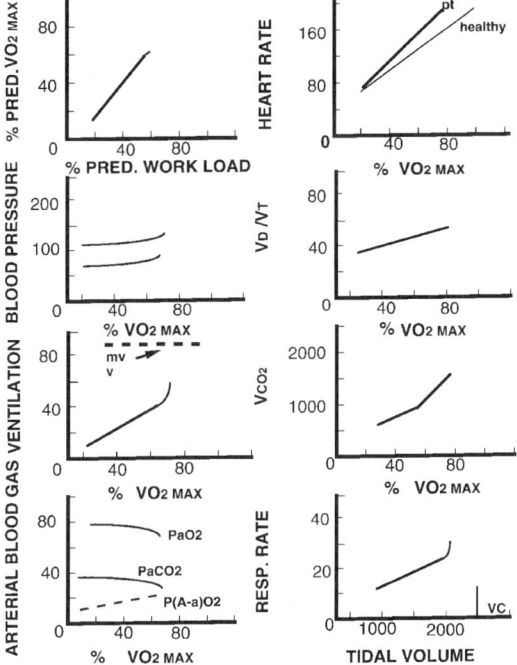

Figure 4

P-18. Examine the radiograph shown in Figure 5 of a 45-year-old man who has a 45 pack/year history of cigarette smoking, who has coughed for 15 years, and has recently noticed some increase in sputum, weight loss, and mild dyspnea on exertion. The most likely diagnosis is:
   a. Lung abscess.
   b. Bronchogenic carcinoma.
   c. Aspergilloma.
   d. Mucous plug and atelectasis.
   e. Tuberculous cavitation.

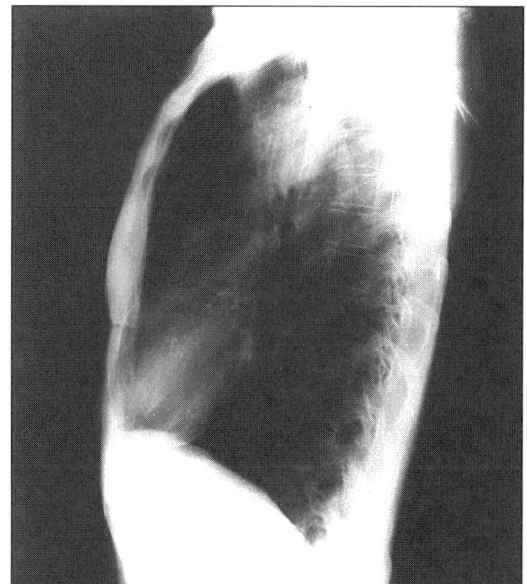

Figure 5b

P-19. When faced with the radiograph shown in Figure 5, you would first:

   a. Perform pulmonary function tests to determine ability to withstand a resection.
   b. Perform metastatic work-up to determine curability by resection.
   c. Establish diagnosis and cell type of tumor.

d. Perform staging mediastinoscopy.

e. Obtain a chest CT, including images of liver and adrenals.

P-20. Examine Figure 6, which is the graphic report of exercise testing in a patient. This represents:
a. Poor physical fitness.
b. Cardiovascular limitation.
c. Ventilatory limitation.
d. Lack of effort.
e. Pulmonary vascular abnormality.

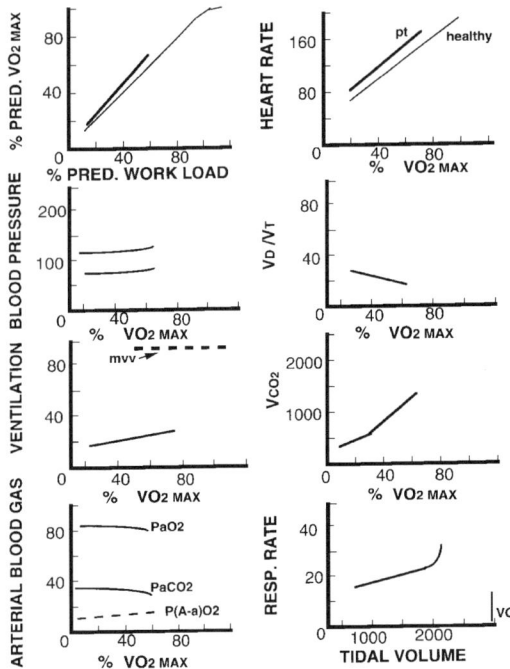

Figure 6

P-21. A 28-year-old woman who is complaining of cough, dyspnea, and weight loss for 6 months has a high-resolution CT scan shown in Figure 7. The diagnosis is:
a. Centrilobular emphysema.
b. Alpha$_1$-antitrypsin deficiency.
c. Churg-Strauss syndrome.
d. Allergic bronchopulmonary aspergillosis.
e. Lymphangioleiomyomatosis.

P-22. A 60-year-old man has a bout of the "flu" with dry cough and progressive shortness

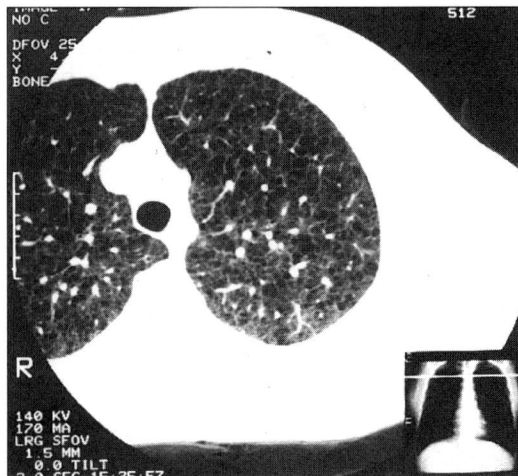

Figure 7

of breath. An open lung biopsy specimen is shown in Figure 8. This is:
a. Cryptogenic organizing pneumonia.
b. Desquamative interstitial pneumonitis.
c. Sarcoidosis.
d. Alveolar proteinosis.
e. Lymphangioleiomyomatosis.

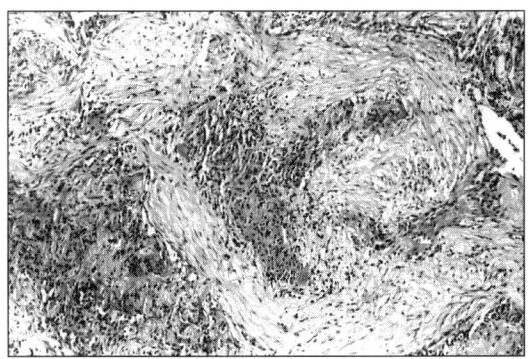

Figure 8

P-23. The diagnosis in the radiograph shown in Figure 9 is likely to be:
a. Tuberculosis.
b. Pancoast's tumor.
c. Aspergilloma.
d. Lung abscess.
e. Coccidioidomycosis.

P-24. After a right pneumonectomy, a patient with a preoperative FEV$_1$ of 2.4 liters

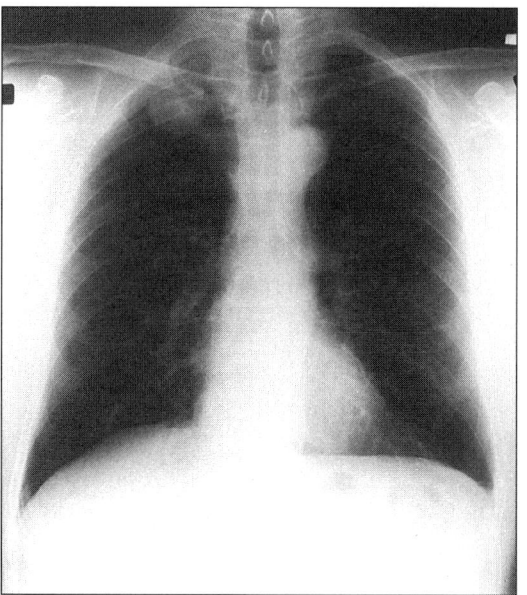

Figure 9

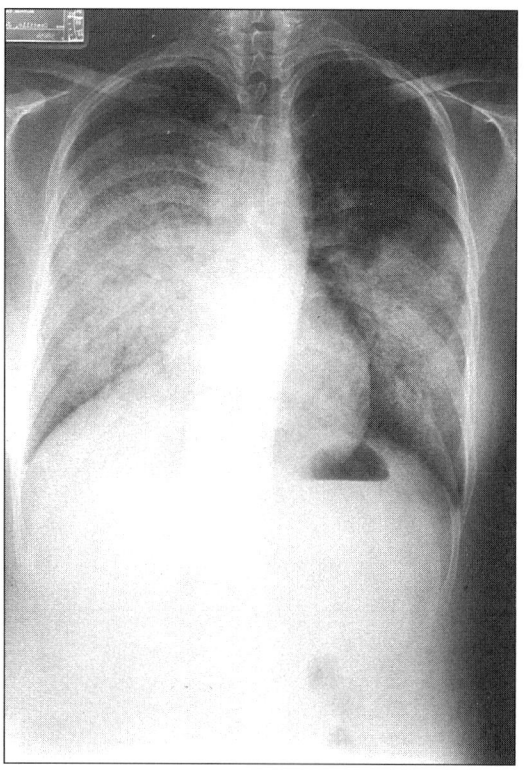

Figure 10

will be left with an FEV_1 of approximately:
a. 600 ml.
b. 960 ml.
c. 1200 ml.
d. 1440 ml.
e. 1600 ml.

P-25. A 22-year-old woman with systemic lupus erythematosus is admitted at sea level complaining of progressive fatigability for 3 months; increasing dyspnea and dry cough for 2 weeks; and some blood-streaked sputum for 4 days. Physical examination revealed a pale, thin female, with no abnormal chest signs and no clubbing. Hb was 5.2 gm, WBC 7200, ESR 70 mm. The chest radiograph is shown in Figure 10. Further laboratory studies indicated urinalysis negative, BUN 20, creatinine 0.7, and sputum demonstrated iron-staining histiocytes. This is likely to be:
a. Congestive heart failure.
b. Idiopathic pulmonary fibrosis.
c. Sarcoidosis.
d. Diffuse alveolar hemorrhage.
e. Multiple pulmonary emboli.

P-26. Further tests showed:

FVC	2.10	(67% pred.)
FEV_1	1.63	(78% pred.)
FEV_1/FVC	0.78	
FRC	1.65	(70% pred.)
TLC	2.70	(72% pred.)
D_LCO	5.5	(35% pred.)
PaO_2	69	
$PaCO_2$	37	
pH	7.42	

This is consistent with:
a. An obstructive defect.
b. Airway hyperresponsiveness.
c. A restrictive defect.
d. Alveolar hypoventilation.
e. A mixed defect.

P-27. A 25-year-old woman, who is a clerk in a wallpaper firm, presents with dyspnea while dressing and while talking and is limited to a wheelchair. She has a history

103

of symmetric polyarthralgias and synovitis and was treated with ASA, nonsteroidal inflammatory agents, and oral gold. She also received d-penicillamine (250–750 mg/day) for 8 months. Several years later, she developed a flu-like illness with low-grade fever and cough. The cough persisted for 6 weeks and responded ultimately to ampicillin and cough suppressants. Later she noted progressive dyspnea, along with dryness of the mouth and eyes. On physical examination, her eyes and oral mucosa are dry, and there are bibasilar rales anteriorly and posteriorly, with no cyanosis or clubbing. Assessment of function showed:

	Before BD		After BD
	Obs	% Pred	
FRC	5.95	180	5.70
RV	4.98	370	4.50
TLC	6.76	131	6.56
FEV_1	0.63	20	0.90
FVC	1.70	47	1.85

This is consistent with:
a. An obstructive defect.
b. Airway hyperresponsiveness.
c. A restrictive defect.
d. Alveolar hypoventilation.
e. A mixed defect.

P-28. The diagnosis is likely to be:
a. Asthma.
b. Hypersensitivity pneumonitis due to gold.
c. Bronchiolitis obliterans and organizing pneumonia.
d. Bronchiolitis obliterans.
e. Sjögren's syndrome.

P-29. A 32-year-old nonsmoking man was admitted to the hospital complaining of a nonproductive cough, chest discomfort, and dyspnea for one year. There were no abnormal physical signs, and laboratory tests were all within the normal range. The chest roentgenogram is shown in Figure 11. The likely diagnosis is:

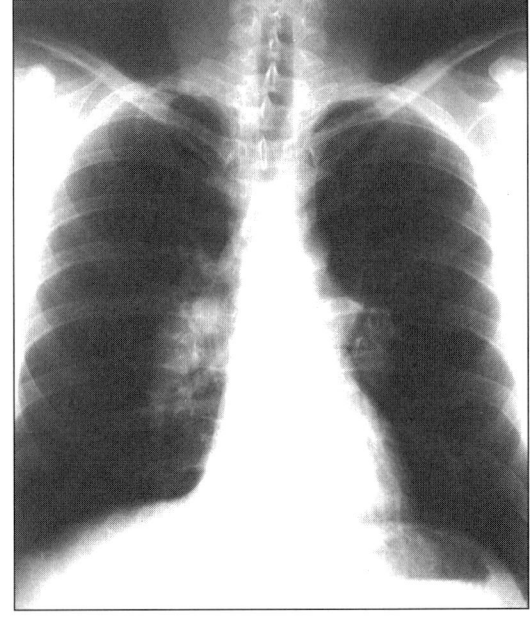

Figure 11

a. Hypersensitivity pneumonitis.
b. Eosinophilic granuloma.
c. Sarcoidosis.
d. Kaposi's sarcoma.
e. Pulmonary non-Hodgkin's lymphoma in AIDS.

P-30. A 34-year-old farmer who has had fever, fatigue, and weight loss over the past 5 weeks presents with the chest film shown in Figure 12. This is likely to be:
a. Tuberculosis.
b. Adenocarcinoma.
c. Lymphomatous carcinoma.
d. Eosinophilic granuloma.
e. Coccidioidomycosis.

P-31. If the sputum is positive for acid-fast bacilli, the optimum treatment is:
a. Isoniazid (INH), rifampin (RF), pyrazinamide (PZA), ethambutol hydrochloride (EMB).
b. Clofazimine, RF, and elective ciprofloxacin.
c. INH and RF.
d. Streptomycin (SM), INH, and RF.
e. SM, RF, and PZA.

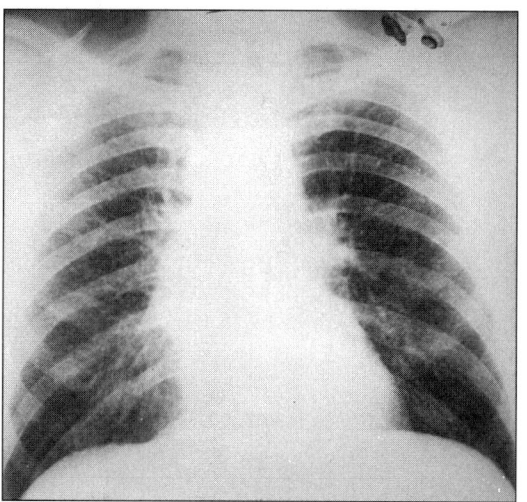

Figure 12

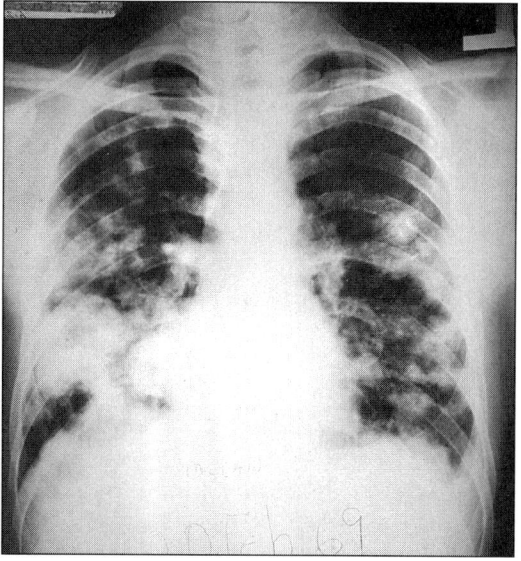

Figure 13

P-32. A young man who is HIV positive is exposed to an individual with infectious, INH-resistant tuberculosis. You would:
   a. Watch carefully for development of signs and symptoms.
   b. Start rifampin and ethambutol hydrochloride or pyrazinamide after active TB is ruled out.
   c. Place on rifampin after active TB is ruled out.
   d. Place a PPD skin test and, if 5 mm or greater, begin rifampin.
   e. Place a PPD and, if negative, have him return in 6 months for a further skin test.

P-33. A 30-year-old man complains of progressively increasing dyspnea and fatigue. The chest roentgenogram is shown in Figure 13. This is:
   a. Cryptogenic organizing pneumonia.
   b. Desquamative interstitial pneumonitis.
   c. Sarcoidosis.
   d. Alveolar proteinosis.
   e. Wegener's granulomatosis.

P-34. In a patient with cough, sputum, and fever, the roentgenogram confirms an infiltrate and reduced volume of the right upper lobe. The acid-fast stain was positive and the patient was placed on chemotherapy,

but the excessive cough and localized wheeze persisted. You would:
   a. Perform fiberoptic bronchoscopy.
   b. Order a CT scan.
   c. Change the antibiotics.
   d. Order sputum cytology.
   e. Administer corticosteroids.

P-35. An elderly man presents with fever and productive cough. Chest film shows bilateral pulmonary infiltrates. Gram's stain of the sputum shows streptococci and many neutrophils. However, the cocci seen are lancet-shaped and congregate in pairs, strongly suggesting *S. pneumoniae*. You now:
   a. Prescribe cefamandole.
   b. Prescribe erythromycin.
   c. Prescribe penicillin.
   d. Prescribe gentamicin.
   e. Perform a transtracheal aspirate before prescribing antibiotics.

P-36. An elderly man presents with fever and productive cough. Chest film shows bilateral pulmonary infiltrates. Gram's stain of the sputum shows neutrophils and faintly-staining small gram-negative coccobacillary forms suggestive of *Haemophilus influenzae*. You now pursue which course of action?

a. Prescribe ampicillin.

b Prescribe penicillin.

c. Prescribe erythromycin.

d. Prescribe gentamicin.

e. Perform a transtracheal aspirate before prescribing antibiotics.

P-37. An elderly man presents with fever, productive cough, and pulmonary infiltrates. The Gram's stain of the sputum shows many epithelial cells and streptococci. You now select which course of action?

a. Prescribe penicillin.

b. Prescribe cefamandole.

c. Prescribe erythromycin.

d. Perform a transtracheal aspirate before prescribing antibiotics.

e. Perform bronchoscopy with BAL before prescribing antibiotics.

P-38. In a patient with pneumonia, a Gram's stain shows many neutrophils, but a paucity of organisms. Which of the etiologic diagnoses listed below is suggested?

a. *Hemophilus influenzae.*

b. *Klebsiella pneumoniae.*

c. *Mycoplasma pneumoniae.*

d. *Legionella pneumophila.*

e. Influenza A.

P-39. A 38-year-old nonsmoking woman was admitted to the hospital complaining of a nonproductive cough, chest discomfort, and dyspnea for one year. She has had several bouts of pneumonia over the past few years. The chest roentgenogram and CT scan are shown in Figure 14. The likely diagnosis is:

a. Hypersensitivity pneumonitis.

b. Eosinophilic granuloma.

c. Sarcoidosis.

d. Chronic eosinophilic pneumonia.

e. Pulmonary non-Hodgkin's lymphoma in AIDS.

P-40. A young man presents with an insidious history of malaise, night sweats, and pro-

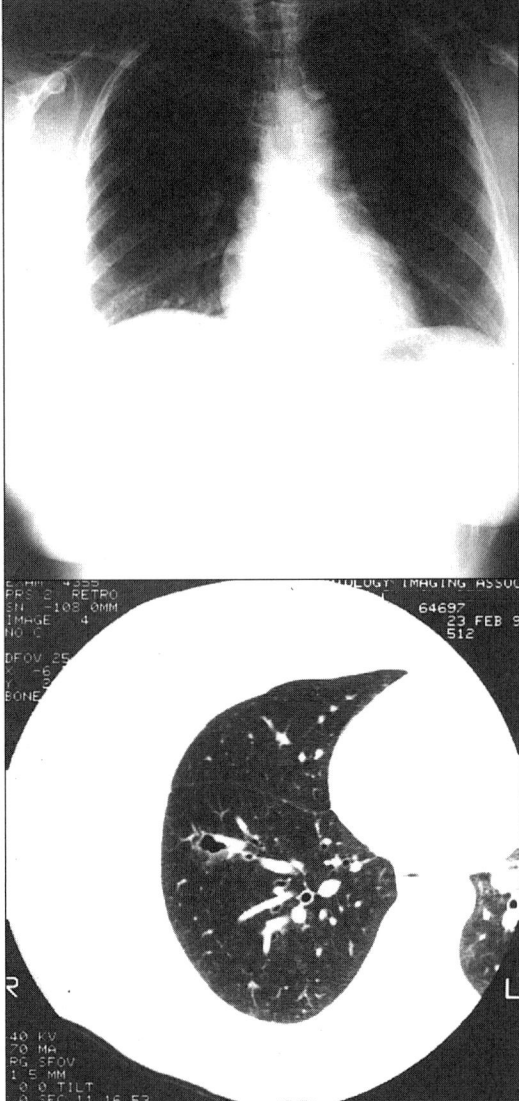

Figure 14

ductive cough. Chest roentgenogram shows bilateral hilar lymphadenopathy and new pulmonary infiltrates. Open lung biopsy reveals spherules packed with endospores. Which of the following is likely to be the pathogen?

a. *Strongyloides.*

b. *Pneumocystis.*

c. *Cryptococcus.*

d. *Coccidioides.*

e. *Histoplasma.*

P-41. A patient presents with a 2.0-cm peripheral lesion in the right lung, demonstrated to be a squamous cell carcinoma by needle biopsy. Pulmonary function tests are virtually normal. Metastatic work-up is negative. Chest CT reveals a 1.5-cm right paratracheal lymph node. The next step should be:

a. Referral to radiation therapy.

b. Mediastinoscopy.

c. Bone marrow biopsy.

d. A frank discussion with the patient that palliative therapy may actually decrease the quality of life.

e. Referral for chemotherapy.

P-42. A 40-year-old man is admitted with cough and hemoptysis. The chest film is shown in Figure 15 and indicates:

a. Bronchogenic carcinoma.

b. Sarcoidosis.

c. Wegener's granulomatosis.

d. Arteriovenous fistulas.

e. Hematogenous metastases.

P-43. The differential diagnosis in the above situation includes all of the following *except*:

a. Tuberculosis.

b. Nitrofurantoin toxicity.

c. Rheumatoid disease.

d. Actinomycosis.

e. Cyclophosphamide toxicity.

P-44. A 35-year-old heavy smoker complains of chronic cough and some dyspnea on exertion. Look at the electron microscopic examination obtained from bronchoalveolar lavage (Figure 16). This shows:

a. An alveolar macrophage in idiopathic pulmonary fibrosis.

b. A Schaumann's body in sarcoidosis.

c. Langerhans' cell in bronchoalveolar carcinoma.

d. Langerhans' cell in eosinophilic granuloma.

e. A lymphocyte in lymphocytic interstitial pneumonia.

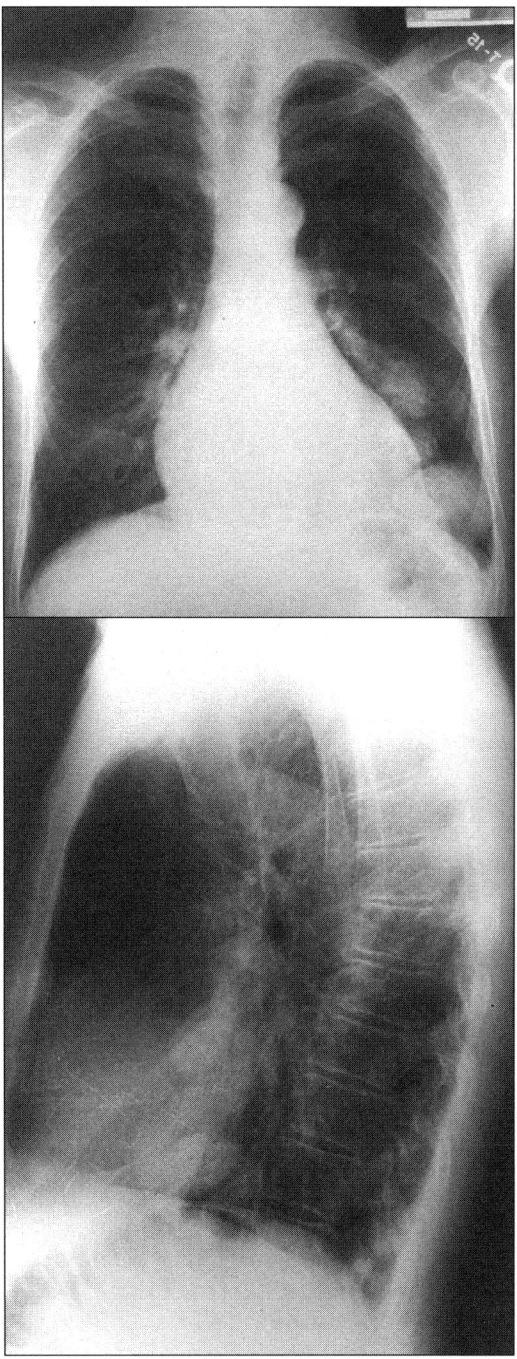

Figure 15

P-45. A 64-year-old woman was admitted for an exacerbation of COPD. The FEV_1 was <1.51 (30 % of predicted). There was bullous disease on the chest film.

107

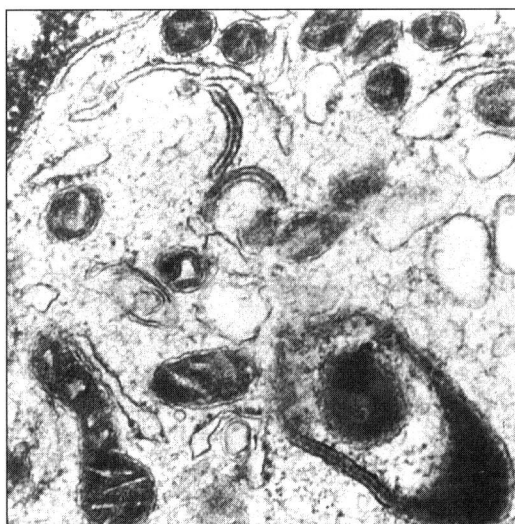

Figure 16

There was no evidence of heart disease. The PaO_2 was 40 mm Hg and $PaCO_2$ 50 mm Hg. She was placed on a ventilator for respiratory failure. The systolic blood pressure fell to 60 mm Hg; 500 cc of NaCl was given and the systolic blood pressure rose to 80 mm Hg. The pulmonary capillary wedge pressure was 20 mm Hg. During suctioning, the systolic blood pressure rose to 140 mm Hg, pulmonary capillary wedge pressure (PCWP) fell to 10–13 mm Hg. While on the ventilator, exhaled volume was recorded throughout the exhalation period. The esophageal pressure during IPPV was 10–11 cm H_2O and decreased to 3–4 cm H_2O when expiratory time was increased. This is most likely the result of:

a. Selective intubation of one of the main bronchi.
b. Pneumothorax.
c. Auto-PEEP.
d. Hemorrhage.
e. Pulmonary embolus.

P-46. A 45-year-old man is brought to the emergency room and is comatose. There is no smell of ethanol on his breath. The pH is 7.15, and the pCO_2 25 mm Hg along with an elevated anion and osmolar gap. There are crystals in the urine. This is consistent with:

a. Diabetic ketoacidosis.
b. Lactate acidosis.
c. Ethylene glycol poisoning.
d. Morphine overdose.
e. Salicylate poisoning.

P-47. A 22-year-old man presents with some hemoptysis following a chest injury from a steering wheel in an automobile accident that happened 4 days ago. He has just had a violent coughing episode after drinking some milk. You suspect:

a. Gastroesophageal reflux.
b. Reflex bronchospasm.
c. Pulmonary embolus.
d. Tracheoesophageal fistula.
e. Aspiration pneumonia.

P-48. You would first:

a. Perform an esophageal contrast study.
b. Perform a bronchoscopy.
c. Perform an endoscopy.
d. Take the patient to the operating room for emergency surgery.
e. Perform esophageal manometry.

P-49. A 21-year-old Hispanic woman is brought to the emergency room at 3:00 a.m. complaining of having awakened at midnight with epigastric pain, and nausea and vomiting. She now has a sore throat. Laryngoscopy reveals no evidence of an epiglottitis or retropharyngeal abscess. The nausea increases, and she begins to develop diplopia and dysphagia. She begins to have difficulty breathing and is put on a ventilator. The prime condition you suspect is:

a. Poliomyelitis.
b. Guillain-Barré syndrome.
c. Myasthenia gravis.
d. Botulism.
e. Tetanus.

P-50. The most informative test is:
 a. Tensilon test.
 b. Rapid repetitive-stimuli EMG.
 c. Stool toxin.
 d. Lumbar puncture.
 e. Blood sugar.

P-51. A 70-kg (154 lb) man with the adult respiratory distress syndrome is being mechanically ventilated with these settings: tidal volume of 650 ml, rate 20 breaths per minute, FIO_2 of 0.50, and positive end expiratory pressure (PEEP) of 20 cm H_2O, which is producing an arterial pO_2 of 80 mm Hg. His blood pressure has decreased from 150/80 to 90/60 over 4 hours. His urine output begins to fall. The mean pulmonary arterial pressure is 35 mm Hg, pulmonary arterial occlusion pressure is 14 mm Hg, cardiac output is 2 L/min. Which of the following statements concerning the interpretation and treatment of this clinical problem is correct?
 a. Blood, sputum, and urine cultures should be obtained and the patient started on broad-spectrum antibiotics.
 b. The occlusion pressure indicates that left ventricular preload is adequate.
 c. PEEP should be reduced.
 d. Dopamine at 10 μg/kg/min should be infused.
 e. The pulmonary arterial occlusion pressure should be remeasured after temporarily discontinuing PEEP.

P-52. A 45-year-old woman with the adult respiratory distress syndrome secondary to acute bronchitis is admitted. She does not respond to 2 hours of treatment with bronchodilators and corticosteroids and requires endotracheal intubation and mechanical ventilation. Within 5 minutes her blood pressure drops from 150/90 to 80/50, heart rate increases from 110 to 150/min, and her urine output decreases markedly. Which of the following would you do first?
 a. An electrocardiogram.

 b. Repeat arterial blood gas measurements.
 c. Measure end expiratory alveolar pressure.
 d. Cultures of blood, urine, and sputum and therapy with broad-spectrum antibiotics.
 e. Reduce the dose and frequency of bronchodilators.

P-53. A 16-year-old girl comes to your office at 5 p.m. complaining of chest pain and shortness of breath, which awoke her suddenly from a nap at 4 p.m. She is 2 weeks postpartum and is holding her screaming infant in her arms. Her social situation is complicated because she is unwed and has recently left her parent's home because of her social situation. Her vital signs are remarkable for a pulse of 96 and a respiratory rate of 22. The physical examination is otherwise unremarkable. The chest roentgenogram is read as normal. Arterial blood gases on room air show a pH of 7.50, pCO_2 of 30 mm Hg, and pO_2 of 80 mm Hg. Your next action would be to:
 a. Refer her to a social worker.
 b. Order a pulmonary angiogram.
 c. Give 5000 units of heparin intravenously and send her to the hospital for a lung scan.
 d. Prescribe aspirin and tell her to call you in the morning.
 e. Prescribe erythromycin, 500 mg every 6 hours.

P-54. A 66-year-old man living at sea level has had a dry hacking cough for 10 years and shortness of breath for 3 years. Over the past year he has noted increasing fatigability and chest tightness. An electrocardiogram is normal. Arterial blood gas analysis reveals a pH of 7.44, pCO_2 of 38 mm Hg, and a pO_2 of 84 mm Hg. In a modified BRUCE protocol exercise test, he goes to stage III without much dyspnea and develops no ischemic changes. Figure 17 shows

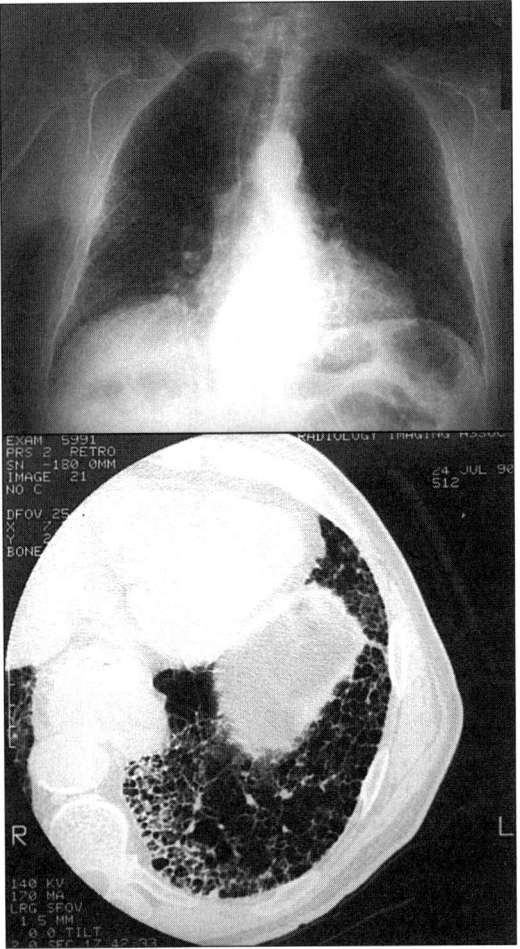

Figure 17

the chest radiograph and high-resolution computed tomography (HRCT). The most likely diagnosis is:

a. Congestive heart failure.
b. Eosinophilic granuloma.
c. Idiopathic pulmonary fibrosis.
d. Alveolar cell carcinoma.
e. Chronic eosinophilic pneumonia.

P-55. A 19-year-old female college student who has been treated for asthma for 6 months comes to see a pulmonologist because of chronic cough and shortness of breath. She had a spontaneous pneumothorax 12 months previously. She claims to smoke few cigarettes, but does smoke marijuana regularly. The chest

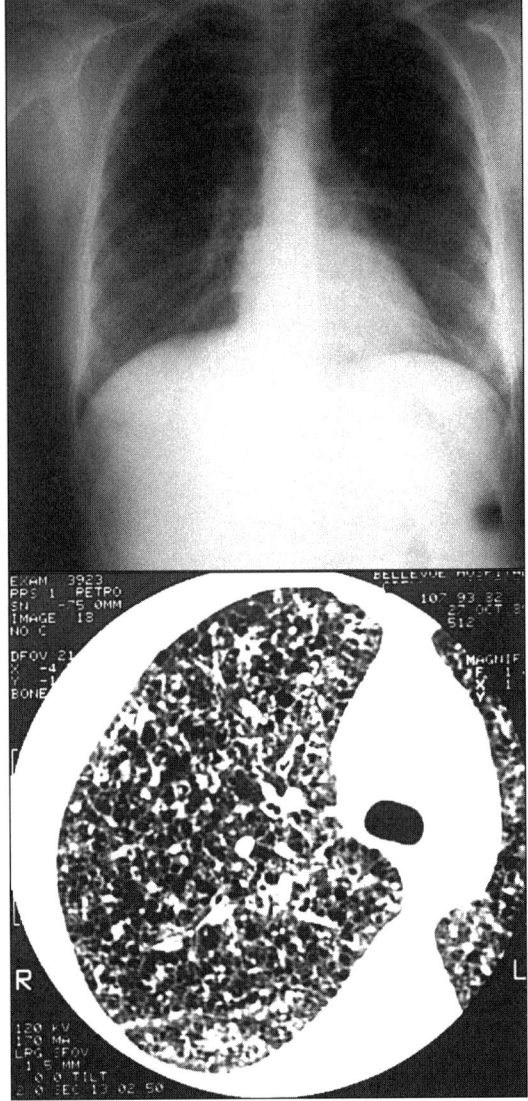

Figure 18

film and HRCT scan are shown in Figure 18. This is likely to be:

a. Churg-Strauss syndrome.
b. Eosinophilic granuloma.
c. Idiopathic pulmonary fibrosis.
d. Allergic bronchopulmonary aspergillosis.
e. Chronic eosinophilic pneumonia.

P-56. An 85-year-old man with a history of 40 pack/year smoking and previous employment as a coal miner and a foundry worker complained of a worsening cough productive of yellow sputum and night sweats as well as increasing dyspnea on exertion for 1 month. He denied any weight loss or hemoptysis. On examination his temperature was 100.4°F, and there were coarse rhonchi with faint expiratory wheezing. There was no digital clubbing. WBC was 11,500 with a normal differential; hematocrit was 41%; arterial pH was 7.45; pCO_2 was 36 mm Hg; and pO_2 was 49 mm Hg. The chest radiograph is shown in Figure 19. The most likely diagnosis is:

a. Silicotuberculosis.

b. Eosinophilic granuloma.

c. Idiopathic pulmonary fibrosis.

d. Alveolar cell carcinoma.

e. Chronic eosinophilic pneumonia.

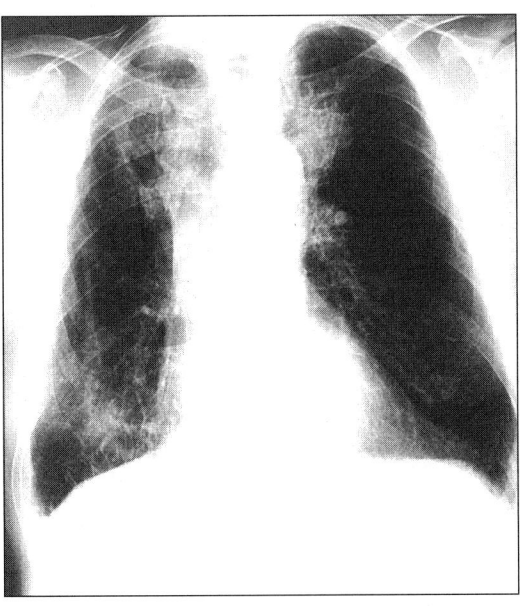

Figure 19

P-57. A 32-year-old woman in the second trimester of pregnancy presents with complaints of pain and swelling in the right thigh. Impedance plethysmography studies of the leg are abnormal, and contrast venography confirms the presence of deep venous thrombosis of the popliteal and superficial femoral veins. Following 10 days of intravenous heparin, the best long-term treatment would be:

a. Warfarin to prolong the prothrombin time to 1.5 to 2.0 times control.

b. Aspirin at 325 mg/day.

c. Warfarin to prolong the prothrombin time to 20 to 25 times control.

d. Heparin given subcutaneously in a dose to prolong the activated partial thromboplastin time to 1.5 times control at the mid-dose interval.

e. Heparin subcutaneously in a dose of 5000 units every 12 hours.

P-58. A 50-year-old man is admitted to the critical care unit with chest pain and EKG findings of acute inferior myocardial infarction. A balloon flotation catheter passed repeatedly cannot be advanced beyond the right ventricle. The catheter is withdrawn. Over the next 2 hours the patient develops hypotension, jugular venous distension, 20 mm Hg pulsus paradoxus, and a pulsatile liver, but the lungs remain clear. The single best method to differentiate tamponade from right ventricular infarction in this patient is:

a. Physical examination.

b. Echocardiography.

c. A balloon flotation catheter to measure right-sided pressures.

d. Electrocardiography.

e. Technetium pyrophosphate scan of heart.

P-59. A 57-year-old man presents to the critical care unit with complaints of chest pain, diaphoresis, and syncope occurring every time he arises from a sitting position. His blood pressure is 80/50, pulse is 120, and respiratory rate is 22. There is jugular venous distension; the lungs are clear to percussion and auscultation. The heart is not enlarged, but some listeners report a soft S_3 gallop. The electrocardiogram shows Q waves with ST elevation in leads II, III, and AVF. There is borderline ST elevation in lead VI. Appropriate initial therapy for this clinical state is:

a. Intravenous furosemide.

b. Intra-aortic balloon pumping.

c. Infusion of physiologic saline.

d. Intravenous nitroglycerin.

e. Intravenous digoxin.

P-60. A 62-year-old man complains of shortness of breath for 6 weeks, tightness of the chest for 5 weeks, and cough with expectoration of dark sputum and fever for 4 weeks. Noted on physical examination were carious teeth, dullness on percussion, amphoric breathing, and coarse crepitations over the right lower chest posteriorly. The chest film is shown in Figure 20. This is:

a. Silicotuberculosis.

b. Eosinophilic granuloma.

c. Lung abscess.

d. Alveolar cell carcinoma.

e. Chronic eosinophilic pneumonia.

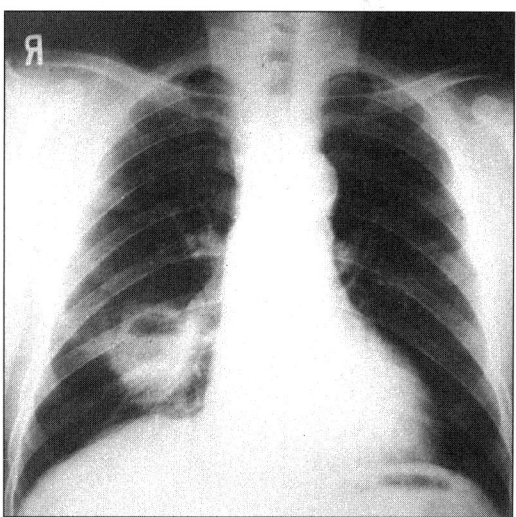

Figure 20

P-61. A lung biopsy was performed in a 30-year-old woman with a pneumothorax, and is shown in Figure 21. The likely diagnosis is:

a. Desquamative interstitial pneumonitis.

b. Bronchiolitis obliterans.

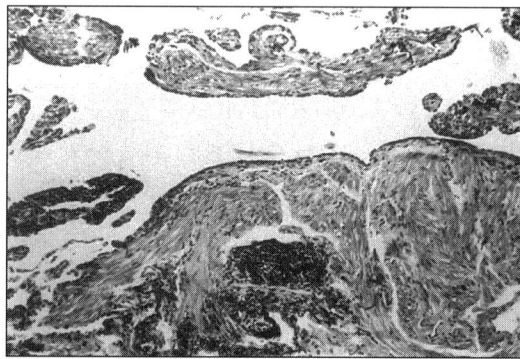

Figure 21

c. Lymphangioleiomyomatosis.

d. Chronic eosinophilic pneumonia.

e. Wegener's granulomatosis.

P-62. A 30-year-old man, who has a history of excessive alcohol intake, appears in the emergency room with a history of chills, fever, cough, and sputum. The chest film is shown in Figure 22. The disorder is probably due to:

a. *Legionella*.

b. *Pneumocystis*.

c. Tuberculosis.

d. *Streptococcus pneumoniae*.

e. *Mycoplasma*.

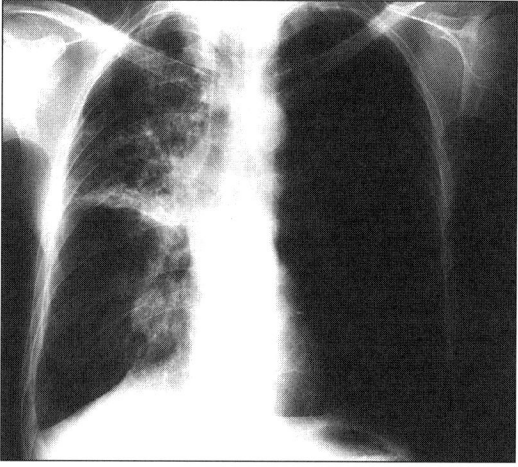

Figure 22

P-63. Examine the lung biopsy in Figure 23. The likely diagnosis is:

a. Desquamative interstitial pneumonitis.
b. Bronchiolitis obliterans.
c. Sarcoidosis.
d. Chronic eosinophilic pneumonia.
e. Wegener's granulomatosis.

b. Mesothelioma.
c. Sarcoidosis.
d. Chronic eosinophilic pneumonia.
e. Rheumatoid disease.

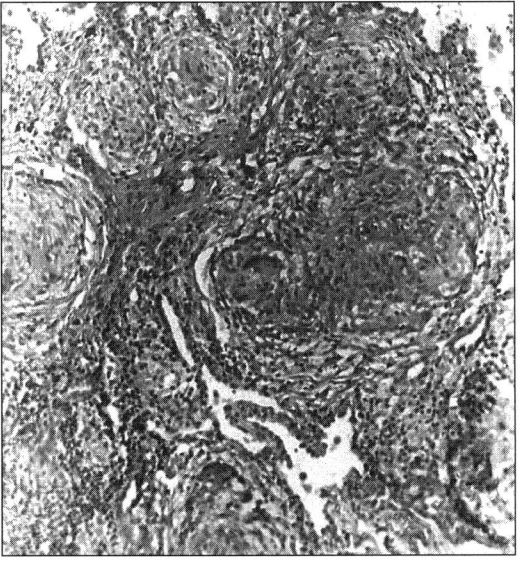

Figure 23

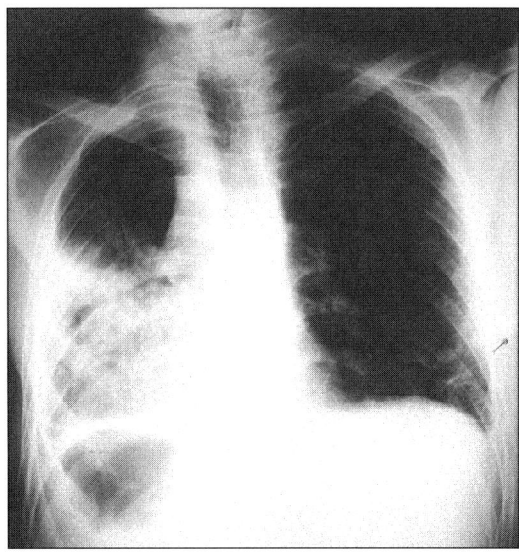

Figure 24

P-64. A 36-year-old hard rock miner, an ex-smoker, spent 4 years as a pipe fitter in the navy and has tiredness, weight loss, cough with expectoration, and left pleuritic chest pain. Examine the following pulmonary function assessment:

	Pred	Obs	% Pred
VC	4150	3430	83
FEV_1	3430	2680	78
FRC	3500	2800	80
TLC	4900	3725	76

This is:
a. Airflow limitation.
b. Restriction.
c. Normal function.
d. Mixed disorder.
e. Poor effort or muscle disease.

P-65. Figure 24 shows the chest roentgenogram in this patient. The most likely diagnosis is:
a. Tuberculosis.

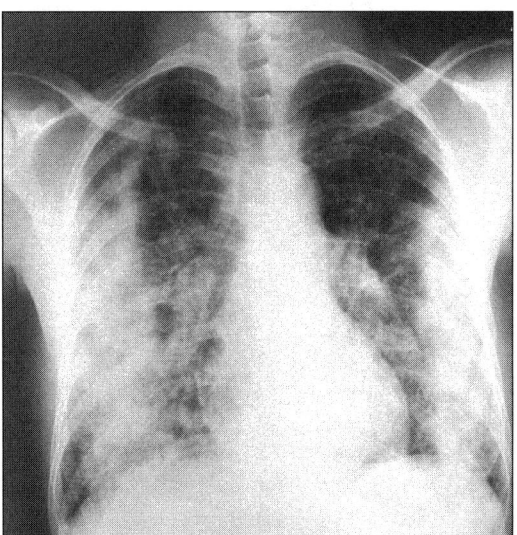

Figure 25

P-66. Figure 25 is the chest roentgenogram of a patient with chronic dyspnea, cough, and expectoration. This is likely to be:
a. Allergic granulomatosis.

b. Cystic fibrosis.

c. Postmeasles bronchiectasis.

d. Chronic eosinophilic pneumonia.

e. Allergic bronchopulmonary aspergillosis.

P-67. Figure 26 is a CT scan of the lungs in a patient who has a history of asthma and has noted increasing cough with expectoration of some "pieces" of white glarey sputum. This is likely to be:

a. Allergic granulomatosis.

b. Cystic fibrosis.

c. Postmeasles bronchiectasis.

d. Hypersensitivity pneumonitis.

e. Allergic bronchopulmonary aspergillosis.

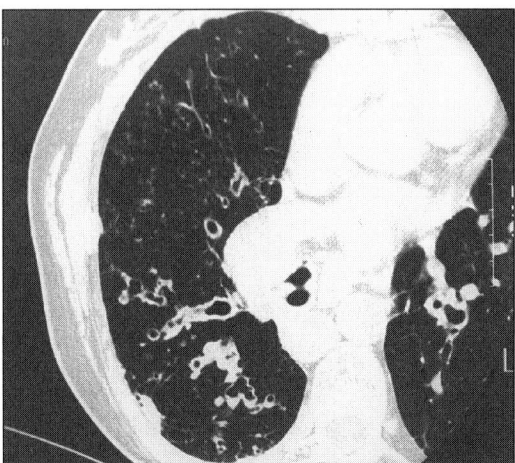

Figure 26

P-68. Figure 27 is the chest roentgenogram of a 20-year-old individual who has had cough and expectoration since early childhood. This is likely to be:

a. Allergic granulomatosis of Churg-Strauss.

b. Cystic fibrosis.

c. Postmeasles bronchiectasis.

d. Hypersensitivity pneumonitis.

e. Allergic bronchopulmonary aspergillosis.

P-69. The disorder in the chest film shown in Figure 28 is likely to be:

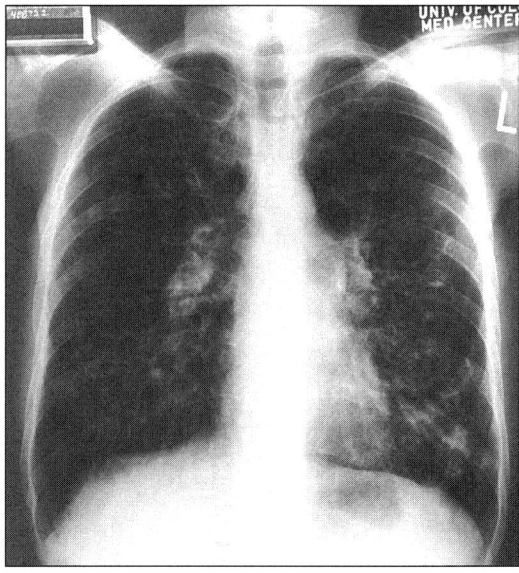

Figure 27

a. Hodgkin's disease.

b. Sarcoidosis.

c. Coccidioidomycosis.

d. Pulmonary hypertension.

e. Bronchiolo-alveolar carcinoma.

P-70. This 32-year-old man, who smoked heavily from age 16 until 2 months ago, developed general malaise followed by acute onset of dyspnea, dry cough, and pain in the right anterior lower chest on cough or deep breathing. In the past he has spent a good deal of time shoveling concrete. On examination he is found to have advanced clubbing of his digits, but he states he has noted this for as long as he can remember. The heart is not enlarged, and there is no jugular venous distension. The PaO_2 was 47 mm Hg, $PaCO_2$ 30 mm Hg, and pH 7.51. During maximal exercise the PaO_2 was 35 mm Hg and $PaCO_2$ was 27 mm Hg. Sputum examination showed only commensal organisms and was negative for acid-fast bacilli. The chest film is shown in Figure 29. The most likely diagnosis is:

a. Coccidioidomycosis.

b. Alveolar proteinosis.

c. Congestive heart failure.

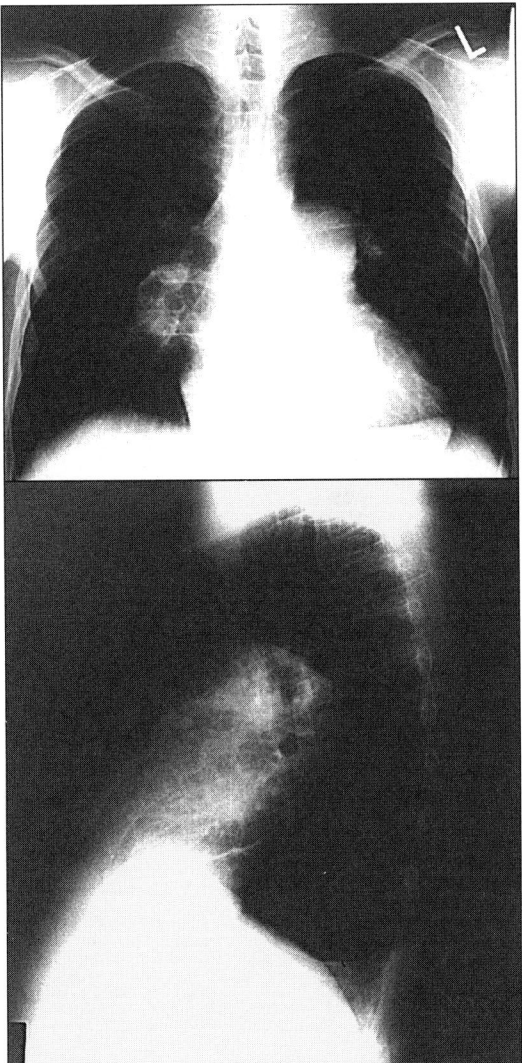

Figure 28

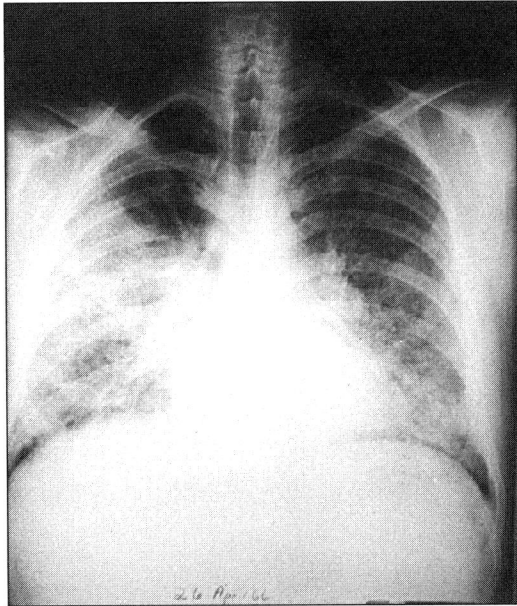

Figure 29

c. Pulmonary edema.
d. Pulmonary embolus and infarction.
e. Silicosis.

P-72. In a patient at sea level whose hemo-globin is 18 gm, oxygen consumption

d. Tuberculosis.
e. *Legionella* pneumonia.

P-71. A 32-year-old hard rock miner with asthma who had suffered a broken tibia and fibula 2 months ago is readmitted complaining of a fainting spell. He has chest tightness and a mild cough with no expectoration. His chest film is shown in Figure 30. This is:
a. Pneumococcal pneumonia.
b. Mucoid impaction.

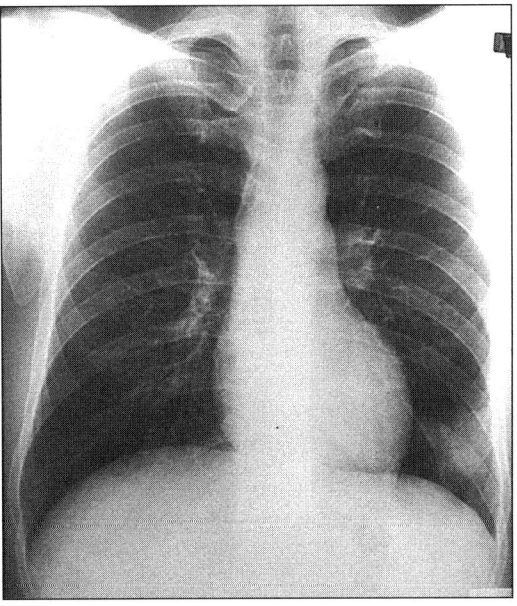

Figure 30

300 ml/min, and cardiac output 5 L/min, the following blood gas values were obtained:

	On Room Air	On 100% O_2
PaO_2	55 mm Hg	200 mm Hg
Arterial O_2 saturation	78%	100%
P(pulm-end cap) O_2	99 mm Hg	695 mm Hg
$PaCO_2$	30 mm Hg	32 mm Hg

The low PaO_2 on room air is most likely to be due to:

a. Diffusion defect.
b. Ventilation-perfusion mismatch.
c. True venous admixture.
d. Alveolar hypoventilation.
e. Dead space type ventilation.

P-73. The calculated percentage of right-to-left shunt is:

a. 10%.
b. 5%.
c. 20%.
d. 30%.
e. 25%.

P-74. Examine the chest roentgenogram of this 65-year-old woman (Figure 31) who complains of dyspnea, weakness, excessive fatigue, some dysphagia, and heartburn. The most likely diagnosis is:

a. Bronchial cyst.
b. Thymoma.
c. Gastroenteric cyst.
d. Teratoma.
e. Esophageal neoplasm.

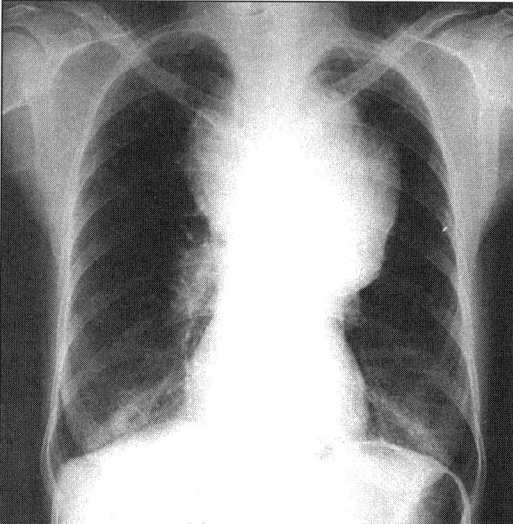

Figure 31

PART 2

ANSWERS

2-1 Basic Principles

B-1. **Answers: a, b, c, d.** In the non-immune host, phagocytosis is facilitated by natural opsonins present in the respiratory tract. Phagocytosis and particle inactivation by pulmonary phagocytes are greatly augmented by specific antibody secreted by effector B lymphocytes and by the secretory products (lymphokines) of sensitized T lymphocytes in the immune host. The alternate pathway of complement activation can be triggered non-specifically by certain microbial polysaccharides in the non-immune host. The resultant generation of C3b, which is fixed to the surface of the organism and interacts with C3 receptors on the surface membrane of polymorphonuclear leukocytes, initiates the process of phagocytosis. Activation of the alternate complement pathway, or direct expression of chemotactic activity by constituents of bacterial cell walls, may stimulate the emigration of monocytes from the circulation, or macrophages from the interstitium, into alveolar spaces and conducting airways. In the non-immune host, the infecting agent initiates a primary immune response and specific antibody or effector T cells do not appear on the scene until days to weeks after the infection has been established.

B-2. **Answer: e.** In primary immunodeficiency disease, such as X-linked hypogamma-globulinemia (Bruton's) and common variable hypogammaglobulinemia, there is a deficiency of all immunoglobulins (occasional normal IgE levels). The most common primary deficiency of IgA occurs in 70% of cases of ataxia-telangiectasia. There may be a deficiency of all immunoglobulins with hypoalbuminemia in nephrosis or amyloidosis, and with malignancies of the reticuloendothelial system. IgM deficiency is common with malignancies of the reticuloendothelial system. Selective IgA deficiency occurs with reaction to drugs such as phenytoins and penicillamine.

B-3. **Answers: b, c, d.** B cells do not come from the thymus. The thymus is the origin of cytotoxic T cells, and it is the place where T cell clones of the "right" phenotype are selected and exported, while those that are inappropriate and might cause autoimmunity, for instance, are eliminated in the thymus. B cells make antibodies that mediate resistance to most bacteria that exist in fluid spaces. IgM, IgE, IgG1, and IgG2 all could be involved in immune responses in the lung. IgA is unlikely to be involved, since it functions primarily on mucosal surfaces and in secretions. CD 8+ cells can kill virally infected targets and cancer cells, and they may prevent autoimmunities, but their major role is probably to turn off immune

117

responses when they are no longer needed.

B-4. **Answers: a, b.** Cytotoxic T cells recognize antigen in the context of class I major histocompatability complex (MHC) antigens, which are the HLA-A, HLA-B, and HLA-C antigens. IL-1 does not mediate T cell effects on macrophages because IL-1 is a macrophage-secreted cytokine that affects T cells. Macrophages do not present antigen to B cells. The correct T–B interaction occurs because the T cell receptor recognizes antigen in the context of class II MHC presented by the correct B cell. B cell help involves both IL-2, for which B cells have receptors, and IL-4, which induces these cells to express immunoglobulin required for antigen-presentation. IL-1 has no known effects on B cells.

B-5. **Answers: a, b, d, e.** C3 plays a pivotal role in the complement cascade, and complete absence of C3 is associated with recurrent *S. pneumoniae*, *H. influenzae*, *Streptococcus pyogenes*, *Klebsiella* and *Neisseria* infections of the meninges and respiratory tract. Immunoglobulin deficiency impairs the opsonization, agglutination, deactivation, and detoxification activities of specific antibody, but T lymphocyte–mediated cellular immune mechanisms are generally intact, so that resistance to viral, mycobacterial, parasitic, and fungal infections is usually normal in the immunoglobulin deficiency states. Primary or idiopathic neutropenia is accompanied by a relative monocytosis, and affected patients have remarkably little difficulty with infections even when absolute neutrophil counts are less than 1500/mm^3, whereas acquired neutropenia predisposes to severe and overwhelming infection with a wide variety of organisms. The majority of affected individuals with selective IgA deficiency are remarkably asymptomatic, perhaps because of compensatory increases in IgG and IgM

levels. There is an inversion of the T4:T8 ratio in bronchoalveolar lavage of patients with AIDS, owing predominately to excessive numbers of T8 cells.

B-6. **Answers: a, d, e.** Specific effector T lymphocytes augment resistance to intracellular microbial organisms and participate in the generation of immune granulomas. In the previously sensitized or immune host, specific T cells appear in tissues in response to antigen deposition, as in the initiation of the delayed hypersensitivity skin reaction to tuberculin antigen by T cell recruitment. IgE binds to mast cells and, on interaction with specific antigen, triggers the release of multiple soluble mediators of immediate hypersensitivity. In the previously unsensitized host, specific antibody and antibody-forming cells will appear in lungs only after days to a week. Conversely, in the immune host, transudation of specific antibody or the influx of specific antibody-forming cells will occur over a very short period of time and promptly enhance phagocytosis and tend to prevent injury or infection. In the previously unsensitized or non-immunized host, periods of days to weeks elapse prior to the appearance of sensitized effector T cells at the site of infection.

B-7. **Answers: a, b, d, e.** Antigen-presenting cells must express class II major histocompatibility complex (MHC) antigens. T cells cannot present antigen since they cannot express class II MHC antigens. All T cells seem to require the interleukin-2 as a growth factor. Interleukin-2 seems to be a differentiation factor for some T cells.

B-8. **Answers: a, b, c, d, e.** The pulmonary macrophages originate as monocytes in the bone marrow. They are released from the bone marrow into the blood and enter the lung from the pulmonary vascular bed. In contrast to polymorphonuclear leukocytes, pulmonary macrophages are long-lived (weeks to months). They can present antigen to lymphocytes and induce immune responses, serve as activated effector cells for specific T cell immunity, and in general modulate pulmonary immune reactivity. Alveolar macrophages have surface membrane receptors for the Fc portions of IgG1 and IgG3 and for C3.

B-9.   **Answers: a, b, d, e.** Hilar lymph nodes have a limiting capsule, contain mature follicles with germinal centers, and are anatomically indistinguishable from extrapulmonary lymph nodes. The concentrations of IgA- and IgE-positive cells in hilar nodes are higher than in other lymph nodes, possibly reflecting the relatively high concentrations of these immunoglobulin isotypes in the mucosa of conducting airways. Immunoglobulin-containing cells of all major classes are present in collections of lymphoid cells adjacent to bronchial glands. Submucosal lymphoid nodules called bronchus-associated lymphoid tissue (BALT) are present directly subjacent to the bronchial mucosa of proximal airways.

B-10.   **Answers: c, d, e.** Immunoglobulin deficiencies can be either congenital (X-linked agammaglobulinemia, selected deficiencies, severe combined immunodeficiency) or acquired (common variable hypogammaglobulinemia). Common variable hypogammaglobulinemia (CVH) is an idiopathic disorder of depressed immunoglobulin synthesis characterized by a variable decrease in all (IgA, IgM, IgG) levels. It is the immunoglobulin deficiency most often associated with bronchiectasis. The respiratory manifestations of CVH include recurrent pyogenic pneumonias, sinusitis, bronchiectasis, empyema, and lymphocytic interstitial pneumonitis.

B-11.   **Answers: a, b, c, d.** After tissue deposition, antigen is taken up by macrophages and processed for presentation to specific antigen-reactive lymphocytes. The macro-

phages engulf, partially degrade, and display relevant antigenic determinants on the surface membrane of the cell. In conjunction with processed antigen, they express class II macromolecular gene products of the major histocompatibility complex (MHC), namely, surface membrane HLA-DR antigens. They also elaborate and secrete soluble mediators, predominately interleukin-1 (IL-1). The mediation of delayed hypersensitivity and cellular cytotoxic reactions is a major function effected by activated T cells.

B-12.   **Answers: a, d, e.** T lymphocytes arise from pluripotential stem cells in the bone marrow and differentiate and mature within the thymus gland. After 3 days, mature antigen-reactive T cells emerge from the thymus and are released into the blood in the form of helper/inducer T lymphocytes (T4 cells) and suppressor/cytotoxic T lymphocytes (T8 cells). In blood, the distribution of T cell phenotypes is approximately T4, 65% and T8, 35%. Different subsets of T4 lymphocytes accomplish delayed hypersensitivity reactions (lymphokine-mediated); helper cells for antibody-producing B cells and for cytotoxic T cells; and inducer cells for suppressor T cells. The major function effected by activated T cells is mediation of delayed hypersensitivity and cellular cytotoxic reactions.

B-13.   **Answers: b, d.** Polymorphonuclear leukocytes are present normally in very small numbers in conducting airways and in alveolar spaces of the respiratory tract; they are virtually absent from normal interstitial spaces of lung parenchyma. Up to one half to 3 times the total circulating pool of polymorphonuclear leukocytes are in the marginating population of cells in the pulmonary vascular bed. Normally, macrophages are less phagocytic than polymorphonuclear leukocytes. After phagocytosis and degradation of particles, polymorphonuclear leukocytes die and are removed by mucociliary clearance mechanisms, or they are ingested and digested by pulmonary macrophages.

B-14. **Answers: b, d.** In delayed hypersensitivity reactions, activated T4 cells, through elaboration of lymphokines, stimulate the influx, accumulation, and activation of a variety of subacute and chronic inflammatory cells. Persistence of this reaction can lead to the formation of immune granulomas. Host cells infected with virus display viral antigens on their surface membranes, and this is recognized by antigen-reactive T8 lymphocytes, which differentiate into virus-specific cytotoxic T cells. Additional cytotoxic mechanisms are mediated directly by natural killer (NK) lymphocytes, as well as lymphocytes that bind to target cells coated with specific antibody. Various subsets of activated T4 cells provide help for antibody production by B cells and for generation of cytotoxic T8 cells.

B-15. **Answers: a, c, d, e.** In the immune host specific antibody and sensitized T cells are available immediately at the site of particle deposition. Antigen is a potent stimulus of sensitized T lymphocytes to secrete a variety of lymphokines. Where preformed specific antibody is present at the site of particle deposition, the interaction of antigen with specific antibody of either the IgG or IgM class results in the formation of immune complexes, and these antigen-antibody complexes are potent stimulators of the classic pathway of complement activation. Phagocytosis and particle inactivation by pulmonary phagocytes are augmented considerably by specific antibody secreted by effector B lymphocytes and by the secretory products (lymphokines) of sensitized T lymphocytes. The magnitude of locally expressed chemotactic activity exceeds that in the non-immune host, and this results in the enhanced influx and accu-

mulation of polymorphonuclear leukocytes.

B-16. **Answers: a, b, c, d, e.** B lymphocytes arise from pluripotential stem cells and differentiate within the bone marrow. Mature B cells, which have immunoglobulin on surface membranes, are released into the circulation and migrate to lymph nodes, spleen, and secondary lymphatic tissues. After antigenic stimulation, B cells proliferate and differentiate into plasmablasts and plasma cells, which secrete specific antibody, and into memory B cells for subsequent secondary anamnestic responses. Antigen that is appropriately presented triggers specific clones of B and T cells to undergo activation and clonal expansion by proliferation. Antigen receptors on T cells are capable of recognizing both antigen and HLA-DR determinants on the surface membranes of antigen-presenting cells, for example, macrophages.

B-17. **Answer: c, d.** Macrophages engulf and process antigen for presentation to antigen-reactive lymphocytes, coordinate cellular interactions, and modulate responses by either enhancing or suppressing lymphocyte proliferation and differentiation. They are stimulated by soluble products of activated T cells (lymphokines) to undergo activation, which enhances their phagocytic, microbicidal, and cytotoxic activities. The phagocytic and cytotoxic activities of macrophages as well as polymorphonuclear leukocytes are enhanced by specific antibody, the soluble product of effector B cells. A variety of environmental factors, including viral infections of the respiratory tract, can depress the phagocytic and bactericidal activities of alveolar macrophages.

B-18. **Answers: a, b, c, e.** The differential diagnosis of diffuse pulmonary disease in the immunosuppressed host includes (1) infections, commonly opportunistic, (2) recurrence or extension of underlying process, (3) adverse drug reactions, and (4) new unrelated process or combinations of the above. Infectious etiologies account for 50–75% of the infiltrates and are associated with a 40–50% mortality. The high mortality rate makes it necessary to use invasive procedures in the evaluation of these patients. In AIDS patients, BAL is 80–85% sensitive in diagnosing PCP. In the non–AIDS-immunosuppressed host, the overall yield in infectious processes is high—about 82–90% in *Pneumocystis carinii* pneumonia and 83–96% in viral pneumonia.

B-19. **Answers: b, c, d, e.** The degree of eosinophilia in asthma does not correlate to the allergic background. Rather, there is a direct relationship between the degree of eosinophilia, and the degree of airway obstruction; the greater the degree of eosinophilia the greater the airway obstruction. Eosinophils are a heterogeneous population of cells evaluated as to their density and function. Eosinophil major basic protein has many functional activities including an ability to cause airway epithelial injury and mediator release, and be cytotoxic to a number of cells. Eosinophils, like polymorphonuclear leukocytes, generate leukotrienes, but eosinophils are characterized by their ability to produce more than the neutrophils.

B-20. **Answers: a, d.** All of the parasites can result in pulmonary infiltrates with eosinophilia. However, the *Schistosoma* species is the only one associated with pulmonary hypertension. This organism invades and obstructs the pulmonary vessels leading to pulmonary hypertension.

B-21. **Answer: c.** The treatment of this disease entity is with diethylcarbamazine. Steroids, quinine, erythromycin, or tetracycline does not cure this disorder.

B-22. **Answers: a, b, c, d, e.** Tropical eosinophilia can be due to infestation with microfilaria, which are introduced through the bite of a mosquito. Eosinophilia develops when the parasite passes through the lungs during its life cycle. Cough, asthma, chest pain, fever, and hemoptysis all may occur. Alteration in pulmonary function can be either obstructive or restrictive in nature.

B-23. **Answer: a.** Only a few studies have investigated pulmonary artery pressure during sleep in COPD. It appears that each percentage fall in oxygen saturation is associated with approximately a 1-mm Hg increase in pulmonary artery pressure, but this is not true in all patients.

B-24. **Answers: b, d, e.** The respiratory muscles are skeletal muscles and are made up of three different fiber types. In the human diaphragm, which is the principal muscle of inspiration, half the fibers are slow oxidative (type I) fibers, a quarter are fast oxidative glycolytic (type IIA) fibers, and a quarter are fast glycolytic (type IIB) fibers. The distribution of fiber types in the other respiratory muscles has not been well studied in the human, but they probably match those of the diaphragm. Contraction of the diaphragm primarily increases the volume of the thoracic cage in a vertical direction, but the transverse diameter also increases because the muscular fibers of the diaphragm run in a vertical direction from their attachment at the costal margins. The descent of the diaphragm during inspiration raises the abdominal pressure and lowers the pressure in the lungs so that air enters, whereas its ascent during expiration lowers the intra-abdominal pressure and raises the pressure in the lungs so that air leaves.

B-25. **Answers: a, d, e.** Functional residual capacity (FRC), i.e., the amount of air present in the lung at end expiration, is relatively constant no matter what respiratory maneuvers are carried out because the pull of the lung in an expiratory direction is counterbalanced exactly by the pull of the chest wall in an inspiratory direction. Airway resistance is lowest at TLC and highest at RV. Compliance of the lungs is the volume change associated with a static pressure change from end expiration to end inspiration. The pressure-volume curve of the lungs is not linear, and the calculated compliance will be different at any lung volume. In fibrosis or lung congestion, lung compliance is reduced.

B-26. **Answers: b, c, d, e.** Resistance to flow is the ratio of the pressure difference across the airways driving flow and the airflow rate (pressure/flow). One can calculate the pressure required to overcome flow resistance in the airways by subtraction of the elastic recoil pressure from the total transthoracic pressure across the lungs. This is the reciprocal of conductance. Flow resistance varies with lung volume because the airways lengthen and dilate during inspiration or at high lung volumes due to the increased traction on the airway walls created by the elastic recoil pressure, and flow resistance will be highest at low lung volumes. When resistance is calculated in a body plethysmograph, one determines the ratio of the box pressure to airway pressure while the airway shutter is closed, and the ratio of box pressure to airflow when the shutter is open. Dividing the slopes of these two ratios:

$$(P_A/P_p)/(Flow/P_p) = Resistance$$

B-27. **Answers: a, b, c, d.** During a forced expiration, the maximal airflow rate achieved at every lung volume is dependent on the pressure (effort) only up to a certain point. At high lung volumes, the airways are widely open so that very high flow rates can be achieved depending on the amount of effort exerted. At mid and low lung volumes, the flow rate increases with effort only up to a certain driving pressure, beyond which the flow rate does not increase because there is dynamic compression of the airways. These maximal expiratory flow rates are the same as those achieved during a forced expiratory vital capacity maneuver at any lung volume.

B-28. **Answers: a, c.** In normal individuals, maximal inspiratory and expiratory flow rates are approximately equal. In a variable lower airway obstruction, expiratory flow is limited to a far greater extent than inspiratory flow. In a fixed airway obstruction, inspiratory and expiratory flow are limited and the oval appearance is classic. In a variable upper airway obstruction, inspiratory flow is limited because the upper airway is narrowed by the negative pressure in it (relative to atmosphere), whereas expiratory flow is good because the positive pressure in the upper airway dilates it. In a carinal obstruction, there is a characteristic initial burst of expiratory flow, and then a plateau that ends abruptly.

B-29. **Answers: b.** Gas tensions are only indicative of the underlying condition if the subject is in a steady state, i.e., CO_2 elimination equals CO_2 production when the blood is drawn. The patient is in a steady state when an arterial blood is drawn if the RQ is within normal limits (.65–.95). An RQ greater than 1.0 suggests alveolar hyperventilation. With a constant ventilation, a fall in respiratory rate means an increase in tidal volume and an increase in alveolar ventilation. In pure alveolar hypoventilation the oxygen in the alveoli comes into equilibrium with the blood in the pulmonary capillary perfusing these alveoli, and the $P(A-a)O_2$ is normal. An abnormality of gas exchange may only be apparent during exertion.

B-30. **Answers: a, b, d.** For flow to occur through the pulmonary capillaries, the perfusing pressure or pulmonary artery pressure must exceed all of the pressures downstream, and there will be no flow if the capillary is closed off because the alveolar pressure is greater than the pulmonary artery pressure (as at the top of the lung). Radioactive techniques have demonstrated that more of the inspired air is distributed to the bottom of the lung than to the top of the lung when one is breathing normally. This is because at the top of the lung, the force of gravity (weight of the lung) and the retractive force of the lung act in the same direction so that the pleural pressure is more negative than at the bottom of the lung, where gravity and the lung retractive force act in opposite directions. As a result of this difference in pressure, areas near the top of the lung are more distended than those near the bottom of the lung (i.e., they are at different portions of their individual pressure-volume curves, and those at the top of the lung are on a flatter part of the curve). During ordinary breathing at FRC, the air spaces at the top of the lung will fill less than those at the base. The matching of blood and gas distribution in the lung ($\dot{V}_A/\dot{Q}$ ratios) is not uniform throughout the lung, even in healthy individuals. The upper zones are overventilated in relation to their perfusion, whereas the lower regions are underventilated in relation to their perfusion. The distribution of blood in the lung is nonuniform. The blood flow is less at the apex than at the base. This is because the distribution of blood flow is profoundly influenced by the surrounding pressures. At the bottom of the lung, the pulmonary artery pressure exceeds the alveolar pressure so that blood flow is greater. For the same reason, raising the pulmonary artery pressure higher than the alveolar pressure will result in blood flow.

B-31. **Answers: c, e.** Diffusing capacity (D_L) can be determined using either oxygen ($D_L O_2$) or carbon monoxide ($D_L CO$). In order to calculate the diffusing capacity

of any gas it is necessary to know the amount of gas that is diffusing across the blood-gas barrier in a minute and the mean difference in partial pressures of that gas between the alveolus and the pulmonary capillary. Thus,

$$D_L O_2 = \dot{V}o_2/P(\overline{A\text{-}c})O_2$$

or

$$D_L CO = \dot{V}co/P(\overline{A\text{-}c})CO.$$

Both "single breath" and "multiple breath steady-state" techniques can be used to estimate diffusing capacity for carbon monoxide. Determination of $D_L CO$ breathing different oxygen levels yields measurement of pulmonary capillary blood volume.

B-32. **Answers: b, d, e.** The saturation of hemoglobin is dependent on the pO_2 in the plasma. In addition, at a given partial pressure of oxygen, oxyhemoglobin will be more saturated (i.e., pO_2 content elevated) when the pCO_2 is lower, pH is higher, and the temperature is reduced. Conversely, the hemoglobin will carry less oxygen when the pCO_2 rises, the pH falls, or the temperature rises.

B-33. **Answers: a, e.** A high ventilation-perfusion ratio indicates that there is ventilation of poorly perfused alveoli. The blood flowing past these alveoli is well oxygenated and excessively depleted of carbon dioxide; hence it is dead space like ventilation. When there is ventilation of poorly perfused alveoli or overventilation of normally perfused alveoli, much of the gas leaving the alveoli has a composition close to that of inspired air — i. e. dead space like ventilation or physiologic dead space.

B-34. **Answer: d.** Alveolar hypoventilation implies that the alveolar ventilation is inadequate relative to the carbon dioxide production. In acute hypoventilation, the PaO_2 falls, $PaCO_2$ rises, and pH falls; there is only a slight consequent increase in bicarbonate (and total CO_2), which may still be in the normal range. If this hypoventilation persists, the kidneys will retain bicarbonate in an effort to restore the normal ratio of bicarbonate to dissolved CO_2 (20:1) so that the bicarbonate and CO_2 content will be elevated and the pH will be restored to the low normal range. The $P(A-a)O_2$ is not increased in pure alveolar hypoventilation, and if it is increased when the $PaCO_2$ is elevated, some other physiologic disturbance must also be present.

B-35. **Answers: b, c, e.** The following are important in this answer:

$$\text{Ventilation } (\mathring{V}_e) = \text{tidal volume } (V_T) \times \text{respiratory rate (f)}.$$

$$V_T = \text{alveolar volume } (V_A) + \text{dead space } (V_D),$$

so that

$$\mathring{V}_e = f(V_A \times V_D) = \mathring{V}_A + \mathring{V}_D.$$
$$\text{Now } pCO_2 = (\mathring{V}CO_2/\mathring{V}_A) \times K.$$

Thus, at a given minute ventilation, an increase in respiratory rate, a decrease in tidal volume, or a rise in CO_2 production will result in a rise in $PaCO_2$. Conversely, an increase in tidal volume (or decrease in respiratory rate) will result in a fall in $PaCO_2$.

B-36. **Answers: a, c, d.** The bicarbonate cannot be measured directly, but the pH, pCO_2, and total CO_2 can be determined. Since, as indicated in the Henderson Hasselbach equation:

$$pH = 6.1 + \log HCO_3{}^-/H_2CO_3$$

and

$$H_2CO_3 = 0.0301 \times PaCO_2.$$

$$\text{Then } HCO_3{}^- = \text{total } CO_2 - (0.0301 \times PaCO_2).$$

Similarly, the bicarbonate can be calculated from $PaCO_2$ and pH. When bicarbonate is ingested, the hydrogen ion concentration falls (pH rises), i.e., there is an alkalemia. The hydrogen ion concentration also falls when the $PaCO_2$ is reduced. In both respiratory alkalemia and metabolic acidemia, bicarbonate is reduced.

B-37. **Answer: a.** Eosinophilic infiltration of the alveolar structures occurs in eosinophilic pneumonia, and in the great majority of cases peripheral blood eosinophilia coexists. Other diffuse pulmonary diseases, such as lymphoma, pulmonary histiocytosis X, IPF, and sarcoidosis may demonstrate eosinophils within lung tissue, although they are certainly not the predominant cell type.

B-38. **Answer: c.** *Klebsiella* pneumonia, postprimary histoplasmosis, aspergillosis with mucoid impaction, and postprimary tuberculosis all have a predilection for upper lobe involvement on the chest roentgenogram.

B-39. **Answer: d.** The upper lobes are generally primarily involved in end-stage sarcoidosis, chronic hypersensitivity pneumonitis, eosinophilic granuloma, and ankylosing spondylitis on the chest roentgenogram.

B-40. **Answer: d.** Alveolar filling on chest roentgenograms is seen in histoplasmosis, chicken pox pneumonia, lipoid pneumonia, and bronchiolo-alveolar carcinoma, but not in coccidioidomycosis, in which multiple pulmonary nodules are the general pattern seen.

B-41. **Answer: e.** The characteristic features of an alveolar filling process are air bronchograms in larger bronchi, acinar rosettes with distal air bronchograms, obliteration or silhouetting of normal structure (heart borders, pulmonary vasculature, and diaphragm), and nodules with ill-defined margins. Interstitial processes, on the other hand, consist of both linear and nodular densities, which have a well-demarcated border and are not associated with distal air bronchograms.

B-42. **Answer: e.** Actinomycosis, primary histoplasmosis, *Streptococcus pyogenes* pneumonia, and pulmonary AV fistula all have a predilection for the lower lobes on the chest roentgenogram.

B-43. **Answer: d.** Lung volume is increased in lymphangioleiomyomatosis, eosinophilic granuloma, chronic hypersensitivity pneumonitis, and diffuse panbronchiolitis (which is virtually only seen in Japan).

B-44. **Answers: a, b, c, d, e.** In the adult the bronchial arteries usually originate from 1–3 trunks arising from the aorta between T3 and T8. The bronchial arteries supply the peripheral lobar bronchi, vasa vasorum of the pulmonary arteries, and in part the esophagus, mediastinum, and pleura. Venous drainage of the bronchial circulation is by both the pulmonary and systemic venous circulations. The bronchial veins drain the major and lobar bronchi and empty into the azygos and hemiazygos veins terminating in the SVC and pulmonary veins. Approximately one third of the bronchial venous circulation returns to the right side of the heart and the remainder to the left atrium.

B-45. **Answers: a. 3, b. 1, c. 5, d. 2, e. 4.** Massive hemoptysis (600 cc in 24–48 hr) is quite uncommon. In a literature review of 456 cases of massive hemoptysis, the causes were as follows: chronic cavitary tuberculosis (44%); inflammatory lung disease—bronchiectasis, fungal, necrotizing pneumonia (37%); lung cancer (7%); lung abscess (6%); bronchovascular fistulas (1%); broncholithiasis (1%); pulmonary contusion (1%); vasculitis (1%); and valvular heart disease (1%).

B-46. **Answer: e.** A pleural effusion may be seen in about 6% of patients with cirrhosis, and it is right-sided in 67% of these. Severe intrahepatic cholestasis may complicate sarcoidosis. The clinical picture mimics primary biliary cirrhosis. Esophageal rupture can result from prolonged vomiting, heavy lifting, childbirth, or defecation. Because the tear is usually located above the gastro-esophageal junction on the left side, the pulmonary manifestations are usually left-sided.

B-47. **Answers: a, b, c, d.** Pulmonary disorders that have been associated with Crohn's disease include granulomatous lung disease, pneumonitis due to sulfasalazine, bronchiectasis, and localized interstitial fibrosis. Bronchoalveolar lavage has demonstrated a high proportion of lymphocytes.

B-48. **Answer: b.** Lower esophageal sphincter pressure is decreased by theophylline, beta agonists, smoking, and alcohol. The FVC and FEV_1 are reduced with gastric but not duodenal ulcer, regardless of smoking history. Theophylline increases gastric acid secretion.

B-49. **Answer: d.** Gastroesophageal reflux can lead to recurrent pneumonia, atelectasis, pulmonary fibrosis, or laryngeal symptoms such as hoarseness, coughing spells, and throat clearing. A history of night cough and nocturnal wheezing is also associated with gastroesophageal reflux.

B-50. **Answers: a, c, d, e.** There are many similarities between sarcoidosis and primary biliary cirrhosis. In primary biliary cirrhosis, serum angiotensin-converting enzyme is elevated, and T-4 lymphocytes are elevated in lavage. However, serum mitochondrial antibodies are positive and the Kveim reaction is negative. Focal biliary cirrhosis should lead to suspicion of cystic fibrosis.

B-51. **Answers: a, b, d, e.** In normal subjects, the extrathoracic trachea is circular as far as the cricoid cartilage, below which its shape changes to a horseshoe, ellipse, or circle. The trachea becomes intrathoracic 1–3 cm above the suprasternal notch and most commonly assumes a round or oval shape, although horseshoe-shaped tracheas are also common. Calcification of the tracheal cartilage is infrequent and usually appears as small densities within the tracheal wall. In "saber-sheath" trachea there is abrupt narrowing of the intrathoracic portion of the trachea at the thoracic inlet associated with sagittal widening, so that the coronal tracheal diameter is less than or equal to one half of the sagittal diameter. The deformity is relatively fixed and uniform throughout its length, and the cartilage is often densely calcified. It is most common in older men with COPD.

B-52. **Answers: c, e.** The microbiology of recurrent pneumonia is mainly *H. influenzae*, *Pneumococcus*, *S. pyogenes*, and *S. aureus*. Once bronchiectasis is established, *S. aureus* and *Pseudomonas* infections predominate. The bronchiectasis associated with common variable hypogammaglobulinemia is diffuse rather than focal. Patients with common variable hypogammaglobulinemia are predisposed to atrophic gastritis with achlorhydria, neoplasia, malabsorption, nodular lymphoid hyperplasia, giardiasis, thymoma and thyroid abnormalities, and noncaseating granulomas in the lungs, spleen, and liver. Therapy consists of both intravenous immune globulin and rotating antibiotics. The intravenous route of administration is more effective than the intramuscular route in preventing infections. Replacement therapy is effective in promoting normal growth in younger patients.

B-53. **Answers: b, d, e.** Lower esophageal pressure increases with inspiration when intra-abdominal pressure also increases. Acid and pepsin secretion, although not markedly increased in subjects with reflux esophagitis, may cause damage to the esophageal mucosa and airways. Short, sudden increases in intra-abdominal pressure may cause reflux episodes, which are more frequent in patients with decreased lower esophageal pressure. Theophylline may aggravate reflux episodes by stimulating acid secretion. Coughing, which acutely increases intra-abdominal pressure, may produce episodes of gastroesophageal reflux.

B-54. **Answers: a, b, c, d, e.** The mean resting lower esophageal sphincter pressure in patients with reflux is lower than that of normal subjects. However, not all patients with reflux esophagitis have decreased lower esophageal sphincter pressure. Further studies have revealed that transient relaxation of the lower esophageal sphincter constitutes one of the major mechanisms responsible for reflux episodes, particularly in the postprandial period. The lower esophageal sphincter pressure can be decreased by dietary factors, smoking, alcohol, and certain drugs such as theophylline and beta-adrenergics.

B-55. **Answer: e.** Several studies have suggested a relationship between chronic bronchitis and ulcerative colitis. The fulminant nature of the bronchitis and the absence of other factors suggest a true association. Hypoxemia in hepatic failure is due to intrapulmonary shunting and to pulmonary edema. Increased intraluminal pressure from heavy lifting, prolonged or recurrent vomiting, forceful childbirth, and defecation can predispose patients to spontaneous esophageal rupture. Because the tear is usually located above the gastroesophageal junction on the left side the pulmonary manifestations are usually left-sided.

B-56. **Answers: a, d, e.** Exercise limitation is reflected in an early plateau in oxygen consumption, i.e., maximum oxygen consumption is markedly reduced. When this is due to ventilatory limitation, the ventilation is elevated at any given work load, and there is an inordinate rise in respiratory rate, i.e., rapid shallow breathing. This is associated with a fall in PaO_2, and rise in $P(A-a)O_2$.

B-57. **Answers: a, e.** In polyarteritis nodosa, consolidation is patchy and fleeting as in Löffler's syndrome. There is no lymph node enlargement in Löffler's syndrome. Pleural effusion is very uncommon in blastomycosis as is chest wall involvement. Pleural effusion is common in *Haemophilus influenzae* infection.

B-58. **Answers: a, b, d.** The TLC and all of the subdivisions of lung volume are reduced in obesity, but the most affected is the expiratory reserve volume. The pressure-volume curve of the lungs is shifted downward, but the slope is normal. This is an example of restriction, and the breathing is generally rapid and shallow.

B-59. **Answer: b, c.** A low ventilation-perfusion ratio implies perfusion of poorly ventilated alveoli or venous admixture–like perfusion.

B-60. **Answer: a.** This indicates a metabolic acidosis, i.e., a low HCO_3^- and pH.

B-61. **Answers: b, d.** Exercise-induced bronchospasm develops in 5–15 minutes after the exercise stops and is generally related to the level of work load and ventilation achieved. It is generally considered that the work load necessary to result in bronchospasm is one that induces at least 85% of the maximum predicted heart rate. The response is exaggerated if the subject is breathing cold air and ablated if one breathes warm moist air or breathes through the nose, which warms and humidifies inspired air. There is often a refractory period after the induction of

bronchospasm, during which a second exercise results in much less or no bronchospasm. One theory for this phenomenon is that the mast cells have released all of their mediators with the first exercise load, and it takes time to renew them. Exercise-induced bronchospasm can usually be ablated by prior inhalation of appropriate amounts of cromolyn or beta-2 agonists, but inhaled corticosteroids are not effective.

B-62. **Answers: a, b.** Retrocardiac or mediastinal densities are due to paraesophageal and contiguous mediastinal inflammation. Late perforations with development of esophago-bronchopleural fistulas occurs in 1–2% of patients. This nearly always fatal complication develops from ulceration and subsequent transmural necrosis of the esophagus and typically occurs 7–14 days after endoscopic variceal sclerotherapy. Barium should be avoided in suspected cases of esophago-pleural fistula, and water-soluble contrast avoided in cases suspected of esophagobronchial fistula. In uncertain cases, water-soluble contrast should be used for diagnosis as the former fistula is more common.

B-63. **Answers: a, c.** At the anaerobic threshold, the delivery of oxygen to the exercising muscles does not meet their demand, so that anaerobic utilization of energy occurs. As a result there is excess carbon dioxide production and excessive lactate accumulates, so that the pH falls. As a result of the increase in CO_2 production without a parallel increase in oxygen consumption, the respiratory quotient rises. Ventilation increases linearly with the carbon dioxide production and disproportionately with the oxygen consumption.

B-64. **Answers: a, b, e.** During moderate exercise ventilation increases, initially by primarily increasing tidal volume, until it reaches about 60% of the vital capacity, and then respiratory rate increases rapidly. The ventilation increases linearly with the work intensity and then, along with the CO_2 production, rises precipitously. Cardiac output also rises linearly, primarily as a result of an increase in heart rate. The oxygen uptake increases linearly until a maximum is reached and then plateaus, with no further increase in oxygen consumption despite increasing load. The vessels in the exercising skeletal muscles dilate and the proportion of the cardiac output going to the exercising muscles increases.

B-65. **Answers: a, b, d.** Either a treadmill or an exercise bicycle can be used to test the response to exercise. The efficiency of the response to exercise is the ratio of power output to oxygen uptake. The normal response to exercise is an increase in tidal volume to about 60% of the vital capacity, so that a patient's tidal volume may easily double. The systolic blood pressure normally rises during exercise, and a fall in systolic blood pressure or a failure to rise is an indication for stopping.

B-66. **Answers: a, b, d.** In a person who is not physically fit, anaerobic metabolism develops early, lactate is produced so that the lactate in blood is elevated, carbon dioxide production rises, and there is a metabolic acidemia. This stimulates the ventilation and the heart rate. The carbon dioxide production exceeds the oxygen consumption at the anaerobic threshold so that the respiratory quotient rises.

B-67. **Answers: a, b, c, d, e.** Hyperleukocytosis is present when the white blood cell count is greater than 100,000 and is usually a feature of myeloproliferative or lymphoproliferative disorders. Elevated leukocyte counts can occur in the chronic leukemias, in which there is proliferation of the mature forms of white cells, or in acute leukemias. Because of the different size, shape, and functional properties

(deformability) of the proliferating white cell, the degree of complications from hyperleukocytosis varies in different leukemias. Even normal, mature granulocytes have prolonged capillary transit time because of their size and stiffness. Myeloblasts are much less deformable and can cause significant stasis in the capillaries of the brain and lung, causing local ischemia as a result of decreased blood flow. Pulmonary leukostasis usually occurs with a white cell count greater than 100,000. The pulmonary manifestations of hyperleukocytosis can range from diffuse alveolar infiltrates to marked hypoxemia despite a relatively normal roentgenogram.

B-68. **Answers: a, d, e.** The development of pulmonary infiltrates in an immunocompromised patient often leads to aggressive and frequently invasive evaluation. The timing and radiographic appearance of the infiltrates are helpful in differentiating infectious from noninfectious etiologies as well as opportunistic from bacterial infections. Parenchymal infiltrates appearing before treatment or within 72 hours of initiating treatment are generally not opportunistic infection. Localized disease occurring either early or late in treatment is likely to be infectious, and the infection is bacterial in the majority. Diffuse disease occurring during treatment is usually noninfectious, but a significant number are opportunistic infections. It is in this group that aggressive, possibly invasive evaluation can be helpful. The use of bronchoscopy with lavage or biopsy in patients who develop diffuse alveolar and interstial infiltrates within 48 hours of treatment generally has a very low yield.

B-69. **Answers: c, e.** Circulating antigen-antibody reactions are involved in type III reactions, not type II. Type II reactions are mediated by antibodies against antigens which are an integral part of a cell or membrane. The granulomatous lesion that typifies the lung lesions in tuberculosis is caused by delayed-type hypersensitivity responses to *Mycobacterium tuberculosis.* C-fixing bacteriolysins increase lysozyme activity and play a role in antibacterial immunity. The major mechanisms in antiviral immunity are cytotoxic T cell–mediated killing of virally infected targets and antibody production, which neutralizes viruses following lytic release and before reinfection. Natural killer cells are not an immune response, per se, since they have neither antigen specificity nor memory. The AIDS virus causes decreased resistance to *Mycobacteria* because it infects CD T4-positive helper T cells, which normally secrete lymphokines that cause increased phagocyte-mediated antibacterial activity.

B-70. **Answer: d.** In pulmonary fibrosis, lung volume is reduced and the elastic recoil is increased (the pressure-volume [P-V] curve is shifted down and to the right, and the shape of the curve is altered, i.e., compliance is decreased). Maximal airflow rates are low because they are being achieved at a low lung volume. Flow resistance is normal, but because the driving pressure is increased (elastic recoil), the flow rates are actually higher than expected at that low lung volume. Indeed, if they are not greater than expected at a particular lung volume under these circumstances, associated airflow obstruction can be inferred.

B-71. **Answer: a.** When the lungs become stiff, the pressure-volume curve of the lungs is shifted downward, and the slope of the curve is reduced. Conversely, when the lungs lose elasticity, the pressure-volume curve of the lungs is shifted upward, and the slope of the curve is increased. When there is airway obstruction with no involvement of the lung parenchyma, the curve is shifted upward, but the slope is normal. Similarly, when there is external chest compression as in obesity, the curve is shifted downward but the slope of the curve is normal.

B-72. **Answer: a.** Although all of these changes in function may be seen in obese patients, the most common finding is a low expiratory reserve volume due to the increased load applied on the lungs by the chest.

B-73. **Answer: a, c.** Obese patients have increased work of breathing due to the external load applied by the chest. Hypoxemia may be present because of altered ventilation-perfusion ratios. However, even in the face of the increased work and an increased CO_2 production, most generally maintain a normal or slightly decreased arterial carbon dioxide tension. They generally breathe rapidly and shallowly. Lung volume is reduced.

B-74. **Answer: a, b, c, d.** The peripheral airways adjacent to the alveoli only contribute about 10–15% of the total airway resistance. When there is nonuniform obstruction in even as much as 50% of the peripheral airways, the overall resistance will rise very little and then will not be recognized by measurements of airway resistance or conductance, maximal expiratory flow rates, or the FEV_1. However, the time constants in the peripheral units (i.e., resistance × compliance) will be nonuniformly distributed so that gas distribution will be altered. On the other hand, since there is no alteration of the parenchyma, the static lung compliance will be unchanged.

B-75. **Answer: a, b, c, e.** Methacholine and, in some cases, histamine inhalation in gradually increasing doses is generally used to assess nonspecific airway reactivity. A fall of 20% of the FEV_1 or 35% of specific conductance is considered positive. Exercise, if carried out at a work load that increases the heart rate to greater than

85% of predicted maximum, will induce a fall in FEV_1 in the majority of patients with asthma. The fall is related to the level of ventilation achieved during the exercise, and voluntary hyperventilation to that level will induce the same result, and this will occur even earlier if cold air is inhaled. Specific agents in the workplace or residence may be responsible for attacks of bronchospasm and may be used to "challenge" the patient.

B-76. **Answer: d.** Gas tensions are only indicative of the underlying condition if the subject was in a steady state, i.e., CO_2 elimination = CO_2 production when the blood was drawn.

B-77. **Answer: a.** If the RQ is within normal limits (.65-.95), it is likely that the patient was in a steady state when an arterial blood was drawn. Concentrations of expired gases allow calculation of O_2 consumption ($\dot{V}O_2$), CO_2 production ($\dot{V}CO_2$), and respiratory quotient (RQ). In a steady state, the RQ is between .65 and .95. A low RQ suggests hypoventilation while the blood was drawn. A high RQ suggests hyperventilation while the blood was drawn. Under these circumstances, blood gas tensions are not an accurate reflection of a gas exchange defect.

B-78. **Answer: b.** Radioactive techniques have demonstrated that more of the inspired air is distributed to the bottom of the lung than to the top of the lung when one is breathing normally. This is because at the top of the lung, the force of gravity (weight of the lung) and the retractive force of the lung act in the same direction so that the pleural pressure is more negative than at the bottom of the lung, where gravity and the lung retractive force act in opposite directions. As a result of this difference in pressure, areas near the top of the lung are more distended than those near the bottom of the lung (i.e., they are

at different portions of their individual pressure-volume curves, and those at the top of the lung are on a flatter part of the curve). During ordinary breathing at FRC, the air spaces at the top of the lung will fill less than those at the base.

B-79. **Answer: d.** As with virtually all conditions or even the general normal population, the highest mortality occurs during the sleep-related hours. Several studies have shown that morbidity (i.e., respiratory failure needing intubation) and mortality in asthma are greatest between midnight and 6 o'clock in the morning. It is possible that sleep exaggerates the circadian increase in airway resistance.

B-80. **Answer: c.** The roentgenogram and often the hemoglobin may be normal even with multiple sites of pulmonary arteriovenous emphysema. The hypoxemia may induce slight hyperventilation so that the $PaCO_2$ is usually low, although with large shunts the $PaCO_2$ is normal, or may be slightly elevated. A simple way to assess the extent of shunt is to have the subject breathe 100% oxygen for about 15 minutes, or until virtually all of the nitrogen is washed out of the lungs. Oxygen is carried in the blood, both in combination with hemoglobin and in physical solution in the plasma. The amount dissolved in the plasma is related to the PaO_2 and at 100 mm Hg is about 0.3 ml/L of plasma. At a PaO_2 more than 500 mm Hg, there will be 1.5 ml O_2/L of plasma. The important aspect about estimating the amount of shunt present is to remember that the hemoglobin may be fully saturated as long as the PaO_2 is greater than 100 mm Hg, and yet a major shunt may be present. A qualitative estimate of the amount of shunt present can be obtained by measuring the PaO_2 while breathing 100% oxygen. A PaO_2 <500 mm Hg while breathing 100% O_2 at sea level indicates a greater than normal amount of shunt.

The amount of shunt can be calculated:

$$\frac{\text{end-pulm.capillary-arterial } O_2 \text{ content}}{\text{end-pulm.cap-mixed venous } O_2 \text{ content}}$$

B-81. **Answers: b, c, d, e.** In orthodeoxia the supine PaO_2 is higher than in the upright position. It is hypoxemia caused by pulmonary vascular abnormalities from chronic liver disease. The pulmonary vascular abnormalities can be of several types: precapillary dilatations 15–160 microns in diameter; true AV communications in the lower lung zones; and pleural based AV "spiders." The cause of the pulmonary vascular abnormalities is unknown.

B-82. **Answers: a, b, c, d, e.** The diagnosis of liver-associated vascular abnormalities requires (1) clinical diagnosis of chronic hepatic dysfunction (dysproteinemias, coagulopathy, chronically elevated LFTs, etc.) from a preexisting condition known to cause liver disease (alcoholic cirrhosis, chronic active hepatitis [CAH], etc.); (2) hypoxemia; (3) demonstration of intrapulmonary vascular "shunting" by a ^{99}Tc-labeled macroaggregated albumin scan (V/Q scan) with immediate scanning of organs in the systemic circulation (brain, liver, kidneys) by contrast enhanced echocardiogram ("bubble echo") or by pulmonary angiography showing "spongy" parenchyma or discrete arteriovenous malformations (AVMs).

B-83. **Answers: a, c, e.** Hypereosinophilia is defined by peripheral eosinophilia ($>1500/mm^3$) that persists for more than 6 months (or death before 6 months with signs and symptoms) in the absence of other known causes of eosinophilia (e.g., allergy, neoplasm, parasite). There is multi-organ system involvement. The persistence of the eosinophilia and the associated organ dysfunction sets hypereosinophilic syndrome apart. Löffler's endocarditis, endomyocardial fibrosis,

and eosinophilic leukemia can all be considered to fall within the spectrum of presentations of hypereosinophilia.

B-84. **Answers: c, d, e.** A 9:1 male predominance has been reported. In the NIH collection of 50 patients the mean age at onset was 33, with 70% of patients presenting between the ages of 20 and 50 years. The extent of organ system involvement ranges from minor skin involvement to life-threatening cardiovascular, hematologic, and neurologic manifestations. There is no "typical" rash of HES; skin lesions are present in 25–50% of patients. Urticaria/angioedema of the face and extremities has been described as has a pruritic maculopapular eruption over the trunk and extremities. Neurologic manifestations include diffuse CNS involvement causing global behavioral and cognitive dysfunction, focal abnormalities related to CVAs and peripheral polyneuropathies.

B-85. **Answers: a, b, d, e.** Characteristically the disorder manifests as endocardial fibrosis with overlying thrombus. The fibrosis leads to pump failure which progresses over days to years. The initial and primary site of injury is believed to be the endocardium. Platelet thrombi develop over the damaged endocardium, resulting in a mural thrombus. The thrombus then organizes and endomyocardial fibrosis develops, resulting in a restrictive cardiomyopathic picture. Thrombosis, fibrinoid change, and inflammatory cell reaction involve small intramural coronary vessels. Thromboembolic events are often present and may dominate the clinical picture.

B-86. **Answers: a, b, c.** Histologically there is mural thrombosis (which contains large numbers of eosinophils), fibrotic thickening of the endocardium, and infiltration of eosinophils into the myocardium. Mitral and tricuspid insufficiency occur when the endocardial fibrosis involves the valve leaflets.

B-87. **Answers: a, d, e.** Eosinophils in peripheral blood may appear large, with hypersegmented nuclei, cytoplasmic vacuolization, and partial degranulation. The eosinophil count at presentation does not predict the extent of organ damage. WBCs may also appear abnormal with immature forms and hypo- or hypersegmented nuclei. Anemia may be present and RBCs may be nucleated or teardrop-shaped.

B-88. **Answers: b, c, d, e.** Pulmonary involvement includes cough, dyspnea, infiltrates, and effusions. The pulmonary disease is generally persistent and may progress to pulmonary fibrosis. There is no evidence of airflow limitation. Neurologic manifestations include diffuse CNS involvement causing global behavioral and cognitive dysfunction. The NIH recommends prednisone 1 mg/kg/d with subsequent taper as disease activity permits. If unresponsive to prednisone, it may be responsive to cytotoxic agents. Hydroxyurea is added to the prednisone.

B-89. **Answers: b, e.** Poor prognostic indicators include WBC>100,000, peripheral myeloblasts, or promyelocytes. Elevated liver function tests and hepatomegaly occur with hepatic involvement. Clinical renal disease is rare. Cardiovascular involvement is generally unresponsive to prednisone. Prognosis is related to the degree of organ involvement, especially cardiac involvement.

B-90. **Answer: c.** There are three basic types of apnea: (1) central apnea in which there is cessation of airflow as well as cessation of any respiratory effort; (2) upper airway obstructive apnea in which there is cessation of airflow but increasing respiratory efforts; (3) mixed apnea in which there is no airflow, and there is a combination of no effort and marked efforts. In a variation of the obstructive apneic episode called either a partial upper airway obstruction or an obstructive hypopnea, airflow is decreased and is associated with normal or greater respiratory efforts. Lastly, hypoventilation, i.e., a decrease in respiratory rate and/or tidal volume associated with an elevated $PaCO_2$ and fall in PaO_2, may develop during sleep. Although this is not a true apnea, patients with hypoventilation can present with the same signs and symptoms as those with sleep apnea. In pure hypoventilation the hypoxemia is less severe than in apneic episodes where ventilation-perfusion imbalances are also present, so that the amount of oxygen desaturation is far out of proportion to the elevated $PaCO_2$.

B-91. **Answers: a, b, c.** Myocardial infarction, inhalation of toxic fumes, and sleep apnea can produce acute pulmonary edema. Myocardial infarction can occur during sleep and obviously produces a cardiogenic pulmonary edema. Toxic fume inhalation produces a noncardiogenic pulmonary edema which can occur at anytime. The sleep apnea syndrome can produce a cardiogenic pulmonary edema due to the hypoxia and cardiac dysfunction that occurs during the apneic episodes. Uncomplicated asthma and interstitial disease do not cause acute pulmonary edema during sleep.

B-92. **Answer: c.** While all of these symptoms are suggestive of the sleep apnea syndrome, the most common symptom is restless sleep, which is present in virtually 100% of the individuals. This may vary from a mild increase in motor activity to severe thrashing and actually falling out of bed. Loud snoring is the next most common feature and occurs in approximately 93–94% of patients, and daytime somnolence occurs in approximately 75–80%. Decreased intellectual capacity, with inability to concentrate and carry out thought processes, occurs in approximately 55–60%. Personality changes are also not uncommon and occur in approximately 45–50% of the patients. Other clinical features include sexual impotency, morning headache, intermittent nocturnal enuresis, and morning nausea.

B-93. **Answers: a, b, d.** Systemic and pulmonary hypertension and erythrocytosis may develop as sequelae of sleep apnea syndrome. Systemic hypertension occurs in approximately 50% of patients who have been diagnosed with sleep apnea. Since the natural history of sleep apnea syndromes is not known, the proportion of patients who will develop pulmonary hypertension, cor pulmonale, and congestive heart failure has not been ascertained. Erythrocytosis is a consequence of the hypoxemia that develops during sleep. Another important sequela of the sleep apnea syndrome, which fortunately occurs rarely, is "unexplained" nocturnal death, which is in all probability related to a cardiac arrhythmia, most likely ventricular fibrillation. All types of arrhythmias can occur, although bradycardia is most common.

B-94. **Answer: d.** Obesity is present in approximately 70% of individuals suffering from the sleep apnea syndrome. However, this means that one in five patients are of normal body weight. Weight loss usually leads to improvement, but it is difficult for these patients to lose and maintain a weight loss.

B-95. **Answer: c.** Several studies have shown that approximately 30% of patients attending hypertension clinics have sleep apnea. Therefore, any patient with hypertension should be questioned about the signs and symptoms suggestive of the sleep apnea syndrome.

B-96. **Answer: b.** Although Cushing's syndrome, acromegaly, and hypogonadism can be associated with the sleep apnea syndrome, hypothyroidism is the most common. In all patients with sleep apnea, thyroid functions should be evaluated. Correction of the hypothyroid state will improve the sleep apnea picture. Iatrogenic Cushing's syndrome due to large steroid dose has been reported to produce sleep apnea. Although premenopausal females have less sleep apnea than males, the whole question of male and female sex hormones has not been fully elucidated.

B-97. **Answer: a.** In the sleep apnea syndrome, sleep stage is shifted away from REM and slow-wave sleep (stages 3 and 4), so that the lighter stages of sleep are more frequent in this syndrome, and REM sleep decreases to about 15% of the night's sleep.

B-98. **Answers: a, b, c.** Obstructive sleep apnea has been shown to occur as a result of obstruction at the nasal, tonsilar, and epiglottal areas. The most common site is the epiglottal area. Occasionally improvement of nasal obstruction will improve the sleep apnea syndrome, and removal of hypertrophied tonsils, even in adults, will alleviate the sleep apnea syndrome.

B-99. **Answer: c.** All have been reported to be successful in treating sleep apnea, but only nasal CPAP has a high success rate, which is approximately 80–90%. Protriptyline hydrochloride, a tricyclic antidepressant, increases the upper airway muscle tone in cats proportionately more than that of the diaphragm, thereby maintaining airway patency, but overall it has a very low success rate in patients. Supplemental oxygen decreases the number and length of apneas and improves oxygen saturation, but at best has a 30–40% success rate. Weight loss will improve the disorder, but initiating and maintaining the weight loss is exceedingly difficult. A nasal pharyngeal airway has a high failure rate because of nasopharyngeal pain and often it does not penetrate beyond the obstruction, which may be as far as the laryngeal area.

B-100. **Answer: b.** Tracheostomy is almost 100% successful in this condition, because the upper airway is being bypassed. However, some patients have marked redundant tissue in the neck area and a drop of the chin toward their chest during sleep can occlude the tracheostomy tube opening. Because the neck is short and fat in many of these patients, an inappropriately performed tracheostomy may be associated with occlusion of the distal end of the tube abutting against the tracheal wall. Uvulo-palatopharyngoplasty has only a 40% success rate in the best of studies. There are no factors that help to predict which patients will respond favorably to the uvulopalatopharyngoplasty. Tonsillectomy in patients with exceedingly large tonsils improves the syndrome, and mandibular advancement is helpful in patients with micrognathia.

B-101. **Answers: a, b, c.** Progesterone and carbonic anhydrase inhibitors are respiratory stimulants that will improve central sleep apnea. Additionally, supplemental oxygen decreases the number of central apneic episodes, probably because improved oxygenation of the respiratory center improves respiratory center control of breathing.

B-102. **Answer: b.** Although apnea and paradoxical respiration can be seen in patients with COPD, the most common cause of hypoxemia is hypopneic ventilation, i.e., a progressive decrease in tidal volume over time with oxygen desaturation. This desaturation is greater than would be expected in pure hypoventilation. The oxygen desaturation due to hypopneic episodes is the greatest during REM sleep in patients with COPD.

B-103. **Answer: a.** Although progesterone, almitrine, and carbonic anhydrase inhibitors improve, to a slight degree, the oxygen desaturation during sleep in COPD, the treatment of choice is supplemental oxygen. Usually a flow rate of 1–3 L/min by nasal cannulae is adequate to overcome the marked oxygen desaturation that can occur.

B-104. **Answer: a.** The history is the most helpful study in evaluating a patient's operative risk because it gives a complete profile of the patient and how he or she has reacted to stress and to other adverse conditions in the past. A history of familial disorders, prior illnesses, prior difficulties with surgical procedures or anesthetics, the presence of allergies or asthma, and the effects of medications, including over-the-counter products, should be included. Physical examination, chest roentgenogram, electrocardiogram, and a liver function profile are useful, but an alert physician will suspect problems from the history alone.

B-105. **Answer: d.** Active immunization results when tetanus toxoid injections are given on the recommended schedule, usually in infancy (with DPT shots) or during military induction. A follow-up booster every 10 years is recommended by the American College of Surgeons. However, any person with a penetrating injury must receive tetanus prophylaxis if previous immunization cannot be documented or if more than 5 years have passed since the last immunization.

B-106. **Answer: d.** A myocardial infarction within 3–6 months of surgery carries a much higher operative mortality risk due to perioperative recurrence. The mortality rate of a perioperative myocardial infarction is as high as 50% and usually occurs in the first postoperative week. There is little difference between risk factors for a subendocardial and those for a transmural myocardial infarction. Emergency procedures that cannot be avoided require careful operative management.

B-107. **Answer: c.** Although patients with pulmonary vascular disease, asthma, carcinoma, or a history of pulmonary embolus

are at increased operative risk, the highest operative risk is for patients with chronic obstructive lung disease. These patients may not be able to generate enough force to cough and clear their airways postoperatively. Atelectasis, pneumonia, and other infections can lead to acute pulmonary decompensation and an inability to be weaned from the respirator.

2-2 Airway Disease

A-1. **Answers: b, c, d.** Unlike polyarteritis nodosum, HepS Ag positivity is uncommon. Three "phases" have been described: an initial allergic phase with allergic rhinitis/atopic disease (which may precede the last phase by 15–30 years), an "asthma" phase, and a final vasculitic phase. An atopic history is present in most, and asthma in nearly all. The patient often presents early as a difficult to control asthmatic. Paranasal sinus disease occurs in >90%. Vasculitis presents usually in the skin, but is seen in the lung, brain, heart, nerves, and uncommonly the kidney.

A-2. **Answers: a, b, c, d.** GI symptoms are present in over 50% of cases. Neuropathy is present in >80%. Cerebral infarction (bleed, ischemic) and cardiac involvement are the usual causes of death. Eosinophils are >10% in >95%. Neuropathy is present in >80% and the ESR elevated in >90% of cases.

A-3. **Answers: b, c, d, e.** Steroids are the mainstay of therapy, with control of reversible airway obstruction, suppression of eosinophil count, and control of

vasculitic manifestations used to determine the dose/length of therapy. The vasculitic phase usually remits before 1 year. Lifelong steroids are not often needed; intermittent therapy is adequate in both. Refractory cases are usually managed with cyclophosphamide, azathioprine, or both. Plasmapheresis adds no benefit. A shorter span between the first two phases and vasculitis carries a poorer prognosis.

A-4. **Answers: a, b, c, d.** Mounier-Kuhn syndrome is a congenital abnormality characterized by atrophy of the elastic and muscular support layers of the airways resulting in tracheobronchomegaly. Protrusion of redundant musculomembranous tissue between rings of cartilage results in deep saccular pouches described as tracheal or bronchial diverticulosis. Weakness of the cartilaginous portions is also frequently present. Typically, the trachea and main bronchi balloon with deep inspiration and collapse markedly with forced expiration or cough.

A-5. **Answers: a, c, e.** Protrusion of redundant musculomembranous tissue between rings of cartilage results in the unusual scalloped or corrugated appearance of the airways. The tracheobronchial changes result in an ineffective cough and pooling of secretions in the airways, and this predisposes these patients to chronic bronchitis, bronchiectasis, and recurrent pneumonias. Additional associated complications include spontaneous pneumothoraces and cor pulmonale.

A-6. **Answers: d, e.** Tracheobronchomegaly is present on the chest film when the diameter of the trachea exceeds 25 mm in any transverse section or 27 mm in the sagittal. For the right main bronchus the value is 21 mm, and for the left, 19 mm. These values represent the mean plus 3 S.D. Nevertheless, bronchoscopy is probably the procedure of choice for diagnosis because the unusual width of the trachea may not be shown clearly or may be overlooked on conventional chest films, and other features besides size are important. Computed tomography is also very useful for confirmation of the diagnosis. CPAP may be useful to help stent the floppy airways open and improve clearance of secretions. Good postural drainage and the early institution of appropriate antibiotic therapy with signs of complicating infection are the mainstays of therapy.

A-7. **Answers: c, d.** Controversy exists in the literature as to whether Mounier-Kuhn syndrome is a congenital or acquired condition secondary to chronic infections and inflammation. A number of features favor the former hypothesis. First, the histologic changes may be seen in the absence of associated inflammation, and MKS is rare compared to the many conditions associated with chronic pulmonary infections. Second, some patients have no history of pulmonary symptoms. In addition, MKS has been associated with other congenital abnormalities of the tracheobronchial tree including tracheal trifurcation, duplica-

tion of the distal trachea, and abnormal branching of bronchi. The Mounier-Kuhn syndrome has also been associated with Ehlers-Danlos syndrome in adults and cutis laxa in children, suggesting the possibility of an inherited defect in connective tissue structure. More severely affected patients are frequently smokers, and the chronic inhalation of irritants may predispose these patients to worse sequelae. Pulmonary function tests usually show increased dead space and tidal volume, and airflow limitation along with an elevated TLC and RV.

A-8. **Answers: a, b, c.** The peripheral airways only contribute about 10–20% of the total airway resistance. When there is nonuniformly distributed obstruction in even as much as 50% of the peripheral airways, the overall resistance will rise little and then will not be recognized by measurements of airway resistance or conductance, or the maximal expiratory flow rates or the $FEV_{1.0}$. However, the time constants in the peripheral units (i.e., resistance × compliance) will be nonuniformly distributed so that gas distribution will be altered. On the other hand, since there is no alteration of the parenchyma, the static lung compliance will be unchanged.

A-9. **Answers: a, d, e.** Methacholine inhalation and, in some cases, histamine inhalation, in gradually increasing doses, are generally used to assess nonspecific airway reactivity. Exercise carried out at a work load that increases the heart rate to greater than 85% of predicted maximum heart rate, which will induce a fall in $FEV_{1.0}$ in the majority of patients with asthma, is also a nonspecific test of airway hyperresponsiveness. The fall is related to the level of ventilation achieved during the exercise and voluntary hyperventilation to that level will induce the same result, and this will occur even earlier if cold air is inhaled. Inhalation of warm moist air frequently prevents exercise-induced bronchospasm. A fall of 20% of the $FEV_{1.0}$ or 35% of specific conductance is considered a positive response.

A-10. **Answers: a, e.** Cases of vitamin A deficiency have been reported in patients with cystic fibrosis and are manifested by increased intracranial pressure and night blindness. Normal blood levels can be maintained by using standard multivitamin preparations containing 5000 to 20,000 IU of vitamin A. Individuals with CF are usually not deficient in the water-soluble vitamins, including the B group and vitamin C, nor do they necessarily lack trace minerals. There are isolated reports of vitamin D deficiency. Patients with CF can demonstrate overt clinical symptoms of vitamin E deficiency including areflexia, gait disturbance, diminished proprioception and ophthalmoplegia. Therefore, vitamin E supplementation is necessary: 200 IU for adults using a water-miscible preparation. Vitamin K deficiency can result from fat malabsorption and from bacterial overgrowth in the gastrointestinal tract due to oral antibiotics. Supplementation of vitamin K should be based on the patient's prothrombin time; in those with an elevated PT, an additional 5 mg per week of vitamin K is sufficient.

A-11. **Answers: a, b, c, d.** Current epidemiologic data supports the concept that cystic fibrosis is inherited in mendelian fashion as an autosomal recessive trait. Siblings of affected individuals, who have two out of three chances of carrying the cystic fibrosis gene, have no way of knowing whether they are indeed carriers. Similarly, they have no way of knowing whether their spouses are also carriers and therefore whether their offspring are at risk of having cystic fibrosis. In Helsinki, in August 1985, Eiberg and associates reported linkage of the cystic

fibrosis gene with the serum enzyme paroxonase, or PON. Three separate groups of investigators have mapped the CF gene to chromosome number 7. Men with cystic fibrosis are nearly always infertile because of maldevelopment of the epididymis, vas deferens, and seminal vesicles—not because of abnormal sperm.

A-12. **Answers: b, d, e.** Pathophysiology of bronchopulmonary fungal hypersensitivity is produced by the spores of various fungi becoming trapped in the viscous mucus of the tracheobronchial tree in patients with asthma. The growing fungus releases antigens that induce a complex immunologic reaction leading to the resulting pathophysiology. Aspergillosis is the best known of these syndromes. The treatment of ABPA consists of oral steroids and follow-up of the blood eosinophil level and serum IgE level. Long-term sequelae include fibrosis, irreversible airway obstruction, upper lobe contraction, and very occasionally aspergilloma.

A-13. **Answer: e.** There are primary and secondary diagnostic criteria for ABPA. The seven primary criteria are asthma, blood eosinophilia, immediate skin test reactivity to *Aspergillus*, precipitating antibodies to *Aspergillus*, increases in serum IgE, history of pulmonary infiltrates, and central bronchiectasis. The secondary criteria include *Aspergillus* in the sputum, history of coughing up brown plugs, and late skin test reactivity to *Aspergillus*.

A-14. **Answers: a, c, d, e.** Alpha$_1$-antitrypsin deficiency is an autosomal recessive disorder. The protein is coded for by a gene on chromosome 14. Each allele on each chromosome expresses its normal or abnormal protein irrespective of combination (autosomal co-dominant) and this forms the basis of the homozygous states (normal MM, abnormal ZZ) and heterozygous states (M or one of its normally functioning variants such as M1, M2, or M3, and S or Z, etc.). A total of 75 alleles are categorized into groups based on the status of the alpha$_1$-protease inhibitor protein in serum: (1) normal (normal serum level, normal function), (2) deficient (level less than 35% of normal but the protein functions somewhat normally), (3) null (no detectable alpha$_1$-protease inhibitor in serum), and (4) dysfunctional (normal level but does not function properly). The protein inhibits neutrophil elastase.

A-15. **Answers: a, c, e.** The Z protein has difficulty in being secreted from the hepatocyte cytosol, and although it has activity against neutrophil elastase, its function is less than normal. The S protein has greater activity than the Z protein. Patients can acutely increase their serum levels in response to stress (infection), neoplasia, pregnancy, or medication (estrogen). Premature development of panacinar emphysema (greater in the lower lobes) occurs in the majority of homozygotes by age 40, but age of onset and severity of disease are somewhat variable. There are case reports of asymptomatic homozygotes over 50 to 60 years old. Tobacco use in conjunction with homozygosity virtually always produces disease (emphysema) by the fourth decade.

A-16. **Answers: d.** There is general agreement on a small increased risk of MZ heterozygotes developing emphysema sooner than their age-matched and smoking-matched MM controls . There is probably no increased risk in the heterozygote who does not smoke. PiMZ smokers have a modestly higher chance of developing clinically significant emphysema than PiMM smokers, and their FEV$_1$ declines on a steeper slope than that of PiMM smokers. The most severely affected individuals are those with the PiZZ variant,

characterized by serum levels <35% normal. Patients with MZ were 2–5 times more common among emphysematous patients than among healthy controls. The Met 358 amino acid residue in the alpha$_1$-protease inhibitor molecule, which is a critical part of the active site of the protein can be oxidized by cigarette smoke, rendering the protein 2000-fold *less* effective in neutralizing neutrophil elastase.

A-17. **Answers: a, c, e.** The dosage of active alpha$_1$-protease inhibitor (derived from human plasma) for homozygotes is 60 mg/kg given intravenously once weekly. This invariably results in protective serum (and therefore alveolar) levels. There are no studies on augmentation therapy for PiMZ phenotype in asymptomatic or symptomatic ex-smokers nor in those who insist on continuing to smoke. Adverse reactions include fever (1%), transient leukocytosis, lightheadedness, dizziness.

A-18. **Answers: a, b, c, e.** Alpha$_1$-protease inhibitor is a glycoprotein of MW 52,000. It is produced mainly by hepatocytes and, to a lesser degree, by mononuclear cells and PMNs. The serum protein diffuses into lung, where it is responsible for >90% of the anti-elastase activity of the lower respiratory tract. The half-life of alpha$_1$-protease inhibitor is 4–5 days. The minimum or threshold level needed in blood to prevent lung destruction by elastases appears to be 11 μM. The Z gene is rare among Blacks and Asians.

A-19. **Answers: a, d.** Cigarette smoke contains free radicals, which oxidize the alpha$_1$-protease inhibitor molecule at a methionine residue, resulting in a much less effective inhibitor of elastase. The phenotype cannot be inferred from the serum level alone, since levels vary significantly among individuals with the same phenotype. About 50% of neonates with ZZ have biochemical evidence of liver disease, and 15% have clinically significant involvement. The liver disease is believed to be due to accumulation of defective A1PI protein in hepatocytes. Liver disease is not seen in null-null deficiency states (thus it is not the absence of inhibitor that harms hepatocytes). In 90% of cases having an abnormal chest roentgenogram, the lung destruction occurs in the lower zones, possibly because there is more blood flow to these regions and thus more blood-borne PMNs.

A-20. **Answer: b.** Clubbing and paranasal sinusitis are virtually universal clinical manifestations of CF. The manifestations and sequelae of CF are truly protean and no organ system is spared. The primary manifestations of CF and the complications can involve the respiratory, gastrointestinal, exocrine, endocrine, renal, hematologic, reproductive, musculoskeletal, and nervous systems. The median survival has increased from less than 2 years in the 1940s to 20 years at present. The normal range of sweat chloride concentrations is slightly higher in adults than in children. *Aspergillus fumigatus* commonly colonizes the tracheobronchial tree in patients with CF and can cause bronchospasm alone or allergic bronchopulmonary aspergillosis. Invasive aspergillosis is rare.

A-21. **Answers: c, e.** Early in the disease process, pulmonary function tests in patients with CF demonstrate a restrictive pattern and later on an obstructive pattern. With severe pulmonary deterioration, there may be a mixed restrictive-obstructive ventilatory defect. Spontaneous pneumothorax is a fairly frequent occurrence (about 16% of adults) in cystic fibrosis. Rectal prolapse, intestinal obstruction, and biliary cirrhosis—and occasionally idiopathic acute pancreatitis—are frequent clues leading to the diagnosis of CF. Approximately 15% of CF children

will have no gross evidence of pancreatic insufficiency. Men with CF do not mature sexually at the same rate as unaffected men. Puberty is often delayed.

A-22. **Answers: none of them**. The risk of a CF mother having a baby with CF is not 1 out of 4; rather, it is 1 out of 40. Assuming the father has no history of CF in his family, his chance of carrying the CF gene as a heterozygote is 1 out of 20. His chance of contributing this gene to the ovum is 1 out of 2, since he can contribute either the normal or abnormal gene carrying chromosome. Since the mother has CF, she carries two copies of the abnormal CF gene and her chance of contributing the gene is 1, so that the risk is $1 \times 1/2 \times 1/20 = 1/40$. Abnormalities in phagocytosis have not been demonstrated except as a consequence of the chronic progressive pulmonary disease. A significant proportion of adults with CF have airway hyper-responsiveness. As many as 25% of adults will also have some degree of exercise-induced bronchospasm. The efficacy of inhaled antibiotics is controversial, and inhaled antibiotics would not appear to be as effective as intravenous antibiotics in the treatment of exacerbations. Individuals with CF usually are not deficient in the water-soluble vitamins, including the B group and vitamin C.

A-23. **Answers: b, c, e.** The microbiology of recurrent pneumonia is mainly *H. influenzae*, *Pneumococcus*, *S. pyogenes*, and *S. aureus*. Once bronchiectasis is established, *S. aureus* and *Pseudomonas* infections predominate. The bronchiectasis associated with CVH is diffuse rather than focal and is diagnosed after exclusion of such conditions as chronic lymphocytic leukemia, lymphoma, multiple myeloma, nephrotic syndrome, and protein-losing enteropathy that may lead secondarily to low immunoglobulin levels. Patients with CVH are also predisposed to atrophic gastritis with achlorhydria, neoplasia, malabsorption, nodular lymphoid hyperplasia, giardiasis, thymoma and thyroid abnormalities, and noncaseating granulomas in the lungs, spleen, and liver. Therapy is with both intravenous immune globulin and rotating antibiotics. The intravenous route of administration is more effective than the intramuscular route in preventing infections. Replacement therapy is also effective in promoting normal growth in younger patients.

A-24.   **Answer: d.** There are no diseases specific to welding, but metal fume fever, polymer fume fever, siderosis, asthma, and pulmonary edema or chemical pneumonia are all associated with welding.

A-25.   **Answer: c, e.** In respiratory bronchiolitis there is accumulation of pigmented macrophages in the respiratory bronchioles. The chest film shows a reticulonodular pattern or it may be normal. Pulmonary function tests reveal a restrictive or mixed pattern. The vast majority of patients are smokers. In addition to pigmented bronchioles there is peribronchiolar fibrosis, type 2 cell hyperplasia, and extension of bronchiolar epithelium into the distal air spaces. Granulation plugs with obliteration of small airways is characteristic of BOOP.

A-26.   **Answers: a, b, c, d, e.** Many drugs, including all of those listed, can produce pulmonary infiltrates with eosinophilia. Other drugs that can produce PIE include aspirin, nonsteroidal anti-inflammatory agents, mephenesin, nitrofurantoin, beclomethasone dipropionate, chlorpromazine, chlorpropamide, carbamazine, tetracycline, para-aminosalicylic acid, azathioprine, gold, isoniazid, streptomycin, tolbutamide, and Dilantin.

A-27.   **Answers: b, d.** Two major factors are found to best explain the increased asthma at night—a fall in circulating levels of epinephrine and heightened

parasympathetic tone. Although there is a reduction in circulating cortisol concentrations, this does not appear to be a major factor as its replacement does not ablate the nocturnal obstruction. The three most common causes of prolonged persistent cough are sinusitis, asthma, and gastroesophageal reflux. Beta agonists and Intal both block exercise-induced bronchospasm, but inhaled corticosteroids do not.

A-28.   **Answers: a, c, d.** There is normally a circadian rhythm in FEV_1. In a patient with a prolonged persistent cough, the three most common causes involve sinusitis, asthma, and gastroesophageal reflux. Two major factors are found to best explain the increased asthma at night—a fall in circulating levels of epinephrine and heightened parasympathetic tone. Although there is a reduction in circulating cortisol concentrations, this does not appear to be a major factor as its replacement does not ablate the nocturnal obstruction. Exercise induced bronchospasm is exacerbated by breathing cold air. Airway cooling can occur and be associated with bronchospasm.

A-29.   **Answers: a, c.** Cephalexin used for 2 years has been shown to reduce colony counts of *S. aureus* and *Haemophilus influenzae* in the sputum, and to reduce the frequency of respiratory exacerbations requiring additional antibiotics and hospitalization. Treatment of *P. aeruginosa* infections is more effective with multiple drug therapy than with a single agent. This is usually accomplished using an aminoglycoside as well as one of the penicillin derivatives, the piperazine penicillins, beta-lactam antibiotics, or third-generation cephalosporins. The dosage of aminoglycoside required to achieve optimal blood levels is often 1.5 to 2 times that calculated for body weight. There are various theoretic explanations for this including a larger apparent volume of distribution and increased renal clearance of the aminoglycosides resulting in shortened half-lives. Intravenous antibiotics are indicated when deterioration is manifested by increased cough, marked fatigue and malaise, anorexia, weight loss, low-grade fever, occasional chills, decreased pulmonary function, or radiographic changes. Commonly, new pulmonary infiltrates are not seen on chest roentgenogram despite obvious decompensation. This should not dissuade the physician from initiating intravenous antibiotics. The efficacy of inhaled antibiotics is controversial, and inhaled antibiotics would not appear to be as effective as intravenous antibiotics in the treatment of exacerbations.

A-30. **Answers: b, c, d.** The most likely diagnosis if a patient develops bronchiectasis, rhinitis, and sinusitis early in life is the immotile cilia syndrome. Situs inversus may accompany the immotile cilia syndrome, and this is called Kartagener's syndrome. Central bronchiectasis is a major manifestation of allergic bronchopulmonary aspergillosis. In the Churg-Strauss syndrome there is allergic rhinitis, asthma, and later a systemic vasculitis. The pathologic findings are granulomas in the lungs, heart, liver, spleen, skin, and nerves.

A-31. **Answers: a, d, e.** In the immotile cilia syndrome there is otitis, sinusitis, bronchiectasis, and in many cases situs inversus. On electron microscopic examination of the cilia, there are abnormalities of the dynein arms and radial spokes. Thus, infertility is more common in males than in females. Situs inversus may also be associated, and this is called Kartagener's syndrome.

A-32. **Answers: a, d.** Williams and Campbell first reported children with soft, compliant bronchi that dilated and collapsed during inspiration and expiration, and

this was accompanied by generalized bronchiectasis. At autopsy there was extensive symmetric deficiency of cartilage distal to the first division of the segmental bronchi, along with thin-walled bronchiectasis. The bronchiectasis is likely to be developmental due to its symmetry and lack of inflammation in adjacent noncartilaginous structures. The condition has been reported in two siblings whose respiratory symptoms developed immediately after birth and who subsequently developed symmetric bronchiectasis, which further suggests a congenital basis for the condition. Most of the patients developed clubbing. Pulmonary function testing shows hyperinflation with obstruction to airflow and a loss of lung elastic recoil (reduced elastance).

A-33. **Answer: c.** Elevation of IgE may occur in atopic dermatitis, parasitic disease such as visceral larva migrans and trichinosis, allergic bronchopulmonary aspergillosis, and a small group of aspergillomas and asthma. IgE is not elevated in eosinophilic pneumonia.

A-34. **Answer: e.** All of the statements describe Löffler's syndrome except that the IgE is not elevated.

A-35. **Answers: a, b, d, e.** The clinical manifestations of ABPA include asthma complicated by recurrent episodes of fever, cough, purulent sputum with plugs, and pulmonary infiltrates. Recurrent episodes may lead to bronchial obstruction with resultant central saccular bronchiectasis. Long-term sequelae include fibrosis, irreversible airway obstruction, upper lobe contraction, and very occasionally aspergilloma. In allergic bronchopulmonary aspergillosis, IgE levels are high.

A-36. **Answers: none of them.** Bronchospasm from aspirin is a pseudoallergy that can occur in patients who do not have nasal polyps. Although this most frequently occurs in patients with rhinosinusitis and/or nasal polyps, it can appear in others. Otitis, sinusitis, and bronchiectasis develop in the immotile cilia syndrome. Situs inversus may also be associated, and this is called Kartagener's syndrome. The most characteristic feature of allergic bronchopulmonary aspergillosis is proximal bronchiectasis. In exercise-induced asthma, factors associated with the development of airway obstruction include mediator release, airway water loss, airway cooling, and the degree of rewarming after exercise. However, lactic acidosis is not involved in the pathogenesis of this problem. Beta-adrenergic treatment in asthma can be associated with down-regulation in hormone receptor function, as noted in studies of the leukocyte and airway smooth muscle. Although beta-adrenergic function is already reduced in asthma, further reductions occur by use of this medication.

A-37. **Answers: c, d, e.** Bronchiolitis obliterans is a nonspecific histologic response of the lung to injury that primarily affects the small conducting airways, usually sparing the interstitium. Extension of granulation tissue organization from the distal alveolar ducts into alveoli is characteristic of bronchiolitis obliterans and organizing pneumonia. Generally, the chest film shows bilateral patchy ground-glass or alveolar opacifications although a miliary pattern is sometimes seen. Bronchiolitis obliterans without organizing pneumonia is probably a common pathologic end point of a wide spectrum of injurious agents and diseases, which include toxic fume inhalation, postinfectious connective tissue disorders, organ and bone marrow transplantation and other causes (idiopathic). Nitrogen dioxide, sulfur dioxide, ammonia, chlorine, phosgene, and cadmium oxide have been associated with bronchiolitis obliterans.

A-38. **Answers: c, d, e.** Bronchiolitis obliterans is a common lower respiratory tract illness in children, often secondary to the respiratory syncytial virus. Bronchiolitis obliterans is rare in adults, but when it occurs it has been associated with *Mycoplasma pneumoniae*. The radiographic pattern is often interstitial, frequently with hyperinflation. Pulmonary function testing may reveal a restrictive and/or obstructive pattern. Individuals exposed to high concentrations of NO_2 can die, within a few hours, of noncardiogenic edema. Patients who survive may present several weeks later with cough, dyspnea, rales, and a miliary or nodular pattern on the chest radiograph. These patients have widespread bronchiolitis obliterans without organizing pneumonia.

A-39. **Answer: d.** Suspicion of cystic fibrosis should be heightened in patients with GI features such as malabsorption, intermittent small or large bowel obstruction, rectal prolapse, or focal biliary cirrhosis. A very high percentage develop sinusitis and nasal polyps.

A-40. **Answers: a, b, c, d, e.** Churg-Strauss syndrome is characterized by pulmonary and systemic necrotizing angiitis, extravascular granulomas, and eosinophilia, which occurs almost exclusively in patients with asthma or an allergic history. The necrotizing angiitis, with prominent eosinophilic infiltrate, characteristically involves both the arteries and the veins.

A-41. **Answer: d.** The disease can develop insidiously following repeated acute episodes or continued antigen exposure, but a patient with chronic hypersensitivity pneumonitis may not have any acute episodes. Hypoxemia, decreased diffusing capacity, and pulmonary function studies consistent with a combined obstructive and restrictive defect are frequently present. Biopsy specimens at this stage reveal bronchiolitis obliterans with distal destruction of alveoli (honeycombing) in association with densely fibrotic zones. As many as 30–40% of farmers have positive serum precipitins without clinical disease. Furthermore, a negative precipitin test does not exclude the diagnosis of hypersensitivity pneumonitis. The chest film shows progressive fibrotic changes with less nodular densities and loss of lung volume with shrinkage of the upper lobes.

A-42. **Answer: d.** This group of diseases is associated with repeated intense inhalation of finely dispersed organic dusts and the formation of antigen-antibody complexes. One form of presentation is an acute reaction following heavy exposure characterized by the abrupt onset (within 4–6 hours) of fever, chills, malaise, nausea, cough, chest tightness, and dyspnea without wheezing that subsides over hours or days. Diffuse fine rales throughout the chest, mild hypoxemia, and a restrictive ventilatory defect accompany these symptomatic episodes. A fleeting, micronodular, interstitial pattern in the lower and mid-lower zone may be identified on chest roentgenogram. Removal from exposure usually results in complete resolution. Pathologically, this stage is characterized by noncaseating interstitial granulomatous pneumonitis.

A-43. **Answer: d.** Bronchiolitis obliterans (occlusion of bronchioles with loose granulation tissue) may occur as a result of viral infections (adenovirus and measles are the important ones), inhalation of toxic substances (oxides of nitrogen, ammonia, sulfur dioxide), and rheumatoid arthritis, in which case it may be related to penicillamine administration, although this has not been proved.

A-44. **Answers: a, b, c, e.** The lung is apparently the only organ involved. All the other statements describe Löffler's syndrome. The etiology is essentially unknown, and it is short-lived.

A-45. **Answers: a, c, e.** The physiology in respiratory bronchiolitis can be normal, but often shows obstruction due to disease of the small airways. If there is associated ILD, a restrictive pattern can predominate. In a case series 4/6 showed restriction while 2/6 showed primarily obstruction. A reduction in $D_L CO$ is common, and 50% will show some O_2 desaturation with exercise testing. Diagnosis usually requires open lung biopsy, but can occasionally be made by transbronchial biopsy in the proper clinical setting, but this is controversial. Treatment is essentially smoking cessation, which is generally associated with complete resolution. In those who continue to smoke, steroids may be of some benefit.

A-46. **Answer: b.** The best preventive treatment consists of chest physical therapy and deep coughing. Additionally, when infections occur it is important to intensify physical therapy and to initiate antibiotics or other types of interventions as indicated.

A-47. **Answers: a, c.** Two major factors are found to best explain the occurrence of increased asthma at night, and these include a fall in circulating levels of epinephrine and also heightened parasympathetic tone. Increases in parasympathetic tone can be translated to increased airway obstruction. Although there is a reduction in circulating cortisol concentrations, this does not appear to be a major factor as its replacement does not ablate the airway obstruction that occurs at night. Airway cooling can occur, but the degree of drop in temperature is too small to account for altered airway function. Although sleep is associated with increased nocturnal symptoms, asthma can occur independent of sleep in the majority of patients.

A-48. **Answers: d, e.** Evidence indicates that aerosolized and parenterally administered beta agonists are equally effective in the treatment of acute asthma. This has been demonstrated by emergency room studies from a number of institutions. Beta-adrenergic treatment in asthma can be associated with down-regulation in hormone receptor function, as noted in studies of the leukocyte and airway smooth muscle. Although beta-adrenergic function is already reduced in asthma, further reductions occur by the use of this medication. In the same regard, there is evidence that patients who have used excessive amounts of beta agonists prior to presenting to the emergency room can respond to inhaled beta agonists. Although the preceding use of beta agonists would be expected to cause down-regulation, inhalation of large doses of beta agonists can overcome this deficit. Studies have repeatedly shown that beta agonists, by either inhaled or parenteral administration, are more effective than intravenous aminophylline in the treatment of acute asthma. The beta agonist, terbutaline, has been shown to cause a drop in serum potassium levels. This is believed to occur as a consequence from catecholamine activation of potassium influx into cells. Sometimes the drop in serum potassium can be striking.

A-49. **Answer: b.** The mechanism of action by which theophylline bronchodilates is not known. Although methylxanthines inhibit phosphodiesterase enzyme activity, the concentrations required to do this are beyond tolerable doses. Enprophylline is a product similar to methylxanthine, but some of its actions are distinct, including an inability to block adenosine-induced bronchoconstriction. This suggests that theophylline's bronchodilating ability may not include the adenosine antagonism. Intravenous methylxanthines are not as effective as beta agonists in the treatment of acute asthma. This is seen even if patients have not been receiving theophylline. Cimetidine interferes with theophylline metabolism. The mechanism by which this occurs is not known. Theophylline has been able to reduce airway hyperreactivity. However, in contrast to other compounds such as cromolyn or inhaled corticosteroids, this modulating activity is minimal.

A-50. **Answer: a, c, d.** Corticosteroids block the phospholipase A2 enzyme and by this method prevent incorporation of phospholipids into arachidonic acid. Corticosteroids increase the peripheral white blood cell count, but this increase is primarily due to a rise in neutrophil, not eosinophil, levels. Inhaled corticosteroid will diminish airway hyperreactivity to histamine. The mechanism by which it occurs is believed to be its ability to reduce airway inflammation. Corticosteroids can affect beta-adrenergic activity by increasing the avidity of the receptor for its agonist. There is also evidence to indicate that corticosteroids may up-regulate the down-regulated beta receptors or cause their regeneration. Corticosteroids given during the first 24 hours of treatment for acute asthma are associated with improvement in airway function over this period of time.

A-51. **Answers: a, b, c.** Although hypertrophy of the mucous glands is the major pathologic feature and there is some goblet cell metaplasia, airflow limitation is due to the mucus secretions present and mural thickening in the larger bronchi, along with the edema and inflammatory changes in the more peripheral bronchioles.

A-52. **Answer: d.** Allergic bronchopulmonary aspergillosis is a syndrome including recurrent pulmonary infiltrates, high IgE levels, and a positive skin test to *Aspergillus*. However, the most characteristic feature of this disease is proximal bronchiectasis. Severe asthma can be present, as can the other factors listed here. However, that which is pathognomonic of this disease is the peculiar bronchiectasis.

A-53. **Answer: d.** In exercise-induced asthma, many factors are associated with the development of airway obstruction. These include mediator release, airway water loss, airway cooling, and the degree of rewarming after exercise. The factor that is most important or the final common pathway has not been elicited. However, lactic acidosis is not involved in the pathogenesis of this problem.

A-54. **Answers: b, e.** The pathophysiology of bronchopulmonary fungal hypersensitivity is produced when the spores of various fungi become trapped in the viscous mucus of the tracheal bronchial tree in patients with asthma. The growing fungus releases antigens that induce a complex immunologic reaction leading to the resulting pathophysiology. Aspergillosis is the best known of these syndromes. Corticosteroids are the treatment of choice.

A-55. **Answers: a, b, c, d, e.** The clinical manifestations of ABPA include asthma complicated by recurrent episodes of fever, cough, purulent sputum with plugs, and pulmonary infiltrates. Recurrent episodes may lead to bronchial obstruction and result in central saccular bronchiectasis. Long-term sequelae include fibrosis, irreversible airway obstruction, upper lobe contraction, and very occasionally aspergilloma.

A-56. **Answer: a.** The treatment of ABPA consist of oral steroids and follow-up of the blood eosinophil level and serum IgE level. This is important because although the patient may subjectively feel better, the eosinophil level and the IgE level are more reliable indicators of the activity of the disorder. If they remain elevated, the disease is not under control. Conversely, if the eosinophil level or IgE level rises during treatment, this forecasts an exacerbation of the disease.

A-57. **Answers: a, b, c.** The pathologic findings are consistent with the clinical findings; altered pathology (i.e., granuloma) is found in the heart, liver, spleen, skin, and nerves.

A-58. **Answers: a, b, c, d.** Steroids are the treatment of choice, but cytotoxic agents may have to be added. The 5-year survival is about 60–65%. Survival is greater the longer the interval between the onset of asthma and the onset of vasculitis.

A-59. **Answer: b.** This destructive lesion, which involves the respiratory bronchioles, is irregular, but the lesions are more common and generally more severe in the upper lobe than in the lower lobe, particularly the posterior and apical segments of the upper lobes.

A-60. **Answer: c.** Panacinar emphysema, which appears to involve the acinus predominantly, is nearly always found in individuals over the age of 70. It tends to occur rather more commonly in the lower zones and at the anterior margins of the lungs.

A-61. **Answers: c, e.** In alpha$_1$-antiprotease deficiency there is widespread severe panacinar emphysema, which is symmetric and is found most commonly in the lower lobes.

A-62. **Answer: b.** Alpha$_1$-protease inhibitor is a glycoprotein of MW 52,000. It is produced mainly by hepatocytes and, to a lesser degree, by mononuclear cells and PMNs. The serum protein diffuses into lung where it is responsible for >90% of the anti-elastase activity of the lower respiratory tract. The half-life of alpha$_1$-protease inhibitor is 4–5 days. The minimum or threshold level needed in blood to prevent lung destruction by elastases appears to be 11 μM. The Z gene is rare among Blacks and Asians.

A-63. **Answers: b, c, d.** The type of emphysema per se does not determine the extent of functional impairment. It is the extent and severity of the pathologic changes and the presence of bronchitis that determine the extent of functional impairment present. The degree of hypoxemia present as well as the degree of obliteration of vascular bed influence the degree of pulmonary hypertension present, but functional impairment per se is not affected by the pulmonary vascular disease.

A-64. **Answer: c.** In simple pneumoconiosis of coal workers, coal containing nodules are associated with enlargement of respiratory bronchioles, which is primarily a process of dilation.

A-65. **Answers: a, c.** BOOP is defined pathologically as granulation tissue plugs within the small airways with complete obstruction of the airways and extension of the granulation tissue or young connective tissue into the alveoli. Other histologic features include intraluminal polyps comprised of connective tissue, fibrinous exudates, alveolar accumulations of macrophages, and inflamed alveolar walls.

A-66. **Answers: a, b, c, d, e.** The histologic findings of BOOP are seen in BOOP secondary to connective tissue disorders, cocaine abuse, drug reactions, HIV infection, myelodysplastic syndrome, or radiation therapy as well as the idiopathic form.

A-67. **Answers: b, c, d, e.** A flu-like illness occurs in one third of cases. On physical examination, end inspiratory crackles are appreciated in two thirds. The mean duration of symptoms at presentation is 3.6 months (versus IPF, 23.8 months). The chest radiograph usually shows bilateral patchy infiltrates, which are often fleeting. Pulmonary function tests reveal a low vital capacity in one half, mild airway obstruction except in cigarette smokers, and a decreased $D_L CO$. BAL usually yields an increase in lymphocytes with or without eosinophils.

A-68. **Answers: a, b, d, e.** The differential diagnosis would include eosinophilic pneumonia, hypersensitivity pneumonitis, acute progressive interstitial pneumonia (Hamman-Rich syndrome), UIP, or organizing infections. Making the distinction between BOOP and the other diseases listed is important, since some are treatable and have a good prognosis while others are associated with a much poorer outcome.

A-69. **Answer: e.** It is unclear why the tracheobronchial tree of cystic fibrosis patients becomes infected with particular organisms. Mucociliary clearance in CF is variable. Some patients have normal or increased clearance and others have diminished clearance. However, the mucociliary clearance in CF is no worse than in chronic bronchitis, and certainly not absent as in patients with immotile cilia syndrome. Abnormalities in complement activity and phagocytosis have not been demonstrated except as a consequence of the chronic progressive pulmonary disease. Serum IgG concentrations are often decreased in children, but pulmonary function is better and colonization with gram-negative bacteria lower than in children with normal IgG levels. Therefore, hypogammaglobulinemia does not account for the bacterial infection in CF.

A-70. **Answers: a, b, c, d.** Four generally accepted criteria for the diagnosis of CF are a positive sweat chloride test (greater than 60 mEq/L) and at least one of the following: chronic obstructive pulmonary disease; exocrine pancreatic insufficiency; or a positive family history. Meconium ileus equivalent occurs in about 24% of cases and should raise suspicion, but it is not a criterion for diagnosis.

A-71. **Answers: a, b, c, d.** Disorders other than CF associated with elevated sweat chloride levels include untreated adrenal insufficiency, pseudohypoaldosteronism, hypothyroidism, hypoparathyroidism, nephrogenic diabetes insipidus, ectodermal dysplasia, type I glycogen storage disease, mucopolysaccharidoses, fucosidosis, malnutrition, Mauriac syndrome, familial cholestasis syndrome, pancreatitis, and hypoproteinemic edema.

A-72. **Answers: a, b, c, d, e.** In the adult population, including those with long-standing disease, the following incidences of the clinical manifestations of CF have been reported: pulmonary disease (97%), pancreatic insufficiency (95%), minor (60%) and major (7%) hemoptysis, nasal polyps (48%), meconium ileus equivalent (24%), intestinal obstruction (21%), pneumothorax (16%), glycosuria (8%), intussusception (5%), cirrhosis (5%), and heat prostration (5%). Clubbing and paranasal sinusitis were virtually universal.

A-73. **Answers: a, b, c.** Cystic fibrosis is the most common fatal inherited disease in Caucasians. It occurs in about 1 in 2000 live births. It is transmitted as an autosomal recessive trait. About 5% of the white population, or 1 out of 20, are carriers of the disease. The incidence of cystic fibrosis in Blacks and Orientals is markedly lower. CF is transmitted as an autosomal recessive trait, but the severity in organ system involvement is variable.

A-74. **Answers: a, c, e.** The CF gene locus has been located on the long arm of chromosome 7. This was accomplished initially using a biochemical and then eventual DNA probe linkage markers. By means of DNA linkage markers, it is possible, in certain circumstances, to detect the CF carrier status in at-risk families and disease status *in utero*. However, at least one affected individual must be linked to the individual of concern to obtain linkage data. Although it is possible to use tightly linked DNA probes near the CF gene to analyze at-risk families, the CF gene has not yet been sequenced or the gene prod-

uct described. The clinical presentation of CF is variable in terms of age of onset, organ system involvement, and rapidity of progression. The manifestations and sequelae of CF are truly protean and no organ system is spared. The primary manifestations of CF and the complications can involve the respiratory, gastrointestinal, exocrine, endocrine, renal, hematologic, reproductive, musculoskeletal, and nervous systems.

A-75. **Answers: d, e.** The life expectancy of patients with CF has improved substantially; the median survival has increased from less than 2 years in the 1940s to almost 20 years now. There are several reasons for this improved survival: better awareness of the clinical manifestations; earlier diagnosis of mildly affected persons; the establishment of CF centers; nutrition and pancreatic enzyme supplementation; aggressive pulmonary toilet; and widespread use of antipseudomonal and antistaphylococcic antibiotics. Although the vast majority of patients are diagnosed in childhood, 20% of those who reach age 18 have been diagnosed after age 15, and a few have been diagnosed between ages 20 and 50. This delay in diagnosis is related both to lack of awareness on the part of the physician caring for the patient and to the mild pulmonary involvement demonstrated in some CF patients.

A-76. **Answers: a, c, e.** In over 98% of the patients with CF, sweat chloride (SC) concentrations are greater than 60 mEq/L; in 1–2%, they are between 50 and 60 mEq/L; and in about 1 in 1000, they are under 50 mEq/L. Therefore, a SC determination less than 60 mEq/L does not exclude the diagnosis of CF if the patient has other clinical features to support the diagnosis. The normal range of SC concentrations is slightly higher in adults than in children. A small percentage of normal adults will have SC determinations between 60 and

80 mEq/L. The SC determination is just as reliable in individuals with chronic obstructive lung disease as it is in other normal adults and children. However, some experts believe that the cut-off for a positive SC determination is greater than 80 mEq/L in an adult. There are several hereditary and rare conditions that can cause a false-positive SC; these include adrenal insufficiency, nephrogenic diabetes insipidus, hypothyroidism, and malnutrition. These conditions are associated with elevated sweat electrolytes, but they usually can be distinguished from CF clinically. False-negative SC levels can occasionally be found in CF patients with edema, but with resolution of the edema, the concentrations return to an abnormal value.

A-77. **Answer: c.** CF children are most commonly infected with *Staphylococcus aureus*. With advancing age of the patient, *Pseudomonas aeruginosa*, particularly the mucoid type, predominates as the major pathogen, either by supplanting the *S. aureus* or as a coinfection. Several series estimate that 88–100% of adult CF patients have *P. aeruginosa* in their sputum, often in combination with *S. aureus* or *Haemophilus influenzae*. Although *P. aeruginosa* can chronically colonize the airways of elderly patients with long-standing, smoking-related chronic obstructive lung disease or postinfectious bronchitis, the presence of this organism, particularly the mucoid form, in any individual should suggest the diagnosis of CF, and be taken as an indication for a sweat test. Aggressive treatment with intravenous antibiotics will often improve the patient's clinical status, but bacteria in the sputum are never fully eradicated. Other common respiratory pathogens in CF patients include various viruses, *Mycoplasma*, *Haemophilus influenzae*, and occasionally *Pseudomonas cepacia*, *Escherichia coli*, and *Klebsiella ozaenae*. *Aspergillus fumigatus* commonly colo-

nizes the tracheobronchial tree in patients with CF and can cause bronchospasm alone or allergic bronchopulmonary aspergillosis. Invasive aspergillosis is rare.

A-78. **Answers: a, c, d, e.** Approximately 2% of adults with CF have a normal chest roentgenogram. In addition, a proportion of adults show only hyperinflation or increased pulmonary markings. Two thirds of CF adults have cystic bronchiectatic changes and honeycombing. The upper lobes are more commonly affected than the lower, and the right lung is more often affected than the left; 10–15% of adults will have normal spirometry. Early in the disease process, pulmonary function tests in CF will demonstrate a restrictive pattern and later on an obstructive pattern. With severe pulmonary deterioration, there may be a mixed restrictive-obstructive ventilatory defect resulting from the parenchymal fibrosis. A progressively compromised FEV_1 is strongly correlated with a poor prognosis.

A-79. **Answers: c, d, e.** Spontaneous pneumothorax is a fairly frequent occurrence (about 16% of adults) in cystic fibrosis. The vast majority of these patients have severe pulmonary involvement antecedent to the pneumothorax with an FEV_1 of less than 50% predicted. The average recurrence rate is nearly 50%, and despite treatment, mortality is 50–60%. This high mortality probably relates more to the severe underlying parenchymal involvement than to the pneumothorax itself. In contrast to the male predominance of spontaneous pneumothorax in the normal population, the male/female ratio in CF is nearly even. Hemoptysis occurs in approximately 7% of adults with CF; it is usually associated with worsening infection and commonly resolves with conservative treatment. Massive hemoptysis is associated with a high mortality. Cor pulmonale commonly accompanies severe pulmonary deterioration, but it can also be seen with less severe impairment and does not occur only as a terminal event. Various manifestations of rhinosinusitis are found in almost all adults with CF. The patients commonly complain of chronic nasal stuffiness, postnasal drip, or rhinitis. Acute sinusitis is rare. Nasal polyposis is far more common in adults than in children and occurs in about 41% of adults.

A-80. **Answers: a, b, c, d, e.** Rectal prolapse, intestinal obstruction, and biliary cirrhosis are frequent clues leading to the diagnosis of CF. Similarly, idiopathic acute pancreatitis also is an occasional presenting finding in CF. In the pediatric age group, the incidence of acute pancreatitis is only 1–5%, but in adults the incidence is much higher. Paradoxically, persons with recurrent pancreatitis often have no gross pancreatic insufficiency. CF is occasionally diagnosed during the work-up for infertility. For instance, evaluation of idiopathic azoospermia, in an otherwise asymptomatic male, may reveal an obstructive azoospermia.

A-81. **Answer: d.** Approximately 15% of CF children will have no gross evidence of pancreatic insufficiency. However, subtle abnormalities can be detected by the bicarbonate stimulation test, duodenal aspiration assays of the digestive enzymes, or pathologic examination of the pancreas. Even though the individual may not complain of frequent bulky foul-smelling stools or crampy abdominal pain, malabsorption may still be present. It may only be demonstrated by failure to gain weight and sequela of the fat-soluble vitamin deficiencies. Therefore, pancreatic enzyme supplements are indicated in these CF individuals despite minimal symptoms of steatorrhea. It has been shown statistically that CF patients with grossly normal pancreatic digestive function have lower sweat electrolyte concentrations and a more favorable pul-

monary prognosis. These individuals lacking evidence of gross pancreatic insufficiency are often prone to recurrent episodes of acute pancreatitis. Patients without pancreatic insufficiency still can develop intestinal obstruction.

A-82. **Answer: e.** Men with CF are nearly always (97–98%) infertile because of maldevelopment of the epididymis, vas deferens, and seminal vesicles, not because of abnormal sperm. These men develop obstructive azoospermia. Men with CF do not mature sexually at the same rate as unaffected men. Puberty is often delayed. The reproductive tract of women with CF is anatomically normal, but these women do not have normal fertility for several reasons. They have anovulatory cycles due to their chronic illness and relative malnutrition. The cervix is often impacted with thick tenacious mucus, which acts as a mechanical obstruction to sperm. This mucus fails to undergo the usual midcycle thinning and increased water content. Some women are plagued by chronic cervicitis, which may also contribute to decreased fertility. Pregnancy has been reported in more than 100 women with CF. Although 88% of these pregnancies resulted in the delivery of a healthy baby, they were complicated by congestive heart failure, poor weight gain, premature delivery, and fetal wastage; 12% of the mothers died within the first 6 months of delivery. The risk of a CF mother having a baby with CF is not 1 out of 4, rather, it is 1 out of 40. Assuming the father has no history of CF in his family, his chance of carrying the CF gene as a heterozygote is 1 out of 20. His chance of contributing this gene to the ovum is 1 out of 2. This is because he can contribute either the normal or abnormal gene-carrying chromosome. Since the mother has CF, she carries two copies of the abnormal CF gene and her chance of contributing the gene is 1. Therefore, the risk is $1 \times 1/2 \times 1/20 = 1/40$.

A-83. **Answers: a, b, c, d, e.** All of these pulmonary entities are common misdiagnoses in individuals with CF. In addition, asthma, chronic bronchitis, bronchiectasis, emphysema, and alpha$_1$-antitrypsin deficiency are occasional misdiagnoses. Although many of these diseases share a common clinical or radiographic similarity to CF, they are usually easily differentiated by history, physical examination, and laboratory investigation.

A-84. **Answers: a, d, e.** Although the efficacy of postural drainage and percussion has never been fully established, the combination of gravity drainage and either percussion or vibration may improve functional status more than gravity drainage alone. Mucomyst is of questionable effectiveness; similarly, normal saline bland aerosols, oral iodines, and glycerol guaiacolate have no proven clinical utility. A significant proportion of adults with CF have a bronchospastic component. As many as 25% of adults will also have some degree of exercise-induced bronchospasm. Therefore, inhaled beta agonists are efficacious in patients with airway hyperreactivity. Exercise may be beneficial in improving mucus evacuation. However, since many CF patients have exercise-induced bronchospasm or severe exercise-induced arterial desaturation, an exercise study should be performed prior to initiating an exercise program. Alternate-day prednisone may reduce hospital admissions and function tests, so that corticosteroids may play a role in improving the functional capacity of individuals with CF.

2-3 Tumors

T-1. **Answers: b, c, e.** There is often profound hypoxia out of proportion to the roentgenogram findings, and PFTs show a restrictive pattern with decreased D$_L$CO. Radiographically, linear, reticular, or nodular shadows radiating from both hila are the classic pattern. Kerley's B lines, adenopathy, and pleural effusions may also be seen. The chest roentgenogram may be normal. Hilar and mediastinal adenopathy is clearly not diagnostic and can be seen in numerous conditions. CT scan shows a characteristic nodular or beaded thickening of bronchovascular bundles, multiple linear densities forming a reticular network, and interstitial lines with a beaded or nodular appearance.

T-2. **Answers: b, d.** The histologic basis of thickened interstitium seen both on roentgenogram and grossly is infrequently caused by pure lymphatic invasion. Instead, a substantial part is due to neoplastic clusters or cords of cells within the lymphatics and the peribronchovascular connective tissue and interlobular interstitium. Tumor cells in the lymphatics can overflow into the surrounding tissues, giving rise to pleural effusions and areas of collapse and consolidation. Intravascular tumor emboli and endarteritis obliterans of the smaller branches of the pulmonary arteries are often seen. The most common clinical manifestation of lymphangitic carcinomatosis is dyspnea, often insidious in nature but progressive and causing great disability. There are three proposed mechanisms by which tumor reaches the intrapulmonary lymphatics: (1) via lymphatics to the thoracic duct or directly to the hilar nodes and then by retrograde spread into the lung, (2) by direct extension through the diaphragmatic lymphatics to the parietal and visceral pleura and later invasion of the pulmonary lymphatics, (3) by hematogenous spread of tumor emboli, which lodge in the smaller pulmonary arteries and subsequently spread through the vessel walls into the perivascular lymphatics. This is probably the most accepted theory at present. The most commonly reported causes of this entity are—in order of frequency—stomach, lung, breast, pancreas, uterus, cervix, prostate, and colon.

T-3. **Answer: c.** The cancer-causing genes that the retroviruses pirate from the host DNA are termed "oncogenes," and the cellular counterparts of viral oncogenes are termed "proto-oncogenes." More than 20 such oncogenes, which are named for the viruses from which they are isolated, have been identified. It has been demonstrated that oncogenes that are quiescent in normal tissue become active or "turned on" in lung cancer. The c-myc oncogene is increased in variant forms of small cell lung cancer. Variant behavior is characterized by shorter doubling times of the tumor, more malignant behavior, and a poor prognosis.

T-4. **Answers: a, b, c, d.** It appears that lung cancer cells can secrete their own growth factors, which serve as constant stimuli for cell division. This has been termed "autocrine" growth. Bombesin is produced in abundance by small cell lung cancer cells and appears to be an autocrine growth factor that stimulates growth. More than 90% of all small cell lung cancers that initially respond to treatment eventually become insensitive to even the highest levels of antineoplastic therapy. Malignant cells are able to evade the body's immune defenses. One way this is accomplished by small cell lung cancer

cells is decreased expression of the class I major histocompatibility antigens.

T-5. **Answers: a, b.** Smoking cessation results in a gradual approach to normal risk for lung cancer over 10 to 15 years. Extrapolation from doubling time observations suggests that by the time a lung cancer is clinically apparent, it has been present for 10 to 20 years. Thus, smoking cessation probably causes a rapid decrease in the formation of new lung neoplasms. However, preexisting carcinomas will continue to be detected for 10 to 15 years. The relative risk of lung cancer for cigarette smokers is approximately 20; that for a nonsmoking asbestos worker is about 5, and since exposure to multiple carcinogens has a synergistic effect, the relative risk of lung cancer is 100. The three major forms of bronchogenic carcinoma probably arise from reserve basal cells of the bronchial mucosa. Adding sputum cytology to chest roentgenographic screening of a high-risk population does not decrease the death rate from lung cancer. Because some lung cancers are diagnosed early, survival is longer, but overall death rate is not affected.

T-6. **Answers: a, c, d.** Microscopic examination of the chromosomes of small cell lung cancer cells has disclosed a consistent loss or deletion of the short arm or "p" portion of chromosome 3 from the region 14 to 23. It is seen only in patients' tumor cells, and not in their normal cells. This region of chromosome 3 appears to be altered in other malignancies, such as renal cell carcinoma, cancer of the ovary, salivary gland tumors, and leukemia. Cigarette smoke condensate has been shown to damage DNA in human lymphocytes.

T-7. **Answers: a, b, e.** The roentgenographic features of alveolar filling disease are acinar rosettes, air bronchograms, diffuse homogeneous consolidation, ill-defined nodular densities, and obliteration of the diaphragm, heart borders, and pulmonary vasculature.

T-8.   **Answer: e.** Adding sputum cytology to chest roentgenographic screening of a high-risk population leads to earlier diagnosis of some lung cancers, so that survival is longer, but overall death rate is not impacted. Superior vena caval obstruction is not as life-threatening as was originally believed. Long-term survival with benign superior vena caval obstruction suggests that the obstruction by itself is not lethal. The Eaton-Lambert syndrome is rare but is typically seen in association with small cell lung cancer, and this diagnosis is made by demonstration of increased muscle potentials with repeated stimulation on EMG, opposite to the findings in myasthenia gravis. The syndrome of inappropriate antidiuretic hormone is the most common endocrine syndrome in small cell lung cancer. Hyponatremia should suggest this histologic diagnosis. Hypercalcemia is suggestive of a non-small cell lung cancer.

T-9.   **Answers: a, b, d, e.** Small cell bronchogenic carcinomas originate in the major bronchi and infiltrate the wall of the bronchus, narrowing the lumen. They metastasize to hilar and mediastinal lymph nodes early, and also readily invade blood vessels and metastasize to distant organs. Uranium miners and workers who are exposed to chloromethyl methyl ether tend to have a high incidence of small cell carcinoma.

T-10.   **Answers: b, c, d, e.** Neurogenic tumors are the most common neoplasms of the mediastinum. Neurogenic mediastinal masses constitute 50–75% of posterior mediastinal masses and rarely present in the anterosuperior mediastinum. Neurilemomas (schwannomas) arise from the axonal nerve sheath. Most neurogenic

tumors among mediastinal masses are benign in adults (<1% mediastinal masses are malignant neural tumors). Pain from bone or nerve erosion and dyspnea or cough from tracheal compression are the most frequently reported symptoms, although most are discovered in asymptomatic patients on routine chest film. Peripheral nerve cell origin tumors are capable of elaborating vanillylmandelic acid and may produce a syndrome of diarrhea, flushing, and diaphoresis.

T-11.   **Answers: a, b, c.** Patients with anterior mediastinal masses abutting the trachea should have preoperative (including mediastinoscopy) supine and erect flow volume loops to exclude airway obstruction in the supine position under general anesthesia. The chromaffin tumors are called pheochromocytomas if hormonally active and chemodectomas if not. Neurilemoma (schwannoma) is the most common neurogenic mediastinal mass. It is usually detected in the third to fourth decade of life. Neurofibromas may occur in the mediastinum of patients with von Recklinghausen's disease, but posterior mediastinal masses discovered in these patients are usually meningoceles.

T-12.   **Answer: a, d.** These tumors are also called "superior sulcus" tumors since they lie in the sulcus or groove made by the subclavian artery in the dome of the pleura and apices of the upper lobes of the lungs. The characteristic clinical features of Pancoast's syndrome include pain in the distribution of C8 through T1–T2, often with weakness or atrophy in the muscles of that arm. Pancoast's syndrome is primarily due to a bronchogenic carcinoma, with about 50% being epidermoid, 30% large or giant cell, and 15% adenocarcinoma. Rare reported causes of Pancoast's syndrome include multiple myeloma, metastases from other malignancies, lymphoma, hydatid cysts, and aspergillomas. Despite their locally aggressive behavior, these tumors are more frequently curable than other presentations of lung cancer.

T-13. **Answers: a, c.** Establishing a tissue diagnosis may be difficult because of the inaccessibility of lesions. In one series bronchoscopy had a yield of only 42%, sputum cytology 47% versus 92% with fine-needle aspirate. By definition, all Pancoast's tumors are T3 lesions because there is extension to the chest wall. Preoperative radiation is the standard of care. Cerebral metastases are especially common with superior sulcus tumors—occurring in 22% of patients in one series. Involvement of the subclavian artery, vertebral body, or rib all adversely affect prognosis but do not preclude long-term survival of up to 30–40% with combined-modality treatment.

T-14. **Answer: e.** Combination therapy with radiation and radical en bloc surgery has provided prolonged survivals and some cures, particularly in localized disease. With radiation, surgery, brachytherapy, and chemotherapy in various combinations the overall 5-year survival has been reported to be 25%. Favorable prognostic features were adenocarcinoma or large cell carcinoma, absence of mediastinal nodes, preoperative radiation, and completeness of resection. The presence of Horner's syndrome adversely affects prognosis but does not preclude long-term survival with combined-modality treatment.

T-15. **Answer: b.** Carcinoid is not found in the trachea. All of the others are.

T-16. **Answer: b.** The natural history of carcinoid is variable, and some patients may live more than 10 years after the development of liver metastases. This has led to valvular replacement in those patients who have significant impairment from endocardial fibrosis, with many reports of patients achieving excellent functional recovery from right heart failure and pro-

longed survival even in the face of liver metastases. All primary lung cancers can present as solitary pulmonary nodules, but this is much more common for non-small cell carcinomas than for small cell carcinoma. Patients with malignant solitary pulmonary nodules tend to have relatively good survival following resection compared to patients with other presentations of lung cancer. Calcification is believed to indicate benignity, but it also occurs in malignant solitary pulmonary nodules, e.g., when a scar carcinoma engulfs a preexisting, calcified, inflammatory lesion. If pathologic specimens are radiographed directly, some calcification can be seen in up to 50% of malignant solitary pulmonary nodules.

T-17. **Answer: b.** Cardiac involvement in carcinoid is common and is a frequent cause of death. ·The hallmark lesion is superficial fibrosis laid down under a normal endothelium. The left side of the heart may be involved, particularly in bronchial carcinoid or when a right-to-left shunt exists. Clinically, tricuspid regurgitation and pulmonic stenosis predominate, leading to right heart failure. Occasionally, a diffuse restrictive cardiomyopathy may be seen.

T-18. **Answer: e.** Cardiac disease is marked by the deposition of endocardial fibrous tissue (smooth muscle cells embedded in mucopolysaccharides, collagen, and microfibrils), which can lead to the combination of pulmonic stenosis and tricuspid regurgitation. Grossly, glistening white-yellow deposits are visible on the tricuspid and pulmonic valves and, to a lesser extent, on the right atrial and ventricular endocardium. Occasionally, a diffuse restrictive cardiomyopathy may be seen. Bronchoconstriction is less common but can be severe during flushing.

T-19. **Answer: c.** Cutaneous flushing is the most common clinical feature and is characteristically erythematous and malar. This may be accompanied by tachycardia and hypertension. Some patients develop purple telangiectasis primarily of the face and neck. Intestinal hypermotility with cramping and explosive diarrhea may occur, but the usual manifestation is chronic diarrhea which, if severe, can lead to malabsorption.

T-20. **Answer: b.** Bronchial carcinoids derive from the Kulchitsky's cells of the respiratory epithelium, a characteristic they share with small cell carcinoma of the lung. The carcinoid syndrome, consisting of intermittent attacks of diarrhea, flushing, and cyanosis, is uncommon with bronchial carcinoid and usually indicates the presence of widespread metastatic disease (especially liver). These tumors may arise from any tissue derived from the embryonic foregut (bronchus, thymus, thyroid, stomach, or pancreas) and the hindgut (often the anorectal region). The treatment of choice for bronchial carcinoid is surgical excision.

T-21. **Answer: d.** Solitary nodule is the most common presenting radiographic manifestation of bronchiolo-alveolar cell carcinoma. Multiple nodules comprise the presenting pattern in 15–25% of cases and consolidation in 30–40% of initial chest films. A characteristic feature of the pneumonic type is the air bronchogram, presumably due to infiltration of bronchial walls without obstruction of them. Hence, atelectasis is uncommon. Pleural effusions are fairly common, occurring on 10–35% of roentgenograms.

T-22. **Answers: a, e.** Carcinoid tumor of the thymus is a specific entity distinct from thymoma and is believed to arise from a population of thymic cells of neural crest origin. In patients with thymic carcinoids in whom the presence of nonforeign carcinoids was excluded, absence of serotonin is universal, and consequently,

carcinoid syndrome has not been observed. This finding may be related to a deficiency in aromatic amino acid decarboxylase, which is necessary for the conversion of 5-hydroxytryptophan to serotonin. However, they have been endocrinologically functional in a substantial number of cases and have usually produced Cushing's syndrome.

T-23. **Answers: c, e.** Atypical carcinoids have greater nuclear atypia and mitotic activity than the typical and an increased incidence of lymph node metastases. Large bowel carcinoids may metastasize but almost never exhibit endocrine effects. Midgut carcinoids have a proclivity to metastasize to the liver but may also involve the bone (often osteoblastic), lung, pancreas, spleen, ovaries, adrenals, and other organs. Some histologically benign-appearing carcinoid tumors metastasize or become locally invasive. Some of the tumors appear histologically as oat cell carcinomas.

T-24. **Answers: a, c, d.** Up to one third of cases presenting with a solitary nodule on chest film are found to have multicentric disease at surgery or autopsy. Several series report an approximate 2:1 upper lobe to lower lobe predominance. Pleural effusion is fairly common, occurring in 10 to 35% of chest films. Cytologic yield from pleural effusions is fairly high, with two series reporting a 62% and 87% yield, respectively. Bone metastases are usually lytic, not blastic. There is less hilar adenopathy than in other lung tumors.

T-25. **Answers: a, b, c.** The incidence of lung cancer in smokers with asbestos exposure is increased 90-fold as compared to nonsmokers without exposure. Of cigarette smokers with asbestosis, 20–35% will develop lung cancer. Nonsmokers with asbestos exposure almost uniformly have severe asbestosis and develop a scar adeno- or bronchoalveolar carcinoma. The presence of a ferruginous body or pleural plaques only supports asbestos exposure and not asbestosis. Ferruginous bodies have been found in the sputum of "nonexposed" city dwellers, and in large autopsy series from industrial cities, ferruginous bodies have been found in 20–50% of persons without known exposure. Asbestosis usually begins in the subpleural lower lobes.

T-26. **Answers: c, d.** The incidence of bronchogenic cancer peaks at 30 to 35 years after asbestos exposure. Asbestos-related carcinoma is predominantly in the lower lobe. Most frequently it is an adenocarcinoma. There is an increased frequency of multicentric and bilateral carcinomas. One study suggests that the risk for developing lung carcinoma appears to correlate more closely with the pathologic burden of asbestos fibers per gram of lung tissue than it does with fibrosis.

T-27. **Answers: a, b, c, d, e.** High-dose chemotherapy followed by autologous bone marrow transplant has been increasingly utilized in patients with Hodgkin's and non-Hodgkin's lymphoma, breast and ovarian carcinoma, small cell carcinoma of the lung, malignant melanoma, and nonseminomatous germ cell tumors.

T-28. **Answer: c.** Bronchoalveolar carcinoma is a well-differentiated form of adenocarcinoma. It arises from several cell lines including alveolar type 2 cells, goblet cells, and the Clara cell. Tobacco use is not considered to be important in its pathogenesis. It often appears in areas of previously scarred lung, e.g., old tuberculosis lesions. The diffuse alveolar filling form of this disease may follow diffuse fibrosing interstitial lung diseases such as idiopathic pulmonary fibrosis or scleroderma lung.

T-29. **Answer: a.** The chest radiograph of alveolar cell carcinoma often differs from that of other diffuse alveolar filling disorders.

Rather than demonstrating a diffuse consolidative pattern, it is characterized by larger alveolar nodules. In 40% of patients with IPF, the rheumatoid factor and/or antinuclear antibody are positive. Infrequently there is bronchorrhea, with a salty taste to the sputum reported. Occasionally nonpulmonary adenocarcinomas (breast and pancreas) may metastasize to the lung, producing an alveolar filling pattern on chest roentgenogram. Recent experience suggests that a transbronchial biopsy that demonstrates the typical features of BOOP obviates open lung biopsy.

T-30. **Answer: d.** Smoking cessation results in a gradual approach to normal risk for lung cancer over 10 to 15 years. Extrapolation from doubling time observations has yielded the estimate that by the time a lung cancer is clinically apparent, it has been present for 10 to 20 years. Thus, smoking cessation probably causes a rapid decrease in the formation of new lung neoplasms. However, preexisting carcinomas will continue to be detected for 10 to 15 years.

T-31. **Answer: d.** All but vitamin A are associated with increased risk of lung cancer. Vitamin A intake may actually protect from the development of lung cancer; individuals with low intake of foods rich in vitamin A are at increased risk for lung cancer.

T-32. **Answer: d.** Exposure to multiple carcinogens tends to have a synergistic effect on lung cancer risk. Asbestos and cigarette smoking are not merely additive (which would give a risk of 25).

T-33. **Answer: d.** Although still a controversial area, most students of lung cancer believe that the three major forms of bronchogenic carcinoma arise from reserve basal cells of the bronchial mucosa. A common cell of origin is supported by the occurrence of tumors containing elements of all three major histologic types of lung cancer. Further support is provided by the observation that genes encoded by the short arm chromosome 3 are lost in all three forms of bronchogenic carcinoma. Conclusive experiments to rule out other cells as the progenitor for lung cancer have not been possible to date.

T-34.   **Answer: a.** Bronchogenic carcinomas are asymptomatic for most of their natural history. Either a new cough or a change in the character of a chronic cough is the most common presenting symptom. Weight loss or malaise is suggestive of extensive disease.

T-35.   **Answer: b.** Although screening has not been proved to be worthless, results with current methods are disappointing. Adding sputum cytology to chest film screening of a high-risk population does not decrease the death rate from lung cancer. Three large studies have examined intensive screening of high-risk populations. All studies were suboptimal in that they did not include an unscreened control population but rather examined different levels of screening intensity. Because some lung cancers were diagnosed early, survival was longer, but overall death rate was not affected. Risk of developing a second primary was up to 5% per year. No studies have determined the optimal frequency for obtaining "routine" chest films. It is more frequent in smokers.

T-36.   **Answer: d.** Although all of the possibilities tend to go with a benign lesion, only dense concentric calcification is highly reliable. Small size or lack of adenopathy obviously does not rule out malignancy. Six months is not a long enough period of stability to definitely exclude malignancy; further follow-up or work-up is warranted. Calcification is highly reliable if it is diffuse, dense, or concen-

tric. A fleck of calcification can occur in a cancer growing adjacent to a scar. Patient age below 35 years does not exclude malignancy.

T-37.   **Answer: c.** Generally, the first step in an organized work-up of a suspicious lung lesion is to establish a tissue diagnosis. Sometimes this can be accomplished by biopsy of a lesion in the liver, skin, or a lymph node and also, the presence of metastatic disease can be established. Because small cell lung cancer is not usually treated surgically, tissue diagnosis of a lesion should precede determination of resectability.

T-38.   **Answer: c.** Although operational morbidity and mortality have decreased, long-term survival from lung cancer has not changed over the past 20 years. Modern staging procedures, including mediastinoscopy, have decreased the incidence of discovery of inoperable disease at thoracotomy from 25% to 5%.

T-39.   **Answer: a.** Superior vena caval obstruction is not as life-threatening as was originally believed. Long-term survival with benign superior vena caval obstruction suggests that the obstruction by itself is not lethal.

T-40.   **Answer: d.** Because of this, aggressive attempts to control the pulmonary primary are justified in patients with a relatively good prognosis. Trials comparing surgery with radiotherapy are now under way.

T-41.   **Answer: a.** The Eaton-Lambert syndrome is rare but typically is seen in association with small cell lung cancer. Diagnosis is made by demonstration of increased muscle potentials with repeated stimulation on EMG, opposite to the findings in myasthenia gravis.

T-42.   **Answer: d.** The syndrome of inappropriate antidiuretic hormone is the most common endocrine syndrome in small cell lung cancer. Hyponatremia should suggest this histologic diagnosis. Hypercalcemia is suggestive of a non-small cell lung cancer.

T-43. **Answer: e.** Bronchogenic carcinoma, bronchiectasis, with or without aspergilloma, tuberculosis (usually from cavitating sources), and pulmonary infarction are commonly considered, but chronic bronchitis is the most common cause of mild hemoptysis; however, this rarely results in massive hemoptysis.

T-44. **Answer: d.** Hilar adenopathy is common in histoplasmosis, coccidioidomycosis, varicella zoster infection, and tropical eosinophilia. Hilar lymph node involvement is uncommon in blastomycosis.

T-45. **Answer: d.** Only two criteria are believed to be reliable predictors of a benign lesion: (1) absence of growth over 2 years, which derives from finding the doubling rates of lung cancers to be within the 1- to 16-month range based on serial chest films, and (2) the presence of certain characteristic patterns of calcification such as dense central calcification, multiple punctate foci of Ca++, bullseye Ca++ (implying granuloma, especially histoplasmosis), and "popcorn" Ca++ (hamartoma). However, Ca++ can also occur in malignant solitary pulmonary nodules, e.g., when a scar carcinoma engulfs a preexisting, calcified, inflammatory lesion (in which case the Ca++ is eccentrically located).

T-46. **Answer: b, d, e.** Rarely found in non-smokers, the classic small cell carcinoma presents as a hilar mass in a patient with a history of heavy tobacco use. It is difficult to accurately diagnose small cell carcinoma from a fine-needle aspirate or transbronchial biopsy; many tumors are atypical and appear more like a carcinoid tumor. Small cell carcinomas that present as peripheral lesions are less likely to metastasize, perhaps because they may represent a different subset of tumor that is less aggressive. The marked difference in survival rates makes an accurate distinction between these two neoplasms important. Often this differentiation can only be made at thoracotomy.

T-47. **Answer: c, d, e.** The mediastinum is an embryologically complex, anatomically diverse, yet extremely compact region. Bounded superiorly by the thoracic outlet, inferiorly by the diaphragm, anteriorly by the sternum, and posteriorly by the vertebral column, it is classically divided into four compartments. The anterior mediastinum is anterior to the pericardial sac and contains the thymus gland, anterior mediastinal lymph nodes, and fat. The superior mediastinum (often combined with the anterior mediastinum) contains the aortic arch and its branches. The middle mediastinum, that area contained within the pericardial sac, includes the heart, the trachea and main bronchi, the hilum, the phrenic nerve, and lymph nodes. The esophagus, thoracic duct, descending aorta, vagus nerve, sympathetic nervous chain, and paravertebral lymphatics are contained within the posterior mediastinum.

T-48. **Answers: c, d.** The most common mediastinal lesions are neurogenic tumors (21%), thymomas (19%), primary cysts (18%), lymphomas (13%), and germ cell tumors (10%). Mediastinal masses are most frequently located in the anterior-superior mediastinum (54%), with the posterior mediastinum (26%) and middle mediastinum (20%) trailing in the polls. In the anterior-superior mediastinum, thymomas occur most frequently (31%) along with lymphomas (23%) and germ cell tumors (17%). Posterior mediastinal lesions are usually neurogenic tumors (54%), bronchial cysts (22%), and enteric cysts (7%). Pericardial cysts (35%), lymphomas (20%), and bronchial cysts (15%) comprise most middle mediastinal lesions.

T-49. **Answers: b, c.** Pericardial cysts are usually seen in the right cardiophrenic angle and are found in the middle mediastinum. Enteric cysts arise from the posterior division of the primitive foregut. Also known as duplications cysts, inclusion cysts, gastric cysts, or enterogenous cysts, they are usually located in the posterior mediastinum. Early and abnormal translocation of endodermal tissue into the mesodermal layer, which ultimately forms the muscular layer of the esophagus, is the presumed mechanism. Although located in the esophageal mucosa, enteric cysts rarely communicate with the esophageal lumen. Anterior-superior mediastinal masses are most likely to be malignant (59%) when compared to middle mediastinal masses (29%) or posterior lesions (16%).

T-50. **Answers: d, e.** The majority of neurogenic tumors are benign in adults; a much greater percentage are malignant in children. Patients between ages 15 and 35 have the greatest proportion of malignant mediastinal neoplasms correlating with the peak incidence of lymphomas and germ cell tumors in this period. The neurogenic tumors are found almost exclusively in the posterior mediastinum and originate from the sympathetic ganglia (ganglioma, ganglioneuroblastoma, and neuroblastoma), the peripheral nerves (neurofibroma, neurilemoma, and neurosarcoma), and the paraganglionic cells (paraganglioma). The development of computed tomography has significantly altered the evaluation of mediastinal masses. CT is relatively accurate in defining the density of a mass, especially in relation to the density of nearby structures such as lung, soft tissue, and bone. Fat in the mediastinum or intrathoracic

fat protruding through a hiatal hernia or the foramen of Morgagni will appear as a mediastinal mass, but can be easily identified on CT. Although CT is sensitive in the evaluation of mediastinal masses, a correct preoperative diagnosis is still made in only 68% of patients, so that histologic examination is still required to make a definitive diagnosis in most cases.

T-51. **Answers: b, c, d, e.** BCNU has been linked to pulmonary fibrosis in over 80 case reports. Incidence figures range from 20–30% of cases in acute or subacute exposure to 100% of cases in latent exposure, making BCNU a more insidious pulmonary toxin than bleomycin. Definite risk factors for BCNU lung toxicity include: (1) total dose, (2) dose/cycle, (3) preexisting lung disease such as COPD, pneumoconiosis, recurrent bronchitis, or pneumonia, and (4) tobacco exposure. Rarely, focal angiitis, necrotizing granuloma, and pulmonary veno-occlusive disease develop.

T-52. **Answers: a, b, c, d.** Pathologically, BCNU pulmonary toxicity causes alveolar epithelial metaplasia with loss of type I pneumocytes and dysplasia of type II pneumocytes, proliferation of fibroblasts and collagen deposition in the alveolar septa, and a proteinaceous alveolar exudate. Evidence of active inflammatory cells is rare, making this a "bland fibrosis."

T-53. **Answers: a, c, e.** Bronchial carcinoids belong to the neuroendocrine (APUD) group of tumors and appear to share with small cell carcinoma a common neuroectodermal stem cell. It is an uncommon low-grade malignancy with a slight female predominance; 70–80% of pulmonary carcinoids arise centrally in a lobar, segmental, or large subsegmental bronchus. Carcinoid tumors located in the periphery of the lung can have a histologic appearance identical to their more central counterparts, but often have a spindle cell configuration. They occur most often in the RUL/RML and lingula.

T-54. **Answers: a, c.** "Atypical" carcinoids may represent a continuum between "benign" typical carcinoids and small cell carcinoma. They account for about 10% of all carcinoids. Lymph node metastasis occurs in 50% of these compared to 5–10% of typicals. The "atypical" label is applied to carcinoid tumors with increased mitotic activity, nuclear pleomorphism and hyperchromasia, increased nuclear/cytoplasmic ratio, areas of increased cellularity with loss of typical architecture, or necrosis. Compared to the typical group, in which 5-year disease-free survival is close to 100%, it is 65–70% in atypicals, and at 10 years, it is 85–90% and 50–55% respectively; 1–3% of patients develop the carcinoid syndrome, most in association with liver metastases, and nearly all with a large tumor burden. In these patients, a high urinary level of 5-HIAA will be seen.

T-55. **Answers: a, d.** A hamartoma is traditionally defined as a non-neoplastic tumor-like developmental malformation composed of tissues that normally constitute the organ in which the tumor occurs, but in which the tissue elements, though mature, are disorganized. Whereas a true hamartoma ceases to grow when the organ in which it is situated stops growing, a neoplasm shows inexorable growth and compresses the surrounding tissue. Pulmonary hamartomas are, in fact, benign neoplasms with their origin in the primitive bronchial mesenchymal tissue, which can differentiate into various tissues. They are perhaps better referred to as mesenchymomas. They consist mostly of cartilage, a fibromyxomatous matrix, and adipose tissue, but may contain smooth muscle, seromucinous bronchial glands, nonspecific chronic inflammatory cells, and even bone and marrow spaces. The male:female ratio is 2 or 3:1.

T-56. **Answers: e.** Hamartomas appear as round, homogeneous opacities in the periphery of the lung; 90% are located peripherally; 10% are endobronchial and are present centrally. They have onset in adult life with a peak incidence in the sixth decade. None has ever clearly been shown to undergo malignant degeneration. However, about 5% of patients may develop synchronous or metachronous lung cancers, and the relative risk is estimated to be six times that of the general population. Calcification is uncommon (5–10%). The endobronchial variant often has little or no cartilage, but mostly adipose tissue surrounded by loose fibrous tissue with intermixed smooth muscle, glands, and myxomatous tissue.

T-57. **Answers: a, b, e.** Thyroid cancer accounts for about 1% of all new malignancies annually. The most common type, papillary, arises from the thyroid follicular cell and is most often seen in young Caucasian females. The lesion is usually unencapsulated and tends to invade lymphatics and spread to local tissue and regional lymph nodes (42% of cases at presentation).

T-58. **Answers: a, c, d, e.** The dominant site for metastatic disease is the thoracic cavity: lungs and mediastinum, followed by bone and soft tissues. The primary form of intrathoracic metastases is diffuse disease with either miliary or multiple parenchymal nodules, or, more rarely, localized pulmonary infiltration often associated with hilar and mediastinal enlargement and pleural effusions. Anywhere from 15–40% of patients will have a clear chest film. Initial therapy consists of total or subtotal thyroidectomy, followed by ^{131}I ablation, which clearly reduces recurrence and mortality. *In vitro* studies also show that differentiated thyroid cancers have TSH receptors and increase adenylate cyclase in response to TSH, so that suppression of TSH by exogenous L-thyroxine has a favorable impact on tumor progression/survival/recurrence. Chance of recurrent disease is high — greatest in first 6 months, but sometimes occurring as late as 10 to 30 years from presentation.

T-59. **Answers: a, c, d, e.** Serial thyroglobulin measurements are the mainstay of surveillance. Thyroglobulin is only produced by thyroid tissue, and elevation of thyroglobulin levels in a patient with prior surgical/radionuclide ablation is believed to be a good marker of recurrent disease. An elevated TG is highly sensitive and specific for the presence of disease. In comparison, total body scan is only 58% sensitive and 29% specific. In one study, 13% of patients with elevated thyroglobulin levels and biopsy-proven metastatic disease had a negative body scan. False-negatives can occur if patients have failed to cease exogenous thyroid supplementation prior to scan, and false-positives (though rare) have been reported in patients with significant pulmonary inflammation (i.e., bronchiectasis).

T-60. **Answer: a.** Thymoma is the most common tumor of the anterior-superior mediastinum. Other tumors in the differential diagnoses of an anterior mediastinal mass include: lymphoma, germ cell tumor, thyroid carcinoma, and bronchogenic cysts.

T-61. **Answers: c, d, e.** Thymoma is primarily a tumor of middle to late life. The mean age at diagnosis is 50 years, and there is no sex predilection. Myasthenia gravis occurs in approximately 35% of patients with thymoma. Conversely, about 15% of patients with myasthenia are found to have thymoma. Hematologic abnormalities are found in 3% of patients. Hypogammaglobulinemia and pure red cell aplasia are the more common paraneoplastic conditions in this category.

T-62. **Answer: e.** Up to 50% of thymomas are undetectable on the PA chest roentgenogram. The clinical stages of thymomas are: stage I—encapsulated without microscopic evidence of invasion; stage II—extension through the capsule and pericapsular fat invasion; stage III—invasion of neighboring structures (pericardium, great vessels, lungs); stage IV—thoracic dissemination or distant metastases. Stage IV is extremely rare. Spindle cell thymomas are frequently associated with hematologic derangements. Surgery is the basic treatment of thymomas. Treatment consists of extensive resection and radiation following resection, except in well-circumscribed stage I disease. Without radiation, relapse rates are 53%, compared to 0–20% in those treated with radiation. The epithelial subtype, along with age >60 years, presence of mediastinal or constitutional symptoms, invasive or metastasizing thymomas, and a size of 15 cm (average size = 8 cm), has a poor prognosis.

T-63. **Answers: a, b, c.** Pathologically, thymomas can be classified based on the predominant cell type: lymphocytic (25–35%), epithelial (40–42%), and mixed (25–35%). The epithelial type (cortical subtype) of thymoma carries the worst prognosis. A fourth type, spindle cell, may be a variant of the epithelial type and usually behaves in a benign fashion. It is this subtype that is commonly associated with red cell aplasia and with hypogammaglobulinemia (referred to as Good's syndrome) and is sometimes associated with manifestations of T cell deficiency. Whereas thymectomy frequently alleviates the symptoms of myasthenia gravis, it only occasionally results in remission of pure red cell aplasia and does not usually improve hypogammaglobulinemia. Although calcification is identified by CT in 20% of thymomas, it cannot be used to distinguish benign from malignant disease.

T-64. **Answer: b.** Embryologically, the thymus derives from endoderm of the third pharyngeal pouches. That portion giving rise to the thymus migrates down to its position in the anterior mediastinum while the superior horns migrate to the neck to become the parathyroid glands. As the endoderm matures into the epithelial framework and its medullary areas, lymphocytes migrate into the gland to became thymocytes. The gland reaches its largest at adolescence (30–40 gm), thereafter involuting and regressing in size, being largely replaced by fat. T thymomas, which are predominantly epithelial in type, tend to be more aggressive than the lymphocytic type. In general, thymomas are considered to be relatively slow-growing tumors. Five- and ten-year survival rates are 85 and 80% respectively for noninvasive disease and 50 and 35% respectively for invasive thymomas. Along with invasive disease, myasthenia gravis and possibly epithelial type histology are poor prognostic indicators.

T-65. **Answers: a, e.** Malignant non-Hodgkin's lymphoma represents the second most common neoplastic complication of HIV infection. Malignant non-Hodgkin's lymphoma occurs in approximately 3% of AIDS patients (75% are gay). Most are intermediate- to high-grade, aggressive B cell lymphomas. A few cases of T cell lymphomas have been reported. The majority of patients have extensive disease (stage III or IV) at diagnosis, with a high incidence of extranodal involvement (65–90%). Common extranodal sites include CNS, bone marrow, GI tract, and liver. The lung is an uncommon site (4–10%). Primary lymphoma without extrathoracic disease has been reported.

T-66. **Answers: a, c, d.** Chest film findings in pulmonary non-Hodgkin's lymphoma are variable, but are similar to those seen in non-AIDS patients. Clinical manifestations of pulmonary non-Hodgkin's lymphoma are nonspecific and include cough, dyspnea, fever, malaise, weight loss, and lymphadenopathy. Unlike pulmonary Kaposi's sarcoma, coexistent opportunistic infections are uncommon in pulmonary non-Hodgkin's lymphoma; however, there may be an increased incidence of bacterial infections (including pneumonia) in HIV-associated non-Hodgkin's lymphoma. Diagnosis is often difficult, with fiberoptic bronchoscopy and transbronchial biopsy having a dismal sensitivity; it is only about 20% in non-AIDS non-Hodgkin's lymphoma.

T-67. **Answers: a, c, d.** Profound suppression of cell-mediated immunity is the hallmark of infection with the HIV virus, and has altered the spectrum and the natural history of neoplasia in certain segments of the population. Kaposi's sarcoma, once a rare and indolent tumor, is now seen in up to 40% of homosexuals with AIDS, and behaves in a much more aggressive fashion. Other tumors frequently associated with AIDS include malignant lymphomas of several histologic types, including Burkitt's lymphomas and Hodgkin's disease, often behaving very aggressively and involving the CNS. Nonspecific lymphocytic alveolitis characterized by lymphocytosis in BAL is seen in up to two thirds of patients without regard of concurrent pulmonary infection. Pulmonary Kaposi's sarcoma lesions are less cellular than the cutaneous ones.

2-4 Interstitial Disease

F-1.　**Answers: a, b, c, d, e.** Pulmonary eosinophilic syndromes are a heterogeneous group of disorders characterized by inflammation of the lung with infiltration of eosinophils. Classification of these syndromes originally by Crofton and amended by Carrington, is broadly as (a) eosinophilic pneumonia (simple/Löffler's, chronic) and (b) tropical eosinophilia.

F-2.　**Answers: b, c, d.** The most likely diagnosis if a patient develops bronchiectasis, rhinitis, and sinusitis early in life is the immotile cilia syndrome. Situs inversus may accompany the immotile cilia syndrome, and this is called Kartagener's syndrome. Central bronchiectasis is a major manifestation of allergic bronchopulmonary aspergillosis. In the Churg-Strauss syndrome there is allergic rhinitis, asthma, and later a systemic vasculitis. The pathologic findings are granulomas in the lungs, heart, liver, spleen, skin, and nerves.

F-3.　**Answers: a, b, e.** Löffler's syndrome is defined in terms of its brevity and mild manifestations. Patients present with cough, malaise, low-grade fever, wheezing, and dyspnea, but most are asymptomatic. The chest film reveals "fleeting" pulmonary infiltrates, which are peripheral, and serum eosinophil count is elevated (usually >6% of differential). Hypoxemia is unusual, and PFTs can show a mild restrictive pattern with decreased D_LCO.

F-4.　**Answers: a, b, c.** Histologic information is limited, but a few biopsies available reveal infiltration of eosinophils and macrophages into the interstitium with edema and collagen disruption. Basement membranes remain intact and immunofluorescence is negative.

F-5.　**Answers: a, b, c, e.** The usual presentation includes high-grade fevers, drenching night sweats, weight loss, and productive cough. Mild hemoptysis may occur. The chest film reveals the classic "photographic negative of pulmonary edema," with fluffy infiltrates in the apices and axillary regions in two thirds of cases. Although the eosinophil count is generally markedly elevated, significant tissue eosinophilia can occur with normal circulating levels. Transbronchial biopsy shows massive filling of airspaces with a mixture of monocytes and eosinophils, some giant cell infiltration, and evidence of small necrotic foci within exudate.

F-6.　**Answers: a, b, c, d, e.** The hallmark of Löffler's syndrome is complete and spontaneous remission of symptoms within 2–4 weeks of onset. In contrast, patients with chronic eosinophilic pneumonia have a disease of much greater severity and duration (mean time to diagnosis 8 months in some series). There are recent reports of patients presenting with acute eosinophilic pneumonia being acutely ill with respiratory distress, high fevers, bilateral pulmonary infiltrates, and severe hypoxemia. In all cases, the diagnosis was made by exclusion of other entities and by eosinophilia on trans-bronchial biopsy and BAL fluid. The mechanism for lung injury remains unclear, but major basic protein, which is toxic to respiratory epithelial cells and can lead to desquamation of bronchial epithelium, is increased in body fluids. The disease has been correlated with a variety of drug/toxin exposures, fungi, and mycobacterial diseases, but is most often idiopathic.

F-7.   **Answers: a, b, c.** Nervous system involvement may occur with sarcoidosis of any stage. It is also not uncommon for patients to develop neurologic manifestations of sarcoid prior to developing signs or symptoms of extraneurologic sarcoid, and when this happens the diagnosis may be elusive. The most common neurologic manifestation of sarcoidosis is facial nerve paralysis (20–30% of patients with neurosarcoid). It can be unilateral or bilateral and is usually transient (with or without steroid therapy). Pathogenesis was thought to relate to compression of the nerve as it passed through an enlarged parotid gland; however, brain stem evoked potentials suggest that the problem is at the brain stem level. The second most commonly involved cranial nerve is the optic nerve. Symptoms include blurred vision, visual field defects, and abnormal pupillary responses.

F-8.   **Answers: a, b, e.** Auditory nerve involvement may result in hearing loss and/or vertigo and is said to carry a poor prognosis. Anosmia may occur either from olfactory nerve involvement or from nasal mucosal disease. Localized granulomatous mass lesions have been reported in every part of the CNS (supratentorial > infratentorial). MRI may uncover granulomas missed on CT. Treatment for these lesions has included steroids +/- other immunosuppressive agents and radiation in resistant cases.

F-9.   **Answers: a, b, c, d, e.** Neuroendocrinologic abnormalities, most commonly diabetes insipidus, have been reported in association with mass lesions (also, hyperprolactinemia and galactorrhea-amenorrhea syndrome). CNS sarcoid may also present with psychiatric manifestations (apathy, memory loss, agitation, hallucination, depression). Cerebellar involvement may result in choreiform movements, hemiballismus, and parkinsonism, but these conditions are rare.

F-10.   **Answers: d, e.** Asymptomatic muscle involvement may occur in 28–80% of patients with sarcoidosis, but symptomatic myopathy is rare. Involvement may be in the form of nodules (least frequent), acute myopathy (in women more often than in men), or, most commonly, chronic myopathy with onset over months to years. Aseptic meningitis is common. The most common CSF finding is pleocytosis (lymphocyte predominance). Approximately 50% will show increased protein and approximately 20% will show decreased glucose. The prognosis for meningitis and cranial neuropathy is better than that for CNS involvement and myopathy. Peripheral neuropathy manifestations such as paresthesias, root pains, weakness/muscle wasting, and decreased or absent deep tendon reflexes most commonly affect the ulnar and peroneal nerves.

F-11.   **Answers: c, d, e.** Respiratory bronchiolitis is a smoking related disorder of first- and second-generation respiratory bronchioles and historically has been viewed as an incidental finding at autopsy or lung resection. It is characterized by the presence of clusters of pigmented macrophages within respiratory bronchioles and adjacent alveoli. Associated findings are mild thickening and fibrosis of involved alveolar septa and the peribronchiolar interstitium. The "dusty brown" macrophages have abundant cytoplasm filled with fine, granular golden brown particles that stain with PAS and Prussian blue stains.

F-12.   **Answers: a, d, e.** Respiratory bronchiolitis is associated with a form of ILD that has some features in common with IPF. It has a lower lung zone predominance and is characterized by an insidious onset of nonspecific respiratory complaints; 80% of patients show patchy reticular or reticulonodular infiltrates on chest film. The differential diagnosis includes EG, DIP, UIP w/IPF, and pulmonary hemorrhage.

F-13. **Answers: b, c, e.** The diagnosis of Goodpasture's syndrome is reserved for patients with combined diffuse alveolar hemorrhage and glomerulonephritis (60–80%) who do not have evidence of a systemic vasculitis but demonstrate antibody directed against basement membrane in circulation bound to tissue. There are also cases (<5%) in which diffuse alveolar hemorrhage occurs without obvious renal disease. However, renal biopsy still demonstrates the linear deposition of IgG directed against basement membrane. Diffuse alveolar hemorrhage occurs in 100% of smokers with Goodpasture's syndrome and in only 20% of nonsmokers. Resumption of smoking or exposure to volatile hydrocarbons and URIs precipitates exacerbations.

F-14. **Answers: b, c, d, e.** Systemic lupus erythematosus is a common (1/2,000 population, female/male 10:1; 1/700 females between ages 15 and 65; 1/245 Black females ages 15–65) multisystem connective tissue disease that affects the lungs in 30–70% of patients. Immunopathologic staining can show subepithelial deposition of DNA, anti-DNA antibodies, IgG, and C3. Pulmonary hemorrhage can be a manifestation of systemic lupus erythematosus. Certain medications (e.g., sulfonamides) and infections can precipitate a lupus flare. Uncommonly, in those with pulmonary hemorrhage, there can be a leukocytoclastic vasculitis.

F-15. **Answers: a, b, c, e.** The pulmonary manifestations of lupus pneumonitis are varied and include (1) pleuritis, (2) pulmonary hypertension, (3) pulmonary emboli, (4) lymphocytic interstitial pneumonitis, (5) diaphragmatic weakness, (6) pulmonary hemorrhage, and (7) lupus pneumonitis.

F-16. **Answers: a, b, d, e.** Lupus pneumonitis can present as either an acute or a chronic process. It may present as diffuse alveolar damage and hyaline membranes. Bilateral pulmonary involvement with pleural effusions are common. Radiographically it most often presents as an alveolar infiltrate with basilar predominance. Acute lupus pneumonitis can be the initial manifestation of the disease. It can lead to chronic disease with progressive interstitial fibrosis.

F-17. **Answers: a, b, c, d, e.** Lymphangioleiomyomatosis (LAM) is a rare and devastating disease that occurs primarily in females of reproductive age, although cases have been reported in postmenopausal women receiving estrogen supplementation. Spontaneous pneumothorax occurs in approximately 50% of patients at presentation and can be recurrent and bilateral. Pleural effusions are common in the course of the disease and are chylous in nature. The chest film can be normal, but usually shows a reticulonodular pattern in the setting of preserved or enlarged lung volumes.

F-18. **Answers: a, c, d.** The pathologic hallmark of LAM is believed to be abnormal proliferation of immature smooth muscle cells in the lung, although extrapulmonary involvement (kidneys, retroperitoneum) can occur. The smooth muscle is not only abundant, but abnormal, with increased glycogen stores, disordered cellular architecture and abnormal structural organization. Primarily, the cells appear to involve pulmonary lymphatic channels, but also involve terminal and respiratory bronchioles and small pulmonary veins. Lymphatic obstruction leads to chylothorax and, rarely, chylous ascites. Obstruction of vessels leads to venous congestion with rupture of small veins and hemosiderosis/hemoptysis with uneven pulmonary perfusion. Despite evidence of a diffuse interstitial process on chest roentgenogram, PFTs typically show normal or increased TLC and RV due to air trapping and hyperinflation.

F-19. **Answer: d.** Maximal expiratory flows are reduced to a greater degree than elastic recoil, indicating that airflow limitation is primarily due to compression of airways rather than emphysema. The myocytes in LAM are postulated to be stimulated by estrogen (worsening of disease with menses, oral contraceptives, and pregnancy), although this has not been demonstrated *in vitro*. Tissue studies reveal presence of both estrogen and progesterone receptors in lung tissue of patients with LAM, which are not present in normal lung and are similar to those noted in uterine tissue. Therapy has generally been disappointing. Steroids, cytotoxics, and irradiation have not been helpful. Data on oophorectomy (surgical or chemical) or on use of progesterone are controversial, anecdotal, and uncontrolled. The largest study from Stanford failed to find benefit from oophorectomy, but found that patients with chylothorax or chylous ascites were most likely to benefit from progesterone. Unfortunately, limited data have failed to show correlation between ER/PR status and clinical response to hormonal interventions, which are the mainstay of therapy.

F-20. **Answers: a, c. e.** Acute beryllium disease is thought to be dose related and occurs predictably in workers exposed to high levels of beryllium fumes or dusts in industrial accidents (>100 µg/m³). It manifests as a toxic, chemical pneumonitis and tracheobronchitis. Radiographic findings can be minimal or severe with an ARDS-like picture. Treatment is with steroids. The disorder usually resolves after the exposure is removed. Long-term sequelae include bronchiectasis and chronic beryllium disease.

F-21. **Answers: b, e.** Although chronic beryllium disease is primarily a pulmonary disease, it also has systemic manifestations (renal stones, hypercalcemia, dermatitis, hepatosplenomegaly, conjunc-

tivitis). Classically there are small round and irregular opacities ("sandpaper") with hilar adenopathy. Pleural disease occurs in 10% of cases.

F-22. **Answers: a, d, e.** Chronic beryllium disease can occur at variable times after exposure. The upper zones are typically most affected. Lymphocytes from peripheral blood have a 70–80% sensitivity. The skin test (patch test) has poor sensitivity; a significant false-positive rate and the risk of sensitization in unsensitized individuals make it unattractive. The prognosis is variable, but most develop progressive pulmonary disease. Treatment is with lifelong steroids.

F-23. **Answers: a, b, d.** Polymyositis has a well-known association with ILD. It appears to be asymptomatic in many based-on-autopsy studies, but the presence of pulmonary fibrosis adds a poor prognosis to the disease (30-month mortality of 40%). Respiratory complaints may be the first major symptoms, but often the prior diagnosis of polymyositis or rheumatologic symptoms preexist. Pleuritic chest pain may be present during the course of the progressive dyspnea. Fatigue from dyspnea may obscure symptoms of muscle weakness. ILD may present at any stage of polymyositis.

F-24. **Answers: b, c, d.** Muscle biopsy confirms most cases of polymyositis, but muscle involvement may be spotty and the diagnosis missed, even though clinically apparent. Anti-Jo 1 antibodies are found in 10–20% of polymyositis patients, with ILD "risk" as high as 50% in these patients. While rarely found in idiopathic ILD, it is not a sensitive marker as 15% of anti-Jo1 negative patients have ILD. BOOP (cryptogenic organizing pneumonia), usual interstitial pneumonia (UIP), and diffuse alveolar damage (DAD) are the major subgroups of ILD in polymyositis.

F-25. **Answers: b, c, d, e.** The alterations in histology of diffuse alveolar hemorrhage with capillaritis consist of neutrophilic invasion of the alveolar walls (interstitium) with fibrinoid necrosis and capillary thrombosis. The neutrophils become fragmented (leukocytolysis), causing accumulation of nuclear dust in the lung parenchyma. As a result, there is loss of integrity of the alveolar capillary membrane with leakage of RBCs into the alveolar space and hemosiderin accumulation in the alveolar macrophages and the lung parenchyma. Other histologic features include organization of the alveolar hemorrhage, type II cell hyperplasia, and monocytic interstitial infiltration. Without capillaritis it is a bland hemorrhage with RBCs and hemosiderin containing macrophages within alveolar spaces and hemosiderin in the tissue. There is no significant alveolar wall inflammation or necrosis, but there is intraalveolar organization and type II cell hyperplasia with minimal mononuclear cell interstitial infiltration. With recurrent episodes, interstitial fibrosis can occur.

F-26. **Answers: a, b, c.** The clinical presentation of diffuse alveolar hemorrhage is usually acute with cough, dyspnea, hemoptysis, fever, and systemic symptoms and signs, when systemic vasculitis is present. However, hemoptysis can be delayed or not be prominent initially. Crack cocaine inhalation, penicillamine usage, and bone marrow transplantation can all cause diffuse alveolar hemorrhage. Trimellitic anhydride—a compound used in the manufacture of paints, epoxy resins, and plastics—causes diffuse alveolar hemorrhage but no renal disease. Kerley's B lines imply underlying mitral stenosis or pulmonary venoocclusive disease as the cause of diffuse alveolar hemorrhage.

F-27. **Answers: b, c.** Serial measurements of the diffusing capacity for carbon monoxide will demonstrate initially high and then decreasing values due to the binding of CO with the readily available intraalveolar hemoglobin. Henoch-Schönlein purpura is an immune complex–mediated disease, and antibody directed against IgA is found in the circulation and tissue. Goodpasture's syndrome occurs in 100% of smokers and in only 20% of nonsmokers. Resumption of smoking precipitates exacerbations. The diagnosis of Goodpasture's syndrome is reserved for patients with combined diffuse alveolar hemorrhage and glomerulonephritis who do not have evidence of a systemic vasculitis but demonstrate antibody directed against basement membrane in circulation bound to tissue.

F-28. **Answers: a, c, d.** In most cases of Goodpasture's syndrome, the lung and renal disease appear simultaneously. The highest incidence is in males between 20 and 30 years of age. In older age groups, the sex distribution equalizes and the disease is more likely to be renal limited. There is a high incidence of histocompatibility antigens HLA-DRw2 (90%) and HLA-B7 (60%). The severity of the renal disease determines the outcome.

F-29. **Answers: a, c, e.** Pulmonary capillaritis with diffuse alveolar hemorrhage, but without the typical pathologic changes in the lung or usual clinical presentation (upper airway disease, cavitating of pulmonary lesions) of WG, occurs in 5%. In the majority of these, the more typical clinical and histologic picture appears later during the course of the disease. Accompanying the diffuse alveolar hemorrhage there is always a focal segmental necrotizing glomerulonephritis, but the appearance of a cutaneous leukocytoclastic vasculitis, arthritis, or episcleritis is less predictable. The typical histology is medium vessel involvement, tissue necrosis, and granulomatous inflammation. WG with pulmonary capillaritis, diffuse alveolar hemorrhage, and renal failure alone cannot be differentiated from systemic necrotizing vasculitis by any clinical, histologic, or serologic criteria. Only the appearance of the typical histology or clinical findings will identify WG.

F-30. **Answers: d, e.** Systemic necrotizing vasculitis (microscopic polyarteritis) is thought to be a variant of polyarteritis nodosa (PAN). However, PAN does not involve the lungs, and has a predilection for the abdominal viscera. Allergic granulomatosis of Churg and Strauss, also considered a variant of PAN, is a medium-sized vasculitis with extravascular granulomatous inflammation and peripheral and tissue eosinophilia. This entity is not associated with capillaritis or diffuse alveolar hemorrhage. It is preceded by a protracted course of asthma and eosinophilia prior to the development of the systemic vasculitis. Pulmonary capillaritis and diffuse alveolar hemorrhage occur in 20–30% of cases of SNV, with focal segmental necrotizing glomerulonephritis being the most consistent finding. Other features of a systemic vasculitis—including cutaneous vasculitis, arthritis, gastrointestinal bleeding from mucosal involvement, episcleritis, peripheral neuropathy, and in a few cases, sinusitis—are seen in variable combinations and often with recurrences.

F-31. **Answers: b, c, d, e.** Diffuse alveolar hemorrhage occurs infrequently with rheumatoid arthritis, scleroderma, and mixed connective tissue disease and is most common in systemic lupus erythematosus. In SLE, diffuse alveolar hemorrhage occurs both with and without pulmonary capillaritis. In either case it is thought to be immune complex mediated, producing a granular deposition of immunoglobulin and complement within the alveolar interstitium. Anti-DNA antibody has also been demonstrated in the lung. Diffuse alveolar hemorrhage most often occurs in an established case of SLE and rarely is it the presenting manifestation. This complication is associated with a 70% mortality due to respiratory failure, a complicating infection, or another systemic manifestation of SLE (renal, CNS). Diffuse alveolar hemorrhage in SLE must be differentiated from acute lupus pneumonitis, an immunologic pneumonia in which the underlying pathology is diffuse alveolar damage and cellular interstitial pneumonia; it is often the presenting manifestation of the disease.

F-32. **Answers: a, b, d, e.** This is a chronic relapsing illness characterized by oral and genital ulceration, iridocyclitis, thrombophlebitis, and a systemic vasculitis consisting of cutaneous leukocytoclastic vasculitis, arthritis, and meningoencephalitis. Immune complexes have been identified in the circulation and affected tissue. The lung is involved in only 5–10% of cases. Diffuse alveolar hemorrhage secondary to pulmonary capillaritis and associated with a focal segmental necrotizing glomerulonephritis with granular deposition of immunoglobulin and complement in both lung and kidney is not the only cause of alveolar hemorrhage. Bronchial and larger pulmonary arterial vessel involvement leads to aneurysm formation, which can cause massive hemoptysis after rupture. In addition, the thrombophlebitis can result in pulmonary arterial occlusion and infarction.

F-33. **Answers: a, b, d.** Henoch-Schönlein purpura is primarily seen in children, but adult cases also present with the purpuric rash and glomerulonephritis. This is an immune complex-mediated disease and antibody directed against IgA is found in the circulation and tissue. Two adult cases of diffuse alveolar hemorrhage associated with pulmonary capillaritis have been reported, and IgA immune complexes were found in the alveolar septa. Pauci-immune glomerulonephritis is a renal-limited vasculitis.

Immune complex-related glomerulonephritis is rarely complicated by diffuse alveolar hemorrhage.

F-34. **Answers: a. b, c, d.** Churg-Strauss syndrome is characterized by pulmonary and systemic necrotizing angiitis, extravascular granulomas, and eosinophilia, occurring almost exclusively in patients with asthma or an allergic history. The necrotizing angiitis, with prominent eosinophilic infiltrate, characteristically involves both the arteries and the veins.

F-35. **Answers: c, d.** Classic polyarteritis nodosa is a systemic disease characterized by necrotizing vasculitis of small and medium-sized arteries. The vasculitis is characteristically focal and segmental, and both acute and healing lesions may coexist in the same patient and in the same vascular bed. About one fourth of patients with necrotizing sarcoid granulomatosis have abnormal chest radiographs, but cavitation does not occur and hilar lymph node enlargement is uncommon. Pulmonary involvement in Behçet's syndrome typically consists of thromboangiitis and multiple aneurysms; the latter may rupture and cause catastrophic hemoptysis. In Wegener's granulomatosis the vasculitis involves pulmonary arteries, pulmonary veins, and sometimes the microvasculature, including capillaries (capillaritis); involvement of the larger vessels is characteristically granulomatous in character, although sarcoid-like non-necrotizing granulomas are unusual.

F-36. **Answers: a, b, d, e.** The diagnosis of idiopathic pulmonary hemosiderosis is basically one of exclusion as neither its clinical nor its pathologic characteristics are pathognomonic. The pulmonary manifestations of hemoptysis and alveolar infiltrates are common to all of the syndromes; therefore, diagnosis rests upon clinical evaluation and pathologic examination of lung and kidney. Idiopathic pulmonary hemosiderosis is predominantly a disease of children and young adults with a female predominance. However, patients as old as 65 have been described. The most common presentation is periodic episodes of cough and hemoptysis with widespread alveolar-filling opacities on chest films. Repeated small episodes can result in interstitial fibrosis, clubbing, and cor pulmonale.

F-37. **Answers: a, b, e.** Pulmonary function tests most often show restricted lung volumes, reduced expiratory flow rates, hypoxemia, and a reduced diffusing capacity. The pathologic picture is nonspecific. Most often there is flooding of alveoli with erythrocytes and hemosiderin-laden macrophages in the alveoli, small airways, and the lung interstitium. Vasculitis, alveolar septal necrosis, and granulomas are absent. Immunofluorescent stains are negative. The most common abnormality is degeneration of type I pneumocytes and hyperplasia of type II cells. This suggests a primary pneumocyte insult rather than vascular injury.

F-38. **Answers: a, c.** IPH is characterized by recurrent bouts of diffuse alveolar hemorrhage without renal or other systemic involvement and therefore is a diagnosis of exclusion. Other causes of diffuse alveolar hemorrhage (i.e., mitral stenosis, connective tissue disease, systemic vasculitis, and Goodpasture's syndrome) must be ruled out. The histology is that of bland alveolar hemorrhage with minimal or no inflammation and hemosiderin accumulation. Electron microscopy reveals abnormalities of the alveolar-capillary basement membrane (i.e., separation, splits, and ruptures). Serum IgA is increased (50%), but IgA immune complexes are not present in the lung. Men predominate 2:1.

F-39. **Answers: a, b, e.** C-ANCA is an antibody causing cytoplasmic staining and directed against proteinase 3, an elastolytic neutral serine protease of both the neutrophil granule and the monocyte lysosome. P-ANCA is an antibody causing perinuclear staining and directed against myeloperoxidase, an enzyme in the primary granule of the neutrophil. C-ANCA is more likely to be elevated if the upper respiratory tract is involved (i.e., classical Wegener's granulomatosis). In those vasculitides with primarily renal disease (i.e., pauci-immune glomerulonephritis), P-ANCA is increased. There is, however, significant crossover in the small vessel vasculitides, and it is not uncommon for both to be increased. Circulating immune complexes are found in Henoch-Schönlein purpura (IgA complexes).

F-40. **Answer: d.** Amyloidosis is a chronic disease characterized by the extracellular accumulation of the B-pleated fibrillar protein amyloid in various organ systems. The biochemical nature of amyloid varies with its underlying cause. Immunoglobulin or light-chain amyloid (AL) is associated with myeloma, and with familial and primary amyloidosis. Amyloid A is found secondary to malignancy and inflammatory or infectious diseases. Systemic deposition of amyloid is often secondary to a number of predisposing conditions, including multiple myeloma, TB, chronic renal disease, cancer, inflammatory bowel disease, and chronic inflammation, or it may be familial. Primary amyloid deposition occurs without an associated disease, and can be widespread or localized. Secondary amyloidosis rarely has pulmonary involvement.

F-41. **Answer: e.** Radiographic features of amyloidosis may include atelectasis, interstitial infiltrates, hilar lymphadenopathy, and multiple cavitating or noncavitating nodules.

F-42. **Answer: a.** Hypersensitivity pneumonitis, or extrinsic allergic alveolitis, is a group of diseases associated with the intense and repetitive exposure to finely dispersed organic dusts. The disease can present in one of two ways. The acute form following heavy exposure is characterized by dyspnea 4–6 hours following exposure and later causes fever, chills, cough, and chest tightness. Removal from exposure usually results in complete resolution over a period of hours to days. The second, or chronic, form resulting from continued antigen exposure may present without any of the symptoms associated with the acute form, but rather more insidiously with fatigue, weight loss, cough, and dyspnea. Analysis of cellular components of BAL fluid reveal increased lymphocytes, particularly CD 8+ T lymphocytes, in nonfibrotic patients as compared to fibrotic ones.

F-43. **Answer: e.** BOOP is defined pathologically as granulation tissue plugs within the small airways with complete obstruction of the airways and extension of the granulation tissue into the alveoli. Other histologic features include intraluminal polyps comprised of connective tissue, fibrinous exudates, alveolar accumulations of macrophages, and inflamed alveolar walls.

F-44. **Answers: a, b, c, d, e.** The histologic findings are seen in the idiopathic form as well as in BOOP secondary to CT diseases, cocaine abuse, drug reactions, HIV infection, myelodysplastic syndrome, or radiation therapy.

F-45. **Answers: b, c, d, e.** A flu-like illness occurs in one third, mild dyspnea in one third, and cough with dyspnea in the remaining third. Hemoptysis and wheezing are rare. On physical examination, end inspiratory crackles are appreciated in two thirds.

F-46. **Answer: d.** The mean duration of symptoms at presentation is 3.6 months. In IPF, it is about 24 months. The chest radiograph usually shows bilateral patchy infiltrates which are often fleeting. Cavities and effusions are present in less than 5%. Chest CT reveals bilateral airspace consolidation and nodular opacities in one half. On HRCT, bronchial wall thickening and dilation can be appreciated. Pulmonary function tests reveal a low vital capacity in one half, no airway obstruction except in cigarette smokers, and a decreased $D_L CO$. BAL usually yields an increase in lymphocytes with or without eosinophils.

F-47. **Answers: a, b, c, d, e.** Classically, the clinical presentation is a subacute prodrome of nonproductive cough, dyspnea, and decreasing exercise tolerance. Pleuritic chest pain, low-grade fevers, and weight loss are also common. Physical examination findings may include generalized rales, clubbing, and cyanosis along with elevated lactate dehydrogenase. Chest radiographs show bilateral symmetric alveolar infiltrates in a "batwing" distribution, but asymmetric, unilateral, nodular patterns or Kerley's B lines have also been noted.

F-48. **Answer: b.** Pulmonary alveolar proteinosis has been reported in patients 6 months to 72 years of age, with average age at presentation being 30 to 50 years. The male:female ratio is 4:1. The cause of the disease is uncertain, but it is divided into "primary" or idiopathic pulmonary alveolar proteinosis and "secondary" pulmonary alveolar proteinosis, which has similar pathologic features and is described in patients with a variety of infections including PCP and hematologic malignancies, and in patients exposed to certain mineral dusts such as crystalline silica, quartz, fiberglass, volcanic ash, and aluminum.

F-49. **Answer: b.** The pathogenesis of excessive deposition of intraalveolar phospholipids actually remains unknown. There are a number of unproven theories including production of the intraalveolar material by desquamated alveolar lining cells, which have released granules and laminated structures into the alveolar content; overproduction of alveolar phospholipids and increased secretion of lamellar bodies into the alveoli; defective mechanisms of alveolar clearance, resulting in prolonged retention of alveolar lipoproteins; imbalance between production and removal of alveolar phospholipids; excessive stress, from the ingested lamellar bodies, on the catabolic capacities of alveolar macrophages; excessive proliferation and desquamation of type II pneumocytes, with resultant intraalveolar accumulation of intracellular substance; and accumulation of lipoprotein substance because of impaired phagocytic function of macrophages.

F-50. **Answers: a, b, c, d, e.** Findings in BAL fluid in pulmonary alveolar proteinosis include few alveolar macrophages; large acellular eosinophilic bodies in a diffuse background of eosinophilic granules and periodic acid–Schiff staining of proteinaceous material; and elevated LDH and shunt fraction.

F-51. **Answers: a, b, c, d.** Tubular myelin has been found in the extracellular alveolar lining layer and is believed to be a breakdown product or extracellular storage form of surfactant. Irregular concentric whorls, known as myelin structures, are found in the alveolar substance. The alveolar material deposited includes phospholipids and proteins. The phospholipids are qualitatively normal with dipalmitoyl lecithin being the primary constituent. Patients are also at high risk of superinfection with bacteria, mycobacteria, fungi, and *Nocardia*.

F-52. **Answers: a, b, c, d.** All of the statements describe Löffler's syndrome except that the IgE is not elevated.

F-53.	**Answers: a, b, c.** Bronchiolitis obliterans with organizing pneumonia (BOOP) or cryptogenic organizing pneumonia is characterized morphologically by buds of organizing granulation tissue (Masson bodies) within respiratory bronchioles, alveolar ducts, and alveoli. Clinically, patients with this histology often have a rather abrupt febrile onset and a course of several weeks of progressive dyspnea, cough, and weight loss. The involved bronchioles are usually respiratory bronchioles. The physiology is typically restrictive with reduced lung volumes and diffusing capacity and relatively normal expiratory flow rates.

F-54.	**Answers: b, c, d.** Bronchoalveolar lavage (BAL) in BOOP demonstrates a marked neutrophilia. In one study neutrophils comprised more than 50% of the cells recovered at BAL. There is usually rapid clinical improvement and a dramatic reduction in the BAL neutrophil count after treatment with corticosteroids. The chest radiograph shows patchy areas of airspace consolidation without hyperinflation. The most distinctive histologic features are patchy distribution of granulation tissue plugs, with uniform temporal maturity of the lesions, and preservation of background architecture. Histologically the lesions have a predominantly peribronchiolar distribution and fibrosis composed of proliferating fibroblasts.

F-55.	**Answers: a. 2, b. 1, c. 1, d. 2, e. 1.** The disease is randomly distributed in IPF. The location of lesions in BOOP are predominantly airspace and peribronchiolar and predominantly interstitial in IPF. The lesions are uniform and appear recent, and the fibrosis is fibroblastic in BOOP. The lesions are of varying ages, and the fibrosis mainly mature (collagen) in IPF. Foamy macrophages are common in BOOP and unusual in IPF.

F-56.	**Answers: b, c, d.** Prednisone (1 mg/kg or 60 mg/day) often results in rapid clinical improvement. Then the dose is decreased to 20–40 mg/day for at least one full year. Recurrence in individuals treated with corticosteroids is usually associated with early cessation of therapy. The salient ultrastructural features of BOOP include acute epithelial injury involving peribronchiolar-alveolar duct/alveolar septal lining cells, epithelial necrosis and denudation of epithelial basal laminae, and proliferation of bronchiolar and alveolar epithelial cells. The chest radiograph shows patchy areas of airspace consolidation without hyperinflation. There is a diffuse patchy ground-glass appearance in about 65% of cases. Unilateral infiltrates, cavities, and pleural effusions have been reported.

F-57.	**Answer: d.** Bronchiolitis obliterans (occlusion of bronchioles with loose granulation tissue) may occur as a result of viral infections (adenovirus and measles are the important ones), inhalation of toxic substances (oxides of nitrogen, ammonia, sulfur dioxide), and rheumatoid arthritis, where it may be related to penicillamine administration, although this has not been proved.

F-58.	**Answers: c, d, e.** Bronchiolitis obliterans is a nonspecific histologic response of the lung to injury that primarily affects the small conducting airways, usually sparing the interstitium. Extension of granulation tissue organization from the distal alveolar ducts into alveoli is characteristic of bronchiolitis obliterans and organizing pneumonia. Generally, the chest film shows bilateral patchy ground-glass or alveolar opacifications although a miliary pattern is sometimes seen. Bronchiolitis obliterans without organizing pneumonia is probably a common pathologic end point of a wide spectrum of injurious agents and diseases, which include toxic fume inhalation, infection, connective tissue disorders, organ and bone marrow transplantation, and idiopathic causes. Nitrogen dioxide, sulfur dioxide, ammonia, chlorine, phosgene, and cadmium oxide have been associated with bronchiolitis obliterans.

F-59. **Answers: c, d, e.** Bronchiolitis obliterans is a nonspecific histologic response of the lung to injury resulting in fibrosis that primarily affects the small conducting airways, usually sparing the interstitium. It is a common lower respiratory tract illness in children, often secondary to the respiratory syncytial virus. Bronchiolitis obliterans is rare in adults, but when it occurs it has been associated with *Mycoplasma pneumoniae*. The radiographic pattern is often interstitial, frequently with hyperinflation. Pulmonary function testing may reveal a restrictive and/or obstructive pattern. Individuals exposed to high concentrations of NO_2 can die within a few hours of noncardiogenic edema. Patients who survive may present several weeks later with cough, dyspnea, rales, and a miliary or nodular pattern on the chest radiograph. These patients have widespread bronchiolitis obliterans without organizing pneumonia.

F-60. **Answer: d.** Spontaneous pneumothorax is a common finding in this entity. Pleural effusion, hemoptysis, and atelectasis are rare.

F-61. **Answer: b.** Although the disease entity is called eosinophilic granuloma, indeed the most common cell on biopsy is the foamy macrophage or histiocyte. The distinctive Langerhans' macrophages have an elongated, convoluted, pale nucleus and contain Birbeck granules on electron microscopy.

F-62. **Answers: a, b, c.** Goodpasture's syndrome (GS) is characterized by immune alveolar hemorrhage and a rapidly progressive glomerulonephritis associated with antiglomerular basement membrane antibody in serum or on immunofluorescent staining of lung or renal tissue. Radioimmunoassays and ELISA assays are highly specific and are, in general, more sensitive than indirect immunofluorescence. In addition to aiding in diagnosis, these assays are also helpful in following response to therapy. The ESR may be elevated but usually not as elevated as in the vasculitides. The syndrome develops predominantly in cigarette smokers.

F-63. **Answers: b, e.** There is a male predominance in Goodpasture's syndrome with a reported ratio ranging from 2:1 to 9:1. Direct immunofluorescence reveals the characteristic linear deposition of IgG, IgM, and IgA along the glomerular basement membrane. Serum complement is normal and ANA is negative. General goals of therapy include removal of the offending Ig from the circulation by plasmapheresis and suppression of further antibody production by treatment with corticosteroids and either cyclophosphamide or azathioprine in concert with plasmapheresis, which is continued until antiglomerular basement membrane antibodies are undetectable or renal function stabilizes.

F-64. **Answers: a, c, d.** Ten to 20% of patients with LIP have Sjögren's syndrome. It is more common in females than in males and the peak age is 40 to 60 years. Lymphocytic interstitial pneumonitis has recently been described in AIDS patients, especially in children. Giant cell formation is common in desquamative interstitial pneumonitis. BOOP is characterized by the presence of lumenal granulation tissue in respiratory granules, alveolar ducts, and alveoli in conjunction with lymphoplasmacytic interstitial inflammatory infiltrates in alveolar ducts and alveoli, and occasionally in respiratory bronchioles.

F-65. **Answers: a, b, c.** Patients with disease in the collagen-vascular disease group develop lesions indistinguishable from IPF. Many patients with IPF have circulating autoantibodies such as rheumatoid factor and antinuclear antibodies. Circulating immune complexes can be detected in a proportion of patients and immunofluorescence shows immunoglobulin and complement in the alveolar walls of some patients in the active cellular phase of the disease. The prognosis is poor, with a median survival of 5 years and only perhaps 15% showing substantial improvement with therapy.

F-66. **Answers: b, d.** The bulk of interstitial cells in IPF are lymphocytes, macrophages, and plasma cells. Neutrophils and eosinophils are generally not striking and are often found in honeycombed spaces. With progression there is distortion of lung tissue and honeycombing, i.e., microcysts, 0.5–2 mm in diameter (dilated bronchioles or bronchiolectasis) separated by dense fibrous tissue, sometimes containing prominent muscle. UIP occurs in smokers and nonsmokers. Cellular interstitial pneumonia is characterized by a mixed round cell infiltrate and may be associated with drug reactions, collagen-vascular disease, and viral infections. Desquamative interstitial pneumonia is characterized by large numbers of hyperplastic alveolar macrophages in the airspaces.

F-67. **Answers: c, d, e.** Desquamative interstitial pneumonia has been reported in asbestosis, in other dust-caused diseases, and following nitrofurantoin therapy. The prognosis of desquamative interstitial pneumonia is considerably better than usual interstitial pneumonia, and responds to steroids better. Characteristically there is a ground-glass pattern of opacification in the costophrenic angle in desquamative interstitial pneumonia on chest radiographs. Lymphocytic intersti-

tial pneumonia is characterized by an exquisite interstitial infiltrate of lymphocytes and/or plasma cells (sometimes the latter predominate). A substantial number (perhaps two thirds) of patients with LIP have a serum gammopathy.

F-68. **Answers: b, c, d.** Eosinophilic pneumonia is characterized by prolonged or recurrent infiltrative lung disease in which eosinophils are the predominant cells. Peripheral eosinophilia is frequently not evident, but eosinophils are markedly increased in the lung on biopsy or bronchoalveolar lavage. Dyspnea, cough, weight loss, fevers, malaise and hemoptysis are the predominant complaints. Therapy is with corticosteroids, and the prognosis is generally good although occasional severe cases of eosinophilic pneumonia have developed acute respiratory failure. The chest film pattern of peripheral infiltrates and clear centrally (i.e., photographic negative pulmonary edema) is characteristic.

F-69. **Answers: a, c, d, e.** In pulmonary fibrosis, lung volume is reduced and the elastic recoil is increased (the pressure-volume curve is shifted down and to the right, and the shape of the curve is altered, i.e., compliance is decreased). Maximal airflow rates are low because they are being achieved at a low lung volume, but flow resistance is normal. Because the driving pressure is increased (elastic recoil), the flow rates are actually higher than expected at that low lung volume. Indeed, if they are not greater than expected at a particular lung volume, associated airflow limitation can be inferred. In a significant number of patients, lung function may be within normal limits, and the only abnormality found is a rise in $P(A-a)O_2$ and fall in PaO_2 during exercise.

F-70. **Answers: a, b, c, d, e.** By far the most common form of CNS involvement in sarcoidosis is cranial neuropathy, usually

VIIth nerve palsy, although involvement of all cranial nerves has been reported. This can be due to either direct granuloma invading the nerve or basilar meningitis. Aseptic meningitis is the second most common CNS abnormality. Hypothalamic insufficiency is the major cause of hypopituitarism. There is usually loss of 2 or more hormones from the anterior pituitary (GH, TSH, FH, and LSH are most common), often in association with abnormal water metabolism. All types of neuropathy have occurred: mononeuritis multiplex, polyneuropathy, or even Guillain-Barré syndrome. Seventy per cent of patients will have a monophasic illness, characterized by a good response to corticosteroids. The other 30% will have a relapsing course, but each relapse tends to be similar to the first episode and usually responds to an increase in corticosteroid therapy.

F-71. **Answers: a, b, c, d, e.** There are six general types of pleuropulmonary manifestations of rheumatoid arthritis: diffuse interstitial fibrosis, pleural effusion, necrobiotic nodules, Caplan's syndrome, pulmonary arteritis and hypertension, and diffuse patchy bronchiolitis obliterans.

F-72. **Answers: b, d, e.** Extraarticular disease occurs in patients with the most severe joint involvement. The majority of patients with pleuropulmonary disease have clinical evidence of rheumatoid arthritis, and in approximately 80%, the sheep cell agglutination or latex fixation tests are positive for rheumatoid factor. The $D_L CO$, maximal elastic recoil pressure of the lungs, and static compliance are normal. Obliterative bronchiolitis may be more common in rheumatoid arthritis patients treated with penicillamine. In "rheumatoid lung disease" patients with rheumatoid nodules have a relatively good prognosis.

F-73. **Answers: a, b, c, d.** About half of all reactions to nitrofurantoin are pulmonary.

Two forms of pulmonary toxicity are generally recognized: an acute hypersensitivity pneumonitis and a chronic fibrotic disease. The mechanism for the chronic form is less understood, but probably involves oxidant injury to the lung, as nitrofurantoin may induce local production of superoxide and hydrogen peroxide in the lung. The chest roentgenogram can be normal but usually reveals parenchymal infiltrates (interstitial more than alveolar) and pleural effusions. The duration of treatment prior to the onset of symptoms is 3–30 days. Some patients report having taken the drug in the past without difficulty. When pulmonary fibrosis occurs in a patient taking nitrofurantoin, duration of therapy has usually been more than 6 months.

F-74. **Answers: b, c, d.** Extrinsic allergic alveolitis is predominantly seen in non- or ex-smokers. The histologic features of allergic alveolitis depend on the stage at which the disease is seen. Acute lesions involve mainly respiratory bronchioles and adjacent vessels, producing an obstructive bronchiolitis. Most biopsies are taken in the subacute phase, and characteristically there is extensive chronic interstitial pneumonia with an infiltrate predominantly of lymphocytes and mixed with a minority of plasma cells. Characteristically, there are scattered giant cells of the foreign body type, and these may contain cleft-like spaces or small doubly refractile particles. There is inflammation of the distal respiratory bronchioles with destruction, distortion, and even obliteration. Bronchiolitis obliterans occurs in 50% of cases.

F-75. **Answers: a, b, c, d, e.** Lymphangioleiomyomatosis is a devastating disease afflicting only women, most of whom are of childbearing age. The disorder is characterized by diffuse cystic changes in the lungs and proliferation of smooth muscle-like cells in perivascular, perilymphatic, alveolar, and peribronchial locations. Lymphatic obstruction can lead to chylous effusions, ascites, and chyloptysis. A diversity of treatments have been attempted with varying, often unsatisfactory, results. By meta-analysis, treatment with progesterone appeared to be helpful in 50% of a small series and Provera, 400 mg IM every month, is recommended.

F-76. **Answers: a, c, d, e.** Hemoptysis results from venous obstruction and resultant hemorrhage. Airflow limitation and recurrent pneumothorax result from the bronchial and distal alveolar lesions. There are cystic thin-walled spaces but not emphysema. The course of the disease is usually that of relentless dyspnea. There is a significantly increased incidence of angiomyolipomas of the kidney in lymphangioleiomyomatosis.

F-77. **Answers: a, b, c, d, e.** Tuberous sclerosis is an autosomal dominant disease characterized by a triad of seizures, mental retardation, and a facial lesion—adenoma sebaceum. The lung pathology in lymphangioleiomyomatosis is virtually indistinguishable from that found in tuberous sclerosis. Nearly 80% of patients with tuberous sclerosis have angiomyolipomas of the kidney.

F-78. **Answer: b.** Chronic beryllium disease tends to follow a more aggressive course than sarcoidosis. The best differentiation between sarcoid and berylliosis rests on immunologic means. The most common method is the lymphocyte transformation test, which confirms the diagnosis of chronic beryllium disease in the proper clinical setting. Lymphocytes sensitized to beryllium undergo blastic transformation with uptake of tritiated thymidine on exposure to antigen. Chronic beryllium disease has a positive lymphocyte transformation test and negative Kveim test. The test can be performed on lymphocytes obtained from peripheral blood or

BAL. BAL lymphocytes often have a stimulation index 10- to 20-fold greater than serum, suggesting a localized specific immune response. The test is unaffected by steroid therapy.

F-79. **Answers: a, b, d.** Unlike sarcoid, chronic beryllium disease rarely presents with isolated hilar adenopathy; extrapulmonary disease is less common; and the Kveim test is negative. As with sarcoid, there is disturbed T lymphocyte function with anergy, decreased T4:T8 ratio peripherally, helper T cell accumulation in the lung, reticulonodular infiltrates with or without hilar adenopathy, and a restrictive ventilatory defect with decreased $D_L CO$.

F-80. **Answer: c.** The inhalation of particles or aerosols of beryllium metal, oxides, or salts may cause either an acute or a chronic syndrome. Whereas acute beryllium disease is a toxic, dose-related disorder limited to the respiratory system, chronic berylliosis is a multisystem disorder; it may progress from acute injury but usually occurs without obvious antecedent events, although stresses such as pregnancy and surgery have been reported to precipitate symptoms in some chronic cases. The differentiation between sarcoidosis and berylliosis is a difficult one. The chest film and abnormalities of function may resemble those of stage II or III sarcoid. Serum immunoglobulins, ACE levels, and lysozyme levels can all be elevated by both processes.

F-81. **Answers: a, c.** *Allogeneic* bone marrow transplantation refers to marrow harvested from a non-twin sibling; *syngeneic* bone marrow transplantation refers to marrow harvested from an identical twin; in *autologous* bone marrow transplant, the patient serves as his/her own donor. The frequency of complications in each is:

Complication	Autologous	Allogeneic	Syngeneic
Idiopathic interstitial pneumonia	Uncommon (4%)	Common (12%)	Common (12%)
Diffuse alveolar hemorrhage	Common (21%)	Uncommon	Uncommon
CMV pneumonitis	Less common (4%)	Common (16%)	Rare
Graft-versus-host disease	None	Common	None

F-82. **Answers: b, c, d, e.** The most common form of pulmonary involvement in connective tissue disease is a chronic interstitial pattern indistinguishable from idiopathic pulmonary fibrosis. Pulmonary lesions are commonly found in patients with progressive systemic sclerosis, the main lesion being interstitial pneumonitis. Pulmonary function tests usually reveal a restrictive pattern with reduced lung compliance and impaired diffusing capacity, often before any clinical or radiographic evidence of lung disease appears. Busulfan, chlorambucil, cyclophosphamide, melphalan, and uracil mustard cause fibrosis in a dose-dependent manner. The patient's age, number of cycles and cumulative dose, history of lung disease, hematologic abnormalities, combination chemotherapy, and, most important, concomitant use of radiation therapy or oxygen exert synergistic or additive effects.

F-83. **Answers: a, b, c.** Bleomycin toxicity should be suspected when the cumulative dose exceeds 150 units. Lung disease is present in 20–50% of patients with cumulative doses of 200–550 units. Of the antibiotics, nitrofurantoin is most likely to produce lung disease. It may cause either an acute, spontaneously resolving pneumonitis associated with peripheral eosinophilia or a chronic interstitial pneumonitis pathologically indistinguishable from idiopathic pulmonary fibrosis. Pulmonary histiocytosis X, or eosinophilic granuloma of the lung, is characterized by granulomatous infiltration of the interstitium and bronchial walls, predominantly by histiocytes. Electron microscopic studies frequently reveal a characteristic X-body within the histiocytes obtained from lung biopsy tissue or bronchoalveolar lavage. Pulmonary lymphangioleiomyomatosis is a rare progressive disease of the lung characterized by hamartomatous proliferation of smooth muscle in perivascular, perilymphatic, alveolar wall, and peribronchial locations. The disease afflicts women of childbearing age. The mean survival in idiopathic pulmonary fibrosis is 4–6 years, although the clinical course is variable.

F-84. **Answer: d.** Spirometry is restrictive. The $D_L CO$ is reduced and is said to correlate with the extent of parenchymal involvement seen on roentgenogram. The degree of fibrosis is dictated by the duration and degree of dust exposure as well as the size of the asbestos contaminants. Bronchogenic carcinoma and mesothelioma are four times more common in patients with a history of significant talc exposure than in the general population. This is speculated to be the result of the asbestos in the talc, rather than the talc itself. The natural history of talc pneumoconiosis is similar to that of other pneumoconioses with slowly progressive pulmonary fibrosis. Radiographic characteristics include parenchymal and pleural abnormalities. Pleural plaque formation probably occurs as a result of the asbestos contamination and not the true talc itself.

F-85. **Answer: c.** In this disorder, lipoproteinaceous bodies are found on BAL. The intraalveolar material consists of glycoproteins and lipids that make up normal pulmonary surfactant. A similar histopathologic picture has been found in acute sandblaster's silicosis. In fact, occupational exposure is found in 50% of cases, most often to silica, asbestos, and cadmium. There is no support for the theory that it results from an increased production of surfactant by alveolar type 2 lining cells. Decreased function of alveolar macrophages has been reported, but this is due to the engorgement of macrophages with the surfactant material rather than a primary macrophage defect. The condition occurs with various hematologic disorders, including Fanconi's anemia, paraproteinemias, acute and chronic myelocytic leukemia, and various other hematologic malignancies.

F-86. **Answer: e.** Bacterial, fungal, and opportunistic infections, most commonly nocardiosis, complicate the condition in 10–20% of cases. Type 2 lining cell hyperplasia of alveolar walls as well as an acellular lipoproteinaceous material fill the alveolar spaces. This material stains positively with periodic acid–Schiff stain, and the diagnosis is established by demonstrating a positive periodic acid–Schiff stain of the intraalveolar material. Eosinophils may be present within lung tissue, but they are certainly not the predominant cell type. Whole lung lavage is effective treatment.

F-87. **Answer: d.** The coexistence of calcinosis, Raynaud's phenomenon, esophageal dysfunction, sclerodactyly, and telangiectasia is indicative of the CREST syndrome. Also, pulmonary vascular involvement may predominate in patients with the CREST syndrome.

F-88. **Answer: d.** The idiopathic variety of eosinophilic pneumonia is characterized by either an indolent progressive form of dyspnea and cough or a more acute form with recurrent fever, cough, and dyspnea. Asthmatic symptoms are often present. The chronic form of eosinophilic pneumonia has a characteristic radiographic presentation, i.e., a peripheral rather than a central distribution of the alveolar infiltrates, the so-called radiographic negative of pulmonary edema. Peripheral eosinophilia is common but may not be present early in the disease.

F-89. **Answer: d.** Eosinophilic pneumonia may follow helminthic infestations, constitute a pulmonary drug reaction, result from allergic bronchopulmonary aspergillosis, complicate the hypereosinophilic syndrome, or represent tropical eosinophilia. The majority of cases, however, are idiopathic and have been referred to in the literature as Löffler's syndrome. The idiopathic variety of eosinophilic pneumonia is more common in women.

F-90. **Answer: b.** Rheumatoid arthritis is associated with pleurisy with or without effusion; interstitial pneumonitis; necrobiotic nodules (nonpneumoconiotic intrapulmonary rheumatoid nodules) with or without cavities; Caplan's syndrome (rheumatoid pneumoconiosis); pulmonary hypertension secondary to rheumatoid pulmonary vasculitis; bronchiolitis obliterans; and drug-induced pneumonitis, especially following gold therapy.

F-91. **Answers: a. 5, b. 4, c. 1, d. 3, e. 2.** In sarcoidosis one finds a BAL lymphocytosis composed of T helper cells and a biopsy revealing noncaseating granulomas. In eosinophilic pneumonia there is an eosinophilic infiltration of the alveolar structures, and in the great majority of cases peripheral blood eosinophilia coexists. In alveolar proteinosis, lipoproteinaceous bodies are found in BAL, and an acellular lipoproteinaceous material fills alveolar spaces. This material stains positively with periodic acid–Schiff stain. In lipoid pneumonia the fluid contains lipid-laden macrophages. In diffuse alveolar hemorrhage there are hemosiderin-laden macrophages.

F-92. **Answers: b, e.** There is a marked difference in activity and composition of monocytes/lymphocytes between the lung and peripheral circulation in sarcoidosis. Cells obtained via BAL have increased lymphocytes and T helper cells;

the suppressor/helper ratio is low. The lymphocytes hyperreact when exposed to mitogens, spontaneously proliferate and secrete IL-1, have increased IL-2 secretion/receptors, are able to stimulate B cell maturation and antibody production, and also secrete macrophage inhibitory factor and monocyte chemotactic factor. The peripheral lymphocytes/monocytes are virtually opposite to those in BAL fluid. One third of sarcoid patients are lymphopenic, there is decreased reaction when exposed to mitogens, decreased IL-1 generation, and defective secretion and action of IL-2.

F-93.   **Answer: c.** Besides idiopathic pulmonary hemosiderosis, other causes of alveolar hemorrhage include anti–basement membrane antibody disease (Goodpasture's syndrome), SLE, other systemic vasculitides, alveolar hemorrhage associated with renal disease, and exogenous agents (d-penicillamine and trimethallic anhydride).

F-94.   **Answers: a, e.** Lymphocytic interstitial pneumonitis has the histologic features of pseudolymphoma with mature lymphocytes and plasma cells infiltrating the interstitium. It is characterized by the absence of involvement of local lymph nodes and extrapulmonary tissues. Associated diseases include AIDS/ARC, SLE, hypo- or hypergammaglobulinemia, chronic active hepatitis, and pulmonary amyloidosis. There is a female predominance; age ranges from 14 months to 77 years.

F-95.   **Answers: a, c, e.** Coal worker's pneumoconiosis often occurs in association with silicosis. Two forms of disease predominate on chest roentgenographic evaluation: simple pneumoconiosis, represented by small opacities (less than 1 cm in diameter) mainly in the upper lung zones; and progressive massive fibrosis (opacities >1 cm in diameter). Pulmonary func-

tion abnormalities occur in simple coal worker's pneumoconiosis only when there is a history of cigarette smoking, regardless of the extent of radiographic involvement. Patients with progressive massive fibrosis may expectorate large quantities of dark sputum (melanoptysis).

F-96.   **Answers: a, b, c, d.** The pleuropulmonary manifestations of systemic lupus erythematosus (SLE) are (1) pleurisy with or without effusion; (2) atelectasis; (3) interstitial pneumonitis (less than 5% of patients) in two forms—acute interstitial pneumonitis (tachypnea, dyspnea, high fever, cyanosis, and potentially fatal pulmonary hemorrhage) and chronic interstitial pneumonia (dyspnea, nonproductive cough, pleuritic chest pain, hypocapnia, impaired diffusing capacity, and a restrictive ventilatory defect); (4) uremic pulmonary edema; (5) diaphragmatic dysfunction with loss of lung volume; and (6) infectious pneumonia. Predominance in females is striking.

F-97.   **Answers: a, b, e.** The idiopathic variety of eosinophilic pneumonia is characterized by either an indolent progressive form of dyspnea and cough or a more acute form with recurrent fever, cough, and dyspnea. Asthmatic symptoms are often present. The chronic form of eosinophilic pneumonia has a characteristic radiographic presentation, i.e., a peripheral rather than a central distribution of the alveolar infiltrates, the so-called radiographic negative of pulmonary edema. The absence of peripheral eosinophilia does not rule out this diagnosis since eosinophilia may not be present early in the disease. The response to corticosteroids is often dramatic.

F-98.   **Answers: a. A, b. S, c. A, d. S, e. A.** Silicosis is found in miners, sandblasters, glass manufacturers, quarry workers, stone dressers, foundry workers, and boiler scalers. Patients with silicosis are highly susceptible to infection by *Mycobacterium tuberculosis* and other atypical mycobacteria. Bilateral pleural thickening along the lower or midthoracic walls, calcified pleural plaques, and hazy infiltrates composed of irregular or linear small opacities, especially in the lower lung zones (asbestosis), are the most common roentgenographic changes. Asbestos is also carcinogenic. Pleural and peritoneal mesotheliomas, stomach and colonic cancers, and bronchogenic carcinoma are recognized complications of asbestosis.

F-99. **Answers: a. S, b. A, c. A, d. S, e. A.** Scleroderma and rheumatoid arthritis occasionally complicate silicosis. Smoking appears to facilitate the damaging effects of asbestos inhalation. Bilateral pleural thickening along the lower or midthoracic walls, calcified pleural plaques, and hazy infiltrates composed of irregular or linear small opacities, especially in the lower lung zones, are the most common roentgenographic changes of asbestosis. Silicosis appears as multinodular rounded densities, predominantly in both upper lung zones. These roentgenographic changes almost always occur before the development of clinical and functional abnormalities. Workers employed in ship building, asbestos mining, and the automotive, insulation, cement, and textile industries are at greatest risk.

F-100. **Answers: a, b, c, e.** Talc is used in a wide variety of industries: rubber, textiles, leather, paint, paper, pharmaceuticals, and of course cosmetics. The lung can clear moderate amounts of talc dust by phagocytosis, ciliary action, or lymphatic drainage, thereby preventing pulmonary tissue damage. This clearing mechanism can be hindered by cigarette smoke, and can be overcome by prolonged exposure to an excessive load of talc. "True" talc (free from most impurities) induces a macrophage-mediated inflammatory response with foreign body reaction in the lung. Fibrous talc (talc naturally contaminated by asbestos) produces this same reaction as well as a more vigorous fibrotic reaction and probably tumorigenesis as well.

F-101. **Answers: a, c.** Talc and asbestos occur in similar geologic strata and are mineralogically related. Quartz (crystalline silica) sometimes contaminates talc and, along with asbestos, is fibrogenic. Talc mined in Vermont contains only traces of quartz and asbestiform minerals. Talc mined in other areas (California, Montana, Texas, North Carolina) contains various amounts of these contaminants. Cosmetic-grade talc is the highest-grade talc and contains the least quantity of asbestos and quartz. The major determinant in the development of talc pneumoconiosis is the dose of exposure (duration and degree) and not the grade of talc.

F-102. **Answers: a, c, d.** Eosinophilic granuloma or pulmonary histiocytosis X describes histiocytic infiltration confined to the lung and/or lytic bone lesions (usually of the ribs, pelvis, and skull) and diabetes insipidus. Peripheral blood eosinophilia is not a feature of this disease. EG most commonly occurs between the ages of 20 and 40 years and almost exclusively in cigarette smokers. Pneumothorax occurs in around 25% of the patients. In adults, the disease is most often confined to the lungs but can be associated with lytic bone lesions and diabetes insipidus. Physical examination is frequently normal, but auscultation of the lungs can reveal scattered wheezes. As opposed to other interstitial lung diseases, inspiratory crackles are rarely present.

F-103. **Answers: a, d.** Radiographically, these patients present with a diffuse, symmetric increase in interstitial pulmonary parenchymal markings. Unlike that in many other ILDs, the interstitial markings are predominantly in the upper and mid lung zones, and there is an absence of volume loss. The development of cavitating nodules progressing to honeycombing can occur in advanced disease. Pleural effusions and adenopathy are rare.

F-104. **Answers: a, b, e.** Evidence of generalized disease, especially cutaneous involvement, is associated with a worse prognosis. High-resolution CT scans further delineate the interstitial changes present in EG and characteristically reveal nodules and thin-walled cysts. Lung volume is normal or increased. Airflow limitation, reduced $D_L CO$, and hypoxemia are common.

F-105. **Answers: a, e.** Gross examination of the lungs in EG often will show blebs or cysts on the lung surface which may explain the frequency of pneumothoraces in these patients. Microscopically, multiple granulomatous lesions are present in the interstitium near the small bronchioles. The histiocyte itself, commonly referred to as the Langerhans' cell, is characterized by a weakly eosinophilic cytoplasm and an irregularly folded and indented nucleus. Intracytoplasmic inclusion bodies called X-bodies or Birbeck granules are seen by electron microscopy. S-100 protein immunostaining differentiates Langerhans' cells from other types of histiocytic cells.

F-106. **Answers: a, b, c, e.** Serum IgG antibodies against cytoplasmic components of neutrophils (ANCA) were first described in patients with segmental necrotizing glomerulonephritis and later in patients with clinical manifestations consistent with Wegener's granulomatosis. Serum titers seem to correlate with disease activity. Two immunofluorescent patterns are described: one associated with diffuse cytoplasmic staining (C-ANCA) and one with perinuclear staining (P-ANCA). If formalin-fixed neutrophils are used as substrate, both C-ANCA and P-ANCA produce identical diffuse granular cytoplasmic staining.

F-107. **Answers: a, b, c, e.** In patients with systemic vasculitis and pauci-immune necrotizing glomerulonephritis, 80–90% of the P-ANCA have specificity for myeloperoxidase. ANCA are found primarily in patients with Wegener's granulomatosis, microscopic poyarteritis nodosa, and idiopathic crescentic glomerulonephritis. The glomerular lesions found in these three diseases are identical—a necrotizing vasculitis with marked extracapillary crescent formation and a paucity of immune complexes. The significant difference among Wegener's granulomatosis, microscopic poyarteritis nodosa, and idiopathic crescentic glomerulonephritis, at least clinically, is the degree of extrarenal involvement.

F-108. **Answers: a, d, e.** The type of ANCA tends to correlate with the distribution of disease. C-ANCA is most commonly seen in vasculitis involving the lung, sinus, and kidney (Wegener's) whereas patients with renal-limited disease are more likely to be positive for P-ANCA. Patients with systemic arteritis including renal and lung involvement, but without classic Wegener's (i.e., no evidence of necrotizing granulomas on lung biopsy) or nonspecific extrarenal symptoms, have an equal frequency of the two. The strong association between pauci-immune necrotizing glomerulonephritis and a positive ANCA allow for presumptive serologic discrimination of this form of GN from the other two major categories of rapidly progressive GN; that due to immune complexes (postinfectious GN, cryoglobulinemia, Henoch-Schönlein purpura, and lupus) and that due to anti–basement membrane disease (Goodpasture's or renal-limited anti-glomerular basement membrane disease). Unfortunately, since the definition and criteria for vasculitis have blurred recently with the creation of many overlap syndromes, the ability to differentiate between the various types of vasculitis based on ANCA subtype is less certain. Clinically evident organ involvement and appropriate biopsies will be the most important criteria for separating those groups.

F-109. **Answers: a, b, c, d.** Glomerulonephritis due to immune complexes are poststreptococcal or postinfectious glomerulonephritis. Cryoglobulinemia, Henoch-Schönlein purpura, and lupus erythematosus may have immune complexes. Goodpasture's or renal-limited anti-GBM disease are due to anti–basement membrane antibodies.

F-110. **Answers: a, b, e.** Whether the presence of a positive ANCA in an appropriate clinical setting is enough to initiate treatment without a biopsy is controversial. Some suggest that a positive ANCA in the face of rapidly progressive glomerulonephritis is adequate basis for initiating treatment without a biopsy. When the lung is involved, the yield of an open biopsy is much greater and usually allows for differentiation between Wegener's and microscopic PAN. Long-term studies support the benefit of combined steroid and cyclophosphamide in Wegener's. With rare exceptions, the ANCA subtype does not change during the course of disease.

F-111. **Answers: a, b.** This condition may present with a flu-like illness, combined with an absence of pulmonary infiltrates or cavitary lesions on radiograph. The P-ANCA is positive, and an open lung biopsy does not reveal any evidence of vasculitis. Long-term studies support the benefit of combined steroid and cyclophosphamide in Wegener's while the benefit of adding cyclophosphamide is not as clear in the other diseases.

F-112. **Answers: a. CSS, b. WG, c. CSS, d. CSS, e. CSS.** Nervous system abnormalities, especially mononeuritis multiplex, are more frequent findings in CSS (75%) than in WG (22%). Anticytoplasmic antibodies (IgG antibodies directed against intracytoplasmic antigens of neutrophils) is a sensitive test for WG, and a changing titer value may be helpful in plotting disease activity and remission. Tissue eosinophilia occurs in CSS, and pleural effusions in CSS are rich in eosinophils as well. CSS patients respond dramatically to steroid therapy alone, whereas WG requires additional immunosuppressive therapy, such as cyclophosphamide, for ultimate control of disease.

F-113. **Answers: a. CSS, b. CSS, c. WG, d. CSS, e. CSS.** Peripheral blood eosinophilia was found in less than 10% of cases of WG and is noted in 94% of cases of CSS at presentation, usually with asthmatic symptoms. The eosinophilia may disappear when vasculitis emerges. Renal failure is the most common cause of death in WG. CSS shows cutaneous disease in more than 70% of cases in contrast to only 13% of patients with WG. Cardiovascular abnormalities are more common in CSS (50%) than in WG (12%), and cardiac failure and myocardial infarction are the most common causes of death in CSS.

F-114. **Answers: a, c, e.** Lymphomatoid granulomatosis is an angiocentric and angiodestructive lymphoreticular proliferation involving the upper respiratory tract, lungs, skin, kidneys, and peripheral and central nervous systems. Although the process is thought to be non-neoplastic and granulomatous, progression to lymphoma occurs in about 15% of cases. Even without overt progression to lymphoma, the 5-year survival rate is less than 50% even in those patients treated with steroids. There are morphologic and clinical similarities between polymorphic reticulosis (PMR) (or midline malignant reticulosis) and lymphomatoid granulomatosis.

F-115. **Answer: d.** The typical lung lesions of Wegener's granulomatosis are necrotizing granulomas combined with vasculitis. The granulomas may be discrete or confluent, forming an irregular geographic pattern. The central zone of necrosis is surrounded by a tight cluster of lymphocytes, plasma cells, and palisading histiocytes. Eosinophils may be present but generally are not prominent. The vascular lesions are essentially a necrotizing angiitis, which may affect some small and large blood vessels and spare others.

F-116. **Answers: a, b, d, e.** Idiopathic pulmonary hemosiderosis is predominantly a disease of children and young adults with a female preponderance. However, patients as old as 65 have been described. The most common presentation is periodic episodes of cough and hemoptysis with widespread alveolar-filling opacities on chest film. Repeated small episodes can result in interstitial fibrosis, clubbing, and cor pulmonale.

F-117. **Answers: a, c, d, e.** Pulmonary capillaritis with diffuse alveolar hemorrhage, but without the typical pathologic changes in the lung or usual clinical presentation (upper airway disease, cavitating of pulmonary lesions) of WG, occurs in 5%. In the majority of these, the more typical clinical and histologic picture appears later during the course of the disease. Accompanying the diffuse alveolar hemorrhage there is always a focal segmental necrotizing glomerulonephritis, but the appearance of a cutaneous leukocytoclastic vasculitis, arthritis, and episcleritis is less predictable. The typical histology is medium vessel involvement, tissue necrosis, and granulomatous inflammation. WG with pulmonary capillaritis, diffuse alveolar hemorrhage, and renal failure alone cannot be differentiated from systemic necrotizing vasculitis by any clinical, histologic, or serologic criteria. Only the appearance of the typical histology or clinical findings will identify WG.

F-118. **Answers: a, b, e.** Most patients present later in life, with a mean age at diagnosis of 57 years. Most present with nonspecific symptoms including fever, nonproductive cough, dyspnea, and chest pain, but 40% are asymptomatic. Chest roentgenogram demonstrates bilateral patchy or nodular infiltrates in 80% of cases, although 20% have single, isolated masses or infiltrates. Cavities have been reported, but are the exception. Organ involvement is limited to the lung in the vast majority of cases, although one case with skin involvement and one case with renal and genitourinary involvement have been reported. Histology reveals a diffuse cellular infiltrate involving alveolar structures, with infiltration of blood vessels and invasion of peripheral airways. The infiltrate consists primarily of mature lymphocytes with lesser numbers of plasma cells and plasmacytoid lymphocytes. "Loose" giant cell granulomas are usually present, but necrosis is the exception.

F-119. **Answers: b, e.** Like allogeneic bone marrow transplant recipients, patients with autologous bone marrow transplants have a high incidence of pulmonary complications (40–60%). However, the spectrum of disease appears to be significantly different. Diffuse alveolar hemorrhage has been previously described in immunocompromised hosts, but it is usually a secondary phenomenon, often seen in association with thrombocytopenia and/or invasive fungal infection. Clinically these patients most often present with dyspnea, nonproductive cough, fever, and patchy alveolar infiltrates. Hemoptysis is rare. The frequency of diffuse alveolar hemorrhage appears to be higher in patients over 40 and in those with solid malignancies (especially melanoma), as well as in renal insufficiency. Diffuse alveolar hemorrhage most commonly occurs within 40 days of transplantation, although there have been case reports of diffuse alveolar hemorrhage occurring 1 to 2 years after autologous bone marrow transplant.

F-120. **Answers: c, d.** Classic polyarteritis nodosa is a systemic disease characterized by necrotizing vasculitis of small and medium-sized arteries. The vasculitis is characteristically focal and segmental, and both acute and healing lesions may coexist in the same patient and in the same vascular bed. About one fourth of patients with necrotizing sarcoid granulomatosis have abnormal chest radiographs, but cavitation does not occur and hilar lymph node enlargement is uncommon. Pulmonary involvement in Behçet's syndrome typically consists of thromboangiitis and multiple aneurysms; the latter may rupture and cause catastrophic hemoptysis. In Wegener's granulomatosis, the vasculitis involves pulmonary arteries, pulmonary veins, and sometimes microvasculature, including capillaries (capillaritis); involvement of the larger vessels is characteristically granulomatous in character, although sarcoid-like nonnecrotizing granulomas are unusual.

F-121. **Answers: a, b, d.** The diagnosis of idiopathic pulmonary hemosiderosis is basically one of exclusion as neither its clinical nor its pathologic characteristics are pathognomonic. The pulmonary manifestations of hemoptysis and alveolar infiltrates are common to all of the syndromes; therefore diagnosis rests on clinical evaluation and pathologic examination of lung and kidney. Idiopathic pulmonary hemosiderosis is predominantly a disease of children and young adults with a female preponderance. However, patients as old as 65 have been described. The most common presentation is periodic episodes of cough and hemoptysis with widespread alveolar-filling opacities on chest film. Repeated small episodes

can result in interstitial fibrosis, clubbing, and cor pulmonale.

F-122. **Answer: e.** Treatment for systemic vasculitis is a combination of corticosteroids and cyclophosphamide. In the NIH experience, 5-year survivals have been 13 months without treatment, 48 months with corticosteroids, and 90 months with steroids and cyclophosphamide.

F-123. **Answers: b, d, e.** Necrotizing sarcoid granulomatosis is four times more common in females. The vasculitis in necrotizing sarcoid granulomatosis affects both the arteries and veins, but is not as destructive as in other forms of necrotizing angiitis. Systemic vasculitis does not occur in necrotizing sarcoid granulomatosis. It is now recognized that lymphomatoid granulomatosis is an angiocentric T cell lymphoma. Bronchocentric granulomatosis is basically a necrotizing bronchitis caused by hypersensitivity to *Aspergillus*.

F-124. **Answers: c, d.** Wegener's granulomatosis is somewhat more common in men, with a peak incidence in the fifth decade. The recognition of the different types of pulmonary angiitis and granulomatosis relies heavily on the correct interpretation of the morphologic features of the disease. Only an open lung biopsy, and not a transbronchial or needle biopsy, should be relied on for the histologic diagnosis of pulmonary angiitis and granulomatosis. The pulmonary lesions of Churg-Strauss syndrome may resemble chronic eosinophilic pneumonia with granulomatous necrosis and vasculitis. Unlike polyarteritis, the necrotizing angiitis, with prominent eosinophilic infiltrate, characteristically involves both the arteries and veins, and the angiitis may affect the systemic and pulmonary blood vessels with equal frequencies.

F-125. **Answers: a, b, c, d, e.** Liebow defined five varieties of pulmonary angiitis and granulomatosis: (1) classic Wegener's granulomatosis; (2) limited angiitis and granulomatosis of the Wegener's type; (3) lymphomatoid granulomatosis; (4) necrotizing sarcoid angiitis and granulomatosis; and (5) bronchocentric granulomatosis. This group of heterogeneous disorders has tissue necrosis and more or less granulomatous inflammatory reaction and angiitis nearly always present in pulmonary vessels and sometimes in systemic vessels as well.

F-126. **Answers: a. 1, b. 3, c. 4, d. 2, e. 5.** In lymphomatoid granulomatosis, initial therapy with oral cyclophosphamide and prednisone is recommended; in benign lymphocytic angiitis, chlorambucil; in Wegener's granulomatosis, cyclophosphamide with prednisone for symptomatic relief; in bronchocentric granulomatosis, resection of the involved lobe or segment; and in allergic granulomatosis, corticosteroids.

F-127. **Answers: a. 1, b. 3, c. 1, d. 2, e. 4.** In lymphomatoid granulomatosis there are multiple nodular densities that wax and wane, and upper airway involvement is not extensive. In benign lymphocytic angiitis and granulomatosis the upper airway and extrapulmonary sites are rarely involved. In Wegener's granulomatosis, upper and lower airway involvement predominate, and there are multiple nodular densities that wax and wane. In bronchocentric granulomatosis, unilateral lesions involving the upper lobe predominate. In allergic granulomatosis, severe progressive asthma is predominant.

F-128. **Answers: a. 3, b. 1, c. 1, d. 2, e. 2.** In lymphomatoid granulomatosis there are atypical lymphoid cells with plasmacytolytic features, while polymorphonuclears and eosinophils are rare. In polyarteritis nodosa the polymorphonuclear is the predominant inflammatory cell. In Wegener's granulomatosis, polymorphonuclears, histiocytes, and the occasional eosinophil are seen. In bronchocentric granulomatosis there are eosinophils, as well as lymphocytes, mononuclears, and multinucleated giant cells. In allergic granulomatosis, eosinophils are the predominant inflammatory cell.

F-129. **Answers: a, b, c, d, e.** Radiographically, most patients have fleeting or persistent infiltrates, nodules, or cavities, and less commonly, diffuse infiltrates, pleural effusions, and atelectasis due to endobronchial obstruction. In general, the limited form of the disease typically has multiple, bilateral, frequently cavitating, thin-walled lesions, especially of the lower lung fields.

F-130. **Answers: a, b, c, d.** Limited Wegener's was first described by Carrington and Liebow, who reported 16 patients with pulmonary lesions classic for Wegener's, but little or no other organ involvement and no glomerulonephritis. The limited form occurs in approximately 15% of patients with Wegener's, and its clinical and pathologic manifestations are identical to the classic form of the disease except for the lack of renal involvement. It carries a better prognosis and has a more favorable response to steroids, a longer duration of remission, and a more prolonged survival even without the use of steroid therapy.

2-5 Vascular Disease

V-1.　**Answers: c, d, e.** Chronic thromboemboli of the major pulmonary arteries (main, lobar, segmental) usually manifests as progressive worsening of symptoms of dyspnea on exertion over months to years. This progression has been thought to be the result of recurrent emboli and/or propagation of an existing clot, in a small minority of cases. Rather, in the majority of patients the progressive clinical deterioration is believed to be related to the single insult and the resulting hemodynamic compromise. Hypoxemia and severe pulmonary hypertension with exercise may lead to progressive RV dysfunction. In addition, hypertensive changes develop in nonobstructed areas of the pulmonary vasculature. Later there may be opening of the foramen ovale or development of small pulmonary AV fistulas.

V-2.　**Answers: b, c, d, e.** One or more segmental or larger unmatched perfusion defects are not specific. Similar findings occur in fibrosing mediastinitis, pulmonary artery agenesis, primary tumors of the pulmonary artery, congenital branch stenosis, and extrinsic compression. This test can help to distinguish between chronic embolism and primary pulmonary hypertension.

V-3.　**Answers: a, b, d.** Hereditary hemorrhagic telangiectasia is the most common disorder associated with pulmonary arteriovenous malformations. Fifteen per cent of patients with hereditary hemorrhagic telangiectasia have pulmonary arteriovenous malformations, and conversely 60% of patients with pulmonary arteriovenous malformations have hereditary hemorrhagic telangiectasia. Secondary causes of pulmonary arteriovenous malformations include chest surgery, trauma, actinomycosis, schistosomiasis, cirrhosis, metastatic carcinoma, and pulmonary hypertension. Hereditary hemorrhagic telangiectasia is an autosomal dominant disorder with a frequency of 1–2/100,000. Three types of angiodysplastic lesions have been described: telangiectasias, arteriovenous malformations, and aneurysms. These defects are believed to be secondary to endothelial cell degeneration, defects in endothelial junctions, and weakness of the perivascular tissue. The most common presenting symptoms in order of frequency include epistaxis, GI bleeding, GU bleeding, and pulmonary hemorrhage.

V-4.　**Answer: e.** Pulmonary symptoms may be absent in up to 50% of patients with pulmonary AVMs. When present, however, the most common symptom is dyspnea, followed by atypical chest pain and, less frequently, hemoptysis or hemothorax. Hypoxemia is relatively common and can be found in 80% of cases at presentation associated with orthodeoxia. Variable chest film abnormalities are detected in the majority of cases and include solitary nodules, masses, or minute diffuse AVMs. Small lesions (1–2 mm) may be subtle on plain films and may not be visualized on plain films or on angiography. Pulmonary hypertension is a rare finding that is reported in less than 1% of cases.

V-5.　**Answers: a, b, c, d.** Some debate still exists in the literature concerning the appropriate management of asymptomatic patients discovered to have pulmonary AVMs. Prior to 1978, surgical resection was the only effective modality for treating these lesions. Since the introduction of embolotherapy, however, this is now believed by many to be the preferred method of treatment. Reported complications are rare, namely air embolism, pleuritic chest pain, and paradoxic embolization. Contrast echocardiography and radionuclide angiocardiography have been reported by some authors to assist in the diagnosis in those patients with micro-AVMs. Alternatively, radionuclide angiocardiography has been reported to be a highly sensitive diagnostic modality and, if negative, excludes the diagnosis. Current radiologic literature recommends embolization of lesions with feeding arteries greater than 3 mm.

V-6.   **Answer: e.** Factors that are associated with an increased incidence of pulmonary infarction include left ventricular failure, the number of lobes with pulmonary emboli, the presence of lung cancer. Although pulmonary embolism is by far the most common cause of pulmonary infarction, other disease states associated with pulmonary infarction include sickle cell anemia, vasculitis, and *in situ* thrombosis secondary to hypercoagulable states. There is no evidence of increased incidence of pulmonary infarction in pulmonary fibrosis.

V-7.   **Answers: a, c, d.** Those with indeterminate or moderate-probability scans have an approximate 40% chance of having a pulmonary embolus, and an angiogram should be performed. The low-probability scan poses the greatest controversy. In retrospective studies, there was a <10% chance of having an angiographically documented pulmonary embolism. However, in the largest prospective study by Hull et al, these were associated with a positive angiogram in 25–40% of cases. The reasons for this discrepancy are not clear, and may have to do with patient selection and definition of "low probability." Should a patient with a high clinical risk for pul-

monary embolus have a moderate- or high-probability lung scan, but a negative pulmonary angiogram, venous studies of the legs should be performed. If these are positive, the patient is treated by anticoagulation. If these tests are negative, a repeat lung scan should be considered. Cough, hemoptysis, previous PE, malignancy, obesity, bed rest, neck vein engorgement, hepatomegaly, hypotension, and fever are significantly associated with mortality, but size of embolus is not.

V-8.   **Answers: b, c, e.** Thromboembolism invariably causes ventilation/perfusion imbalance. Some have suggested that low $\dot{V}/\dot{Q}$ ratios account for all of the hypoxemia while others have indicated that virtually all of the $P(A-a)O_2$ is due to shunt. The anatomic basis for this shunt is unknown. The opening of normally closed intrapulmonary AV anastomoses or foramen ovale is theoretically possible. Cavitation following pulmonary infarction may be due to either superinfection or bland necrosis of the infarcted area; 80–90% of cases of pulmonary infarction with cavitation show evidence of superinfection based on sputum cultures or autopsy histopathology. Superinfection may occur by endobronchial or hematogenous spread. Complications of pulmonary infarction with cavitation include pneumothorax, abscess, and empyema formation. The resolution of angiographic and hemodynamic signs of pulmonary emboli occurs on the average in 10–21 days. The time to resolution and completeness of resolution depends on factors including the patient's age, cardiac status, and the size of the embolus.

V-9.   **Answer: a.** Pulmonary embolism may lead to pulmonary edema in the absence of left ventricular disease because of transudation of fluid in unobstructed vessels secondary to increased capillary hydrostatic pressure (overperfusion pulmonary edema); decreased plasma oncotic pressure due to fluid overload; alteration in microvascular permeability due to regional ischemia/hypoxia; or release of vasoactive mediators after pulmonary embolism such as prostoglandins, serotonin, or histamine.

V-10. **Answer: b.** The morphologic findings are virtually indistinguishable from those of obstructive emphysema. There is bronchitis, bronchiolitis, bronchiolitis obliterans, and dilatation and destruction of lung parenchyma. The condition does not always affect just one lung to the exclusion of the other. It may occur in various anatomic distributions, including one or two lobes of one lung and one lobe of the other. There is often a history of acute lower respiratory tract infection during childhood, and occasionally in adulthood. Several investigators have shown either definitive or highly suggestive evidence of adenoviral pneumonia as the responsible agent for the condition. The peripheral parenchyma is poorly ventilated via collaterals maintaining lung expansion.

V-11. **Answer: d.** The clinical presentation is variable. Most patients are asymptomatic, some complain of dyspnea on exertion, and others have repeated lower respiratory infections. PFTs reveal reduction in VC and mild reduction in flow. $D_L CO$ (single-breath method) is also often reduced. ABGs at rest are normal, but hypoxemia may occur with exercise. When cor pulmonale occurs it is usually a result of intercurrent disease in the contralateral lung (e.g., bronchitis). On fluoroscopy or the appropriate roentgenograms one sees a mediastinal shift to the contralateral side during exhalation.

V-12. **Answers: a, c, d.** The unilateral hyperlucency is caused by decreased blood in the affected lung (not necessarily by increased volume). The hilum on the affected side is small but present. The volume of the affected lung depends on the age of the patient at the time of the infectious insult. The younger the patient at the time, the smaller the fully developed lung, since the insult prevents further maturation. An expiration chest film reveals the greatest differences in the two lungs: increased volume of air and decreased blood in the affected lung contrasted with the opposite in the contralateral lung. The differential diagnosis is finite and includes proximal interruption of a pulmonary artery (PA agenesis) and pulmonary thromboembolism (either acute or chronic—unresolved). The $\dot{V}/\dot{Q}$ scan in Swyer-James syndrome reveals diminished perfusion diffusely not focally, and the ventilation scan reveals delayed distribution and clearance of gas.

V-13. **Answer: b.** Patent foreman ovale is a potential route for a right-to-left shunt in conditions resulting in higher right atrial than left atrial pressure. This can occur with (1) Valsalva maneuver, (2) use of PEEP, (3) pulmonary embolus, (4) pulmonary artery hypertension, (5) COPD, (6) valvular pulmonic stenosis, and (7) right ventricular myocardial infarction.

V-14. **Answers: a, b, c.** Primary pulmonary hypertension consists of three pathological patterns: thromboembolic occlusion of small muscular arteries (*in situ* versus embolic), medial hypertrophy with or without "plexiform" lesions, and venoocclusive disease. There is an association with cirrhotic liver disease. The National Registry has shed new light on the epidemiology, as the male/female ratio is only 1:1.7. The $D_L CO$ is usually markedly decreased but does not correlate with the degree of hypertension.

V-15. **Answer: e.** Based on careful pathologic studies, this disorder can be broken down into: primary pulmonary hypertension, chronic thromboembolism, chronic pulmonary venous hypertension, and pulmonary veno-occlusive disease.

Pulmonary schistosomiasis is a cause of pulmonary hypertension. Plexogenic pulmonary lesions are seen in primary pulmonary hypertension. Thromboembolic pulmonary hypertension is characterized by thrombi in various stages of evolution with thickened vessel media but rarely any evidence of muscular hypertrophy.

V-16. **Answers: a. 4, b. 2, c. 2, d. 3.** Full-dose intravenous heparin remains the mainstay of treatment for established pulmonary embolism and has a proven survival benefit. Urokinase and streptokinase, plasminogen activators with proven thrombus-dissolving capacity, enhance 24-hour angiographic and lung scan resolution in comparison to heparin alone. In addition, both agents significantly reduce pulmonary artery pressures at 24 hours. Both agents are used in early treatment of massive pulmonary embolism with or without shock. Pulmonary embolectomy may be considered in massive pulmonary embolism with shock and deterioration despite maximum medical management.

V-17. **Answer: c.** Low-dose subcutaneous heparin leads to a significant survival benefit in postoperative patients. Full-dose intravenous heparin remains the mainstay of treatment for established pulmonary embolism and has a proven survival benefit. Two well-controlled studies have demonstrated that continuously infused intravenous heparin causes less bleeding than does bolus intravenous heparin. Sufficient heparin should be administered to maintain the activated partial thromboplastin time (or similar clotting test) at two times the control value. The duration of anticoagulation in the patient with no obvious predisposition is unclear but probably should be at least 6 weeks of full-dose anticoagulation (heparin followed by warfarin).

V-18. **Answers: b, d.** Interestingly, pulmonary infarction is more common in the setting of smaller emboli obstructing distal vessels as opposed to larger more proximal emboli. Overall, pulmonary infarction is thought to be uncommon because the lung parenchyma has three potential sources of oxygen: the pulmonary arteries, the bronchial circulation, and the airways. This may account for its occurrence predominantly in patients with underlying cardiopulmonary disease, in whom there may be baseline compromise in tissue oxygenation. The symptoms most commonly encountered in pulmonary infarction include pleuritic chest pain (57%) and hemoptysis (20%). The radiographic features of pulmonary infarction are homogeneous densities in a segmental distribution, which are often preceded by elevation of the ipsilateral hemidiaphragm with a wedge-shaped peripheral infiltrate (Hampton's hump). The pleural fluid is usually exudative with more than 10,000 RBCs.

V-19. **Answers: c, d, e.** Early in a pleural effusion associated with pulmonary infarction there appears to be a polymorphonuclear predominance, but later in the course there is a lymphocyte predominance. Greater than 50% of patients suspected of having a pulmonary embolus have normal angiograms. Similarly, more than 50% of patients suspected of having deep venous thrombosis have normal venograms, and more than 50% of patients with pulmonary emboli have clinical evidence of deep venous thrombosis.

V-20. **Answer: b.** Pleural effusions tend to be small and unilateral, appearing soon after symptoms begin and reaching maximal volume early in the course. Infected infarction following pulmonary embolus is a known but uncommon cause of empyema. Anaerobes are frequently found on culture. An increase in effusion after appropriate therapy for 2–3 days, suggests recurrent emboli, hemothorax, or superinfection/empyema.

V-21. **Answer: c.** The chest film and often the hemoglobin may be normal even with multiple pulmonary arteriovenous shunts. A simple way to assess the extent of shunt is to have the subject breathe 100% oxygen for about 15 minutes, i.e., until virtually all of the nitrogen is washed out of the lungs. Oxygen carried in the blood, both in combination with hemoglobin and in physical solution in the plasma, is related to the PaO_2. The important point to remember is that a major shunt may be present even though the hemoglobin is fully saturated, i.e., $SaO_2=100\%$ and the PaO_2 is greater than 100 mm Hg.

V-22. **Answers: a, b, c.** Exercise limitation is reflected in an early plateau in oxygen consumption, i.e., VO_2 max is markedly reduced. The supply of energy to the exercising muscles is generally inadequate to meet their demand, so that there is early anaerobic metabolism and the respiratory quotient is high. The cardiac output may not rise appropriately, and the blood pressure may fall. Ventilation is increased disproportionately, primarily because of an increased respiratory rate. As a consequence, the dead space/tidal volume ratio does not fall and may even rise.

V-23. **Answers: c, d.** Patent foreman ovale is a potential route for paradoxic embolism and in conditions resulting in higher right atrial than left atrial pressure, a right-to-left shunt. The Valsalva maneuver is one such situation. Right ventricular infarction usually presents as an inferior or posterior infarction with clear lung fields and jugular venous distention, frequently complicated by hypotension and high-grade AV block. Elevated RA pressure may open a previously closed foreman ovale, producing a right-to-left shunt and profound arterial hypoxemia not explained by pulmonary vascular congestion and not responsive to 100% oxygen. PEEP increases right-sided pressures and may increase the shunt. Vasodilators, which decrease pulmonary artery pressures, often decrease left atrial pressure and result in an increased interatrial pressure gradient.

V-24. **Answers: a, c.** The incidence of the syndrome as well as mortality vary with the number and type of bone fractured. Fractures of both femur and tibia carry a higher mortality (20%) than does fracture of the femur alone (9%), which in turn has a worse prognosis than isolated tibial fracture (3%). Pathophysiologically, there are probably two mechanisms involved. First, mechanical disruption of large fat stores and venous drainage of bone marrow may result in direct embolization of fat droplets to pulmonary vasculature. Second, biochemical destabilization of plasma lipids in severely stressed (traumatized) patients may produce intravascular fat droplets capable of sequestration in the lung. Complement activation is a sensitive (100%) but nonspecific (40%) predictor, whereas frozen clot section assays for fat are probably neither sensitive nor specific for the diagnosis. A long-term sequela of fat embolism from any cause is osteonecrosis.

V-25. **Answer: b.** A variety of pulmonary lesions are seen with Behçet's syndrome, including pleurisy, pulmonary fibrosis, tuberculosis, airflow obstruction, recurrent pneumonitis, aneurysms, *in situ* thromboses, and pulmonary hypertension.

V-26. **Answers: c, d, e.** The differential diagnosis of postcapillary hypertension includes left ventricular dysfunction, mitral stenosis and regurgitation, atrial tumors, pulmonary veno-occlusive disease, large pulmonary vein *in situ* thrombosis, congenital heart anomalies such as cor triatriatum, anomalous pulmonary drainage, and fibrosing mediastinitis.

V-27. **Answer: a, e.** In sickle cell disease there is an absolute lymphocytosis. The SaO_2 is decreased at a given PaO_2. The spectrum of infectious disease in sickle cell disease does not suggest impairment of cell-mediated immunity. The clinical course of acute chest syndrome is longer than that of bacterial pneumonia. Exchange transfusion is beneficial in treatment of acute chest syndrome if the clinical situation appears to be deteriorating.

V-28. **Answer: a, b, c, e.** Pleural effusion is a well-known complication of fluid overload of any cause, and this is associated with increased pulmonary capillary permeability. Interstitial fibrosis is a common finding at autopsy in renal failure. The lungs are the most common site of soft tissue calcification. Susceptibility to pulmonary tuberculosis is increased.

V-29. **Answer: a, b, c, d, e.** Pulmonary edema secondary to upper airway obstruction has been well described in children with croup and epiglottitis. The pulmonary edema is usually manifested after relief of the obstruction; however, cases have been reported in which the pulmonary edema developed prior to relief of the obstruction. The mechanism of pulmonary edema secondary to upper airway obstruction is multifactorial: (1) Inspiration against an obstruction can generate a marked negative intrapleural pressure resulting in decreased pulmonary capillary perivascular pressure, which would favor hydrostatic transudation of fluid into the interstitium. If this is prolonged the integrity of the capillary wall may be disrupted. (2) Increased venous return with increased preload as well as afterload.

V-30. **Answer: e.** In sickle cell disease there is microvascular obstruction of the pulmonary circulation by rigid red blood cells. The disease is characterized by a heightened susceptibility to pulmonary infection, and recurrent pulmonary infiltrates in multiple lobes. The disorder is characterized by substitution of valine for glutamic acid at position 6 of beta globulin subunit of hemoglobin tetramer. There is an absolute increase in both T4 and T8 cells, but the T4:T8 cell ratio is not increased.

V-31. **Answer: a.** Pulmonary venous hypertension causes redistribution of the vascular pattern with distension of upper lobe vessels and narrowing of lower lobe vessels, signs of interstitial edema (septal edema Kerley's A and B lines), perivascular edema (manifested by loss of definition of pulmonary markings), patchy alveolar hemorrhage, and deposition of hemosiderin.

V-32. **Answers: d, e.** Myxomas occur mostly in the 4th and 5th decade. In contrast, malignant fibrous histiocytomas affect younger women. No ethnic predilection is seen. Myxomas histologically are hypocellular, nonvascular tumors without necrosis and with rare mitosis. Pulmonary vein occlusion from a rare left atrial tumor is a rare example of postcapillary pulmonary hypertension.

V-33. **Answers: a, b, d.** Congenital pulmonary arteriovenous malformations (AVMs) are often multiple and in 15% of cases are associated with Rendu-Osler-Weber syndrome (hereditary hemorrhagic telangiectasias); 50% of patients with Rendu-Osler-Weber syndrome have pulmonary AVMs. Congenital AVMs are usually not recognized until the second or third decade of life but have been reported in all age groups. Acquired AVMs can occur after trauma, in longstanding liver disease, with carcinoma, or in schistosomiasis infections. Pathologically these lesions have a feeding vessel emanating from the hilum and a draining vessel leading to the right atrium.

V-34. **Answers: a, e.** Pathologically these lesions have a feeding vessel emanating from the hilum and a draining vessel leading to the right atrium. There can be multiple feeding and draining vessels. The lesions tend to have a lower lobe predominance and are often subpleural or interlobular. The afferent limb can include contributions from the bronchial arteries in addition to the expected pulmonary artery. Clinically there is a clear female preponderance (about 2:1); 50% of patients have dyspnea due to a right-to-left shunt with an associated low PO_2 and O_2 saturation; 50%; have epistaxis without associated Rendu-Osler-Weber syndrome.

V-35. **Answers: b, d, e.** Chronic hypoxia, when present, does not lead to the development of pulmonary hypertension. More worri-

some complications include cerebral abscesses, endocarditis, systemic emboli, hemoptysis (which can be massive), rarely spontaneous hemothorax (with pleuritic pain), and high-output congestive heart failure. Physical signs often present are cyanosis, clubbing, and a continuous murmur over the lesion (bruit). Diagnosis requires the recognition of a feeding and draining vessel and can be made on chest film. The lesion can also manifest as a coin lesion and has variably been described as resembling a bunch of grapes. The sharp margins of vascular structures are characteristic. Rapid-sequence CT scanning and angiography are more definitive tests.

2-6 Pleural Disease

PL-1. **Answer: b, c, e.** Pleural fluid eosinophilia is rare, although not unheard of, with tuberculous pleurisy and is unusual with a malignant pleural effusion despite the high incidence of pleural space hemorrhage. When air or blood is not present, parasitic disease, fungal infection, and drugs such as nitrofurantoin may be incriminated. Pleural fluid basophilia is rare but, when present, suggests leukemic involvement of the pleura. Mesothelial cells are predominant in transudative pleural effusions and are found, to a variable degree, in exudative effusions. The presence of more than 5% mesothelial cells virtually rules out tuberculous pleurisy.

PL-2. **Answers: b, d, e.** A milky pleural effusion that remains opaque following centrifugation rules out a large number of leukocytes. Differentiation between a chylothorax and a chyliform pleural effusion is accomplished by measurement of pleural

fluid triglyceride concentrations. The diagnosis of a chylothorax can be made presumptively if the triglyceride concentration is greater than 110 mg/dl. If the triglyceride concentration is less than 50 mg/dl, the patient does not have a chylothorax. Concentrations between 50 and 100 mg/dl represent a gray zone, and lipoprotein electrophoresis should be performed to determine the presence or absence of chylomicrons (presence is diagnostic of chylothorax). Chromosomal analysis can complement cytologic examination in the diagnosis of malignant pleural effusions, particularly if cytologic examination proves negative in lymphoma, leukemia, or mesothelioma.

PL-3. **Answers: a, b, c.** It has been suggested that relief of dyspnea following thoracentesis is related to reduction in the size of the thoracic cage, which allows the inspiratory muscles to operate on a more advantageous portion of their length-tension relationship. Unilateral pulmonary edema is most likely to occur in settings where large alveolar-pleural pressure gradients are created following removal of moderate to large amounts of fluid. This most commonly occurs in the setting of malignancy and with a trapped lung. A grossly bloody effusion in the absence of trauma is most likely to be due to malignancy. A whitish pleural effusion is due to either chyle or cholesterol, or to a large number of leukocytes. Anchovy-colored fluid results when an amebic liver abscess ruptures into the pleural space.

PL-4. **Answers: a, d.** Most effusions with elevated LDH levels have a higher percentage of LDH-4 and LDH-5 than in the corresponding serum. A rheumatoid factor titer in pleural fluid of ≥1:320, or equal to or greater than the serum rheumatoid factor, is suggestive of rheumatoid pleurisy. The chance of finding LE cells in pleural fluid appears to increase if the fluid is allowed to stand at room temperature for several hours before it is examined by Wright's staining. A pleural fluid antinuclear antibody (ANA) titer of ≥1:160 or a pleural fluid/serum ANA ratio of 1.0 or greater is suggestive, but not diagnostic, of lupus pleuritis. Pleural fluid complement levels, whether total hemolytic complement or complement components, are low in most patients with lupus pleuritis or rheumatoid pleurisy.

PL-5. **Answers: b, d.** On average, 50–60% of cases have a history of asbestos exposure, but the range is 0–99 %. The issue is complicated because of difficulty in obtaining a history of asbestos exposure. Autopsies show a wide prevalence of asbestos bodies in the general public (90% of urban dwellers). Most occupations at risk are held by men so that the male:female case ratio is from 2 to 6:1. There is a long latency period from exposure to tumor development (peak incidence is 35–45 years later), and so the typical patient is 50 to 70 years old, although cases do occur in children. In heavily exposed individuals there is an 8–10% risk of developing malignant pleural mesothelioma. The risk of developing bronchogenic carcinoma is 25%.

PL-6. **Answers: a, c, e.** The risk varies with the type of asbestos fiber. Amphiboles (crocidolite in UK, amosite in US) are worse than chrysotile (the most common commercial asbestos). The geometry (e.g., length-diameter and straight versus curved characteristics) of a fiber may affect how well a fiber is deposited in the lungs when it is inhaled, and whether or not the fiber is dissolved when deposited. Chrysotile is not readily deposited, and it seems to dissolve over time, whereas amphiboles persist indefinitely. Asbestos fibers cause mesothelial proliferation *in vitro* and are incompletely phagocytosed, leading to continuous release of O_2 radicals and lysosomal enzymes.

PL-7. **Answers: a, d, e.** Hematogenous spread to liver, brain, and bone is a common finding at autopsy. Malignant pleural mesothelioma is locally invasive and can involve ribs, lung, pericardium, diaphragm, heart, and contralateral lung. Needle biopsy is positive in 25–39%, but the biopsy tract through the skin may be invaded by tumor in 20% of cases. The pathology is epithelial (50%), sarcomatous (20%), or mixed "biphasic"(30%). Distinction from metastatic adenocarcinoma is based on histology if the tumor is biphasic; intracellular neutral mucin on PAS-diastase stain excludes malignant pleural mesothelioma. Malignant pleural mesothelioma has a characteristic pattern of staining for keratin (immunohistochemistry) and demonstrates characteristic long microvilli on the cell surface. The mean survival is 6–14 months, with a 50% one-year survival.

PL-8. **Answers: a, c, e.** The most common symptoms are dyspnea, chest pain, and weight loss. The chest film usually shows a large, unilateral effusion on the right (60%), left (35%), or bilaterally (5%). Pleural plaques or interstitial fibrosis are evident in 20%. Pleural fluid is typically a serosanguineous exudate. Cigarette smoking does not increase the risk of malignant pleural mesothelioma.

PL-9. **Answers: a, b.** Pleural biopsy specimens reveal fibrosis, nonspecific inflammation, and occasionally dilated lymphatic channels. None of these features is pathognomonic of yellow nail syndrome. Typically, the pleural fluid is exudative, the protein is often greater than 4.0 and LDH is always elevated, with normal pH, normal glucose, and white blood cell counts less than 100 K/ml with a lymphocytic predominance (≥80%). A distinct retardation in nail growth is present. The cuticle may be absent, and there is a tendency for the nail to form a hump.

PL-10. **Answers: b, c, e.** The face, lower extremities, and hands are most often involved, and ascites has been rarely described. When present, pleural effusion is usually bilateral, and spontaneous resolution is infrequent. Chronic bronchitis, bronchiectasis, sinusitis, pneumonia, pleuritis, and empyema can be associated with the classic yellow nail syndrome triad. Abnormal ciliary motility is not a pathophysiologic mechanism of recurrent sinopulmonary infection. Pulmonary function testing has most frequently shown mixed obstructive and restrictive physiology, but restrictive and normal airflow patterns have also been demonstrated.

PL-11. **Answers: a, b, d.** The yellow nail syndrome is a combination of yellow nails, chronic lymphedema, pleural effusions, and recurrent sinopulmonary infections. The syndrome may occur with any combination of these features. Lymphangio-

graphic studies performed in a limited number of patients with yellow nail syndrome have demonstrated deficient, hypoplastic, and varicose lymph trunks in the involved extremity. Impaired lymphatic drainage as a consequence of the deficient lymphatic vessels produces the edema and effusions characterizing this syndrome. Pleural fluid albumin kinetics support the notion of impaired lymphatic drainage rather than overproduction. Nail changes may herald the onset of the syndrome by months or years. The median age of onset is 40 years, with a 2:1 female predominance.

PL-12. **Answer: b.** Pleural effusion in rheumatoid arthritis is a serous exudate that is predominantly lymphocytic. It occurs almost exclusively in men. It may antedate signs and symptoms. A low glucose concentration is characteristic. It is usually unilateral, on the right more often than on the left.

PL-13. **Answers: a, b, c, e.** Complications of chylothorax are predominantly related to the removal of chyle with secondary deficiencies in its constituents, i.e., protein and fat malnutrition and immune deficiency related to lymphopenia. Traumatic chylothoraces are usually managed nonoperatively because the majority of effusions will resolve spontaneously. A milky appearance can also be seen in some nonchylous effusions, due either to large numbers of lymphocytes (as in empyema) or to elevated levels of cholesterol—a "pseudochylous" effusion. Pleuritis and fever are rare because chyle is not an irritant for the pleural surface. Although they are the sine qua non of chylous effusions, chylomicrons are actually only a small component of chyle in the thoracic duct. The presence of a chylomicron band on lipoprotein electrophoresis is proof of chylous effusion, whereas the more easily measured triglyceride level is nearly as definitive.

PL-14. **Answers: b, c.** The basic mechanisms underlying chylothoraces of various causes is disruption of the thoracic duct. Simple obstruction (e.g. ligation) is not enough because of extensive collateral lymphatics. An effusion with triglyceride greater than 110 has a greater than 99% chance of being chylous. Conversely, if the triglyceride level is less than 50, there is a less than 5% chance that the effusion represents a chylothorax. Levels in between generally require lipoprotein electrophoresis for diagnosis. The glucose level in chyle is not different from the plasma level. Characteristics of the fluid include an alkaline pH, total protein between 2.2 gm/dl and 6 gm/dl, low LDH, and a cellular differential composed almost entirely of lymphocytes. Lymphocyte subset analysis shows less than 5% of the total cells to be B lymphocytes.

PL-15. **Answers: a, b, c.** The most common cause of chylothorax is mediastinal malignancy, usually lymphoma. In the absence of trauma, the patient should be presumed to have mediastinal malignancy, unless proved otherwise. Approximately 20% of the cases follow thoracic surgery, and 5% are related to trauma— penetrating and blunt. Other causes include congenital and idiopathic, LAM, intestinal lymphangiectasia, subclavian vein cannulation, aortography, and even nephrotic syndrome. Although generally milky white, odorless, and alkaline, chylothorax can be bloody, turbid, or even serous. Furthermore, not all milky pleural effusions are due to chylothorax, and milky fluid can stain negative for fat and still be chylous. The glucose level in chyle is not different from the plasma level. The cholesterol/triglyceride ratio is usually <1.

PL-16. **Answers: b, c.** The thoracic duct usually ascends from the abdomen into the chest cavity along the right paravertebral gutter to the level of the fifth thoracic vertebra.

It then crosses over to the left paravertebral gutter until it reaches the left subclavian vein. Normally, chyle flow is between 1500 and 2500 cc/day. Hence, chylothorax tends to be large. The pattern and volume of chyle flow vary depending on the level of activity, diet, and the nutritional status of the patient. Disruption of the duct below the fifth thoracic vertebra usually leads to right-sided effusions whereas disruption above that level more commonly causes left-sided or bilateral effusion.

PL-17. **Answers: b, c, d.** In the exudative stage, the pleural fluid contains primarily PMNs, normal glucose, and normal pH. In the fibrinopurulent stage, infection has developed in the fluid, and it contains PMNs, bacteria, and cellular debris, and fibrin deposition begins on visceral and parietal pleura. Glucose and pH decrease, and LDH increases. In the organization stage fibroblasts grow and produce a "pleural peel"; 35% of empyemas develop in the absence of pneumonic infection (25% from trauma or postoperatively; 10% spontaneous). The initial intervention is placement of a chest tube into the dependent part of the pleural fluid as soon as possible after diagnosis. Decortication is indicated only for continued pleural infection and not to remove thickened pleura, which has been demonstrated to gradually resolve without intervention. If after 6 months the thickening persists and is associated with PFT abnormalities, decortication may be considered.

PL-18. **Answers: b, c, e.** Classically, effusions are considered to be a manifestation of primary TB in young patients. However, this pattern is changing. More recent reports demonstrate that not only has the disease become one of older adults, but there is also a significant incidence of tuberculous pleural effusion as a manifestation of reactivation disease. Simple effusions are thought to develop when sub-pleural caseous material ruptures into the pleural space. This fluid is usually a serous exudate with few if any infecting organisms. It is believed that a delayed hypersensitivity reaction develops to tubercular proteins and this results in effusion. The pleural fluid is almost uniformly exudative and shows a lymphocyte predominance but not always. Glucose is typically >50 mg/dl, LDH>1000. Pleural fluid adenosine deaminase levels can be used to diagnose tuberculosis with sensitivity of 99% and a specificity of 89%. False-positives were found in lung cancer, lymphoma, empyema, mesothelioma, and rheumatoid arthritis.

PL-19. **Answers: b, d, e.** A negative PPD when the patient is seen early does not rule out the diagnosis. When repeated, the test is generally positive. Sputum is usually negative unless there are infiltrates. Pleural effusion with more than 10% eosinophils is seldom TB. The effusion usually resolves in 6 weeks. Treatment is the same as for pulmonary TB and usually involves a two- or three-drug regimen (INH, rifampin) for 12–18 months. Markedly symptomatic patients with pleurisy can be effectively treated with 40 mg/day of prednisone.

PL-20. **Answers: b, c, d.** A black fluid suggests *Aspergillus* involvement of the pleura. A putrid odor is diagnostic of an anaerobic empyema. An ammonia odor suggests urinothorax. Pleural effusions are frequently subpulmonic and bilateral in the nephrotic syndrome. Pleural effusions in peritoneal dialysis occur usually within 48 hours of initiating dialysis.

PL-21. **Answers: c, d.** Exudative effusions are caused by inflammation of the pleura and by impaired lymphatic drainage of the pleural space, and thus are associated with either a capillary protein leak or decreased protein removal from the pleu-

ral space. In the acute stages, the inflammatory exudates generally have high leukocyte counts with a predominance of polymorphonuclear leukocytes. However, in the subacute or chronic stages, these effusions may have low cell counts with a predominance of mononuclear cells. Exudates have a pleural fluid/serum total protein ratio greater than 0.5, a pleural fluid/serum LDH ratio greater than 0.6, and pleural fluid LDH greater than two thirds the upper limits of normal of the serum.

PL-22. **Answers: a, c, e.** The total leukocyte count in pleural fluid is virtually never diagnostic; however, counts greater than 50,000/µl usually are found only in parapneumonic effusions, usually empyema. Chronic exudates in malignancy and tuberculosis usually have less than 5000 leukocytes/µl. The parapneumonic effusion is the most common exudative effusion with greater than 10,000 leukocytes/µl, but this degree of cellular response can be seen with pancreatitis, postcardiac injury syndrome, and pulmonary infarction.

PL-23. **Answers: a, c.** When only the LDH is elevated, a malignancy or a parapneumonic effusion should be considered. Transudative pleural effusions have pleural fluid total protein concentrations less than 3.0 gm/dl. However, on occasion, patients with congestive heart failure treated with diuretic therapy may have pleural fluid protein concentrations between 3.0 and 4.0 gm/dl. The pleural fluid/serum protein ratio is greater than 0.5 in exudates. Tuberculous pleural effusions generally have protein concentrations above 4.0 gm/dl, whereas parapneumonic effusions have a wide range from 2.5 to more than 6 gm/dl. In general, patients with complicated parapneumonic effusions tend to have higher protein concentrations; however, in the individual case, this point cannot differentiate uncomplicated from complicated effusions. Up to 10% of malignant pleural effusions are transudates.

PL-24. **Answer: a, d, e.** When the pleural fluid is grossly purulent, a pleural fluid leukocyte count often is less than anticipated because many of the polymorphonuclear leukocytes have undergone lysis, and the debris from these cells accounts for the purulence of the fluid. Diseases in which the patient presents soon after the onset of symptoms—such as pneumonia, pulmonary embolism, and pancreatitis—usually are associated with polymorphonuclear predominant effusions. Pleural fluid lymphocytosis, particularly lymphocyte counts of 85 or 90% of the total cells, is highly suggestive of tuberculous pleurisy. However, other diagnoses such as lymphoma and sarcoidosis need to be considered. Carcinomatous pleural effusions will have more than 50% lymphocytes in two thirds of cases. Greater than 10% eosinophils suggests a benign, self-limited pleural effusion associated with air or blood in the pleural space such as following hemothorax, pulmonary infarction, or pneumothorax.

PL-25. **Answers: b, d, e.** A large number of plasma cells in pleural fluid suggests multiple myeloma with pleural involvement. A low pleural fluid glucose (less than 60 mg/dl or a pleural fluid/serum ratio of less than 0.5 is found in rheumatoid pleurisy (85% incidence), empyema (80%), malignant effusion (30%), tuberculous pleurisy (20%), lupus pleuritis (20%), and esophageal rupture. In tuberculous pleurisy, lupus pleuritis, and malignancy, the glucose concentration is generally in the 30 to 55 mg/dl range. A pleural fluid pH less than 7.30 with a normal blood pH is found with the same diagnoses that have a low pleural fluid glucose. Pleural fluid acidosis has been found with esophageal rupture, empyema, rheumatoid pleurisy, malignancy, tuberculous

pleurisy, and lupus pleuritis. In the setting of pneumonia and a parapneumonic effusion, a pleural fluid pH less than 7.10, usually in association with a glucose less than 40 mg/dl and an LDH more than 1000 U/L, suggests the need for chest tube drainage.

PL-26. **Answers: b, c, d.** A pH less than 7.30 predicts a short survival time in a malignant pleural effusion. An increased pleural fluid amylase or a pleural fluid/serum ratio greater than 1.0 is seen in acute pancreatitis, pancreatic pseudocyst, esophageal rupture, or malignancy. Patients with acute pancreatitis may have pleural effusions with high amylase levels. These effusions resolve over several days to weeks as the acute pancreatitis subsides. Patients with esophageal rupture develop high pleural fluid amylase levels; the amylase is of salivary gland origin. LDH levels higher than 1000 U/L suggest either a complicated parapneumonic effusion or rheumatoid pleurisy.

PL-27. **Answers: a, c, d, e.** Pathogenesis in the large effusions is most likely to be a defect in the tendinous diaphragm, usually <2 cm, providing a conduit for ascitic fluid. Diagnosis is best established by intraperitoneal injection of technetium colloid but simultaneous sampling of peritoneal and pleural fluid after intraperitoneal injection of technetium colloid, while creating pneumoperitoneum and observing for a hydropneumothorax, and thoracoscopy have also been performed. Transport via diaphragmatic lymphatics may also be important. Treatment should begin with salt/water restriction and diuretics, but this is often ineffective. Chest tube placement should be done with careful attention to volume loss; and chemical pleurodesis should be performed and the tube removed the same day.

PL-28. **Answers: a, b.** Treatment involves therapy aimed at the ascites (sodium restriction, diuretics, large-volume taps). Thoracentesis should be reserved for diagnostic purposes except for acute symptomatic relief. In general, CT thoracostomy should be avoided. There is one report suggesting that pleurodesis may be effective, but in general pleurodesis is unsuccessful.

PL-29. **Answers: a, c, d.** Pleural effusions occur in 5–10% of cirrhotic patients with ascites. Although rare, pleural effusions also occur in cirrhotic patients with minimal or absent ascites. Pleural effusions due to cirrhosis with or without ascites are always transudates, except for the rare unexplained bloody effusion seen with cirrhosis. The majority of effusions are right-sided, but bilateral and left-sided effusions are also seen. They are usually large.

PL-30. **Answer: b.** BAPE is the earliest manifestation of asbestos-related pleuropulmonary disease usually occurring within the first 10–20 years following initial exposure. Most patients are asymptomatic, with effusions being discovered on a routine chest radiograph. About 20% of patients have chest pain. The pleural effusion is a small, unilateral bloody exudate that may contain eosinophils. The effusion resolves over several months but may be recurrent or may progress to severe pleural fibrosis.

PL-31. **Answer: d.** Tuberculous pleural effusions are serous exudates that are predominantly lymphocytic. The tuberculin skin test may be negative in early cases. There is a strong tendency for subsequent active pulmonary disease to develop if the patient is not treated. This condition is less common in children than in adults. The effusion is rarely bilateral.

PL-32. **Answer: d.** Pleural effusion is commonly associated with staphylococcal pneumonia, *Streptococcus pyogenes* infection, actinomycosis, and *Haemophilus influen-*

zae pneumonia.

PL-33. **Answers: a, b, d.** The effusion tends to occur as the symptoms of pancreatitis are resolving or weeks to months after an episode of pancreatitis. In over 80% of cases the etiology of pancreatitis is alcoholic, and the remainder are due to trauma. Cases of pancreatic pleural effusions due to pancreatic carcinoma have been described. The effusion is usually large. More than 25% have an associated ascites. The pleural effusion is exudative with an amylase value that is much higher than the serum amylase.

PL-34. **Answer: d.** Pancreatic amylase is elevated in acute pancreatitis, chronic pancreatitis with pseudocysts and pancreatic abscess: salivary amylase is elevated in esophageal rupture.

PL-35. **Answers: a, c.** The effusion occurs at the time of acute pancreatitis in 3–15% of patients. Sixty per cent of effusions are left-sided, 30% right-sided, and 10% bilateral. The clinical syndrome is dominated by abdominal symptoms, and the pleural effusions are usually asymptomatic. The effusions are generally small with a pH >7.20, normal glucose, a PMN-predominant exudative effusion, and elevated amylase.

PL-36. **Answers: a, b, c, d, e.** With bowel rest, hyperalimentation, and repeated thoracentesis or chest tube drainage, 40–70% of chronic pancreatic effusions and ascites will resolve in 2–3 weeks. Frequently a chest tube is required due to rapid fluid accumulation and respiratory embarrassment. Both chest tube drainage and repeated thoracentesis have been complicated by empyema. If the effusion fails to resolve, surgery is recommended owing to an increased risk of pleural infection and lower rate of spontaneous resolution with continued conservative therapy. Surgical therapy is directed at drainage of the pseudocyst with or without distal pancreatectomy.

PL-37. Answers: b, d. Closed-needle pleural biopsy is typically nondiagnostic in pleuropulmonary Kaposi's sarcoma owing to the nonhomogeneous distribution of the lesions and the relative sparing of the parietal pleura. Thoracotomy with open lung and visceral pleural biopsy offer the only avenue to antemortem diagnosis of pleural involvement. Autopsy often reveals lymphatic obstruction of lung parenchymal tissue and mediastinal lymph nodes. Radiation therapy has been effective in treating cutaneous and oropharyngeal KS lesions and may play a role in relieving lymphatic obstruction. Attempts at local control of pleural disease using tube thoracostomy with tetracycline sclerosis have been unsuccessful.

PL-38. Answers: a, e. The pleural effusions are typically a serosanguineous exudate with a mononuclear cell predominance. Glucose, amylase, and pH values are generally normal. Chylous effusions have been described and are due to lymphatic obstruction of lung parenchymal tissue and mediastinal lymph nodes.

PL-39. Answers: c, d, e. Typically, cutaneous Kaposi's sarcoma precedes visceral involvement. The disease is rare in IV drug users, hemophiliacs, and the pediatric AIDS population. The radiographic appearance of Kaposi's sarcoma of the lung, uncomplicated by opportunistic infection, has been reported to include unilateral or bilateral hilar or mediastinal adenopathy (most common finding), diffuse interstitial or interstitial-alveolar infiltrates, and pleural effusions.

PL-40. Answers: a, b, e. It is generally agreed that the cell of origin is the pluripotential angioblast, and cytomegalovirus may have a role in the stimulus to sarcomatous change. In contrast to non–AIDS-related Kaposi's sarcoma, which metastasizes to visceral organs in only 20% of cases, AIDS-related Kaposi's sarcoma disseminates commonly, and pulmonary involvement occurs in 20–25% of cases. Raised, violaceous nodules may be visible in the tracheobronchial tree at bronchoscopy, and in addition, both pleural and parenchymal involvement occur.

PL-41. Answers: c, d, e. Classically, the pleural fluid characteristics closely resemble those of the ascitic fluid, and most often they are transudates. Even when they are similar, the pleural fluid tends to be slightly more exudative than the ascitic fluid. With respiration (negative intrathoracic, positive intra-abdominal pressures), diaphragmatic defects probably exhibit a ball-valve phenomenon, which allows passage of peritoneal fluid into the pleural space but not vice versa. Frank exudates occasionally occur in the presence of transudative ascites. This may relate to a lesser influence of portal hypertension on the mechanics of pleural fluid water and solute resorption versus that of ascitic fluid. Bloody effusions with clear ascites are reasonably common and are likely to be due to rupture of small venous vessels which course over and through diaphragmatic defects. Owing to the unidirectional flow, ascites is unaffected.

PL-42. Answer: a, b, c, d. The etiology of these effusions has been debated over the years. Small effusions may in part be due to azygos vein hypertension and increases in lymphatic flow and pressure in association with hypoalbuminemia. However, the majority of effusions (especially moderate to large ones) are due to diaphragmatic defects, which are probably congenital and tend to occur in the tendinous portion of the diaphragm.

PL-43. Answers: a, b, e. Pleural effusions secondary to ascites occur in 5–10% of patients with cirrhotic ascites and often present as massive effusions. These are typically right-sided; however, left-sided effusions occur in roughly 20% of reported cases. Although most ascitic pleural effusions occur in the setting of obvious and often tense ascites, there have been many reports of massive effusions without clinically apparent ascites. Pleural effusions secondary to ascites may be indicative of Meigs' syndrome.

PL-44. **Answers: a, b, c, d, e.** Spontaneous pneumothorax occurs in chronic obstructive pulmonary disease, tuberous sclerosis, lymphangioleiomyomatosis, eosinophilic granuloma, Marfan syndrome, and hydatid disease.

PL-45. **Answers: a, c, d.** Chyle is composed largely of proteins (albumin and globulins), lymphocytes, electrolytes, and lymph from the lower extremities. Chylomicrons from the jejunal mucosa comprise only a small percentage of the thoracic duct lymph. An effusion with triglyceride >110 has <1% chance of not being chylous. Conversely, if the TG level is <50, there is only <5% chance that the effusion represents a chylothorax. The glucose level in chyle is not different from the plasma level. Lymphocyte subset analysis shows <5% of the total cells to be B lymphocytes, and the T4:T8 ratio is approximately 1.5 (peripheral blood ratio is closer to 2:1).

PL-46. **Answers: a, b, c, d, e.** Chylothorax is the accumulation of thoracic duct lymph or "chyle" in the pleural space. Normally, the amount of chyle flow is 1500–2500 cc/day. The pattern and volume of chyle flow varies depending on the level of activity, diet, and the nutritional status of the patient. The most common (50%) cause of chylothorax is mediastinal malignancy, usually lymphoma. Approximately 20% of the cases follow thoracic surgery and 5% are due to trauma — penetrating and blunt. Other causes include congenital and idiopathic, LAM, intestinal lymphangiectasia, subclavian vein cannulation, delivery, aortography, and even nephrotic syndrome. Although generally milky white, odorless, and alkaline, chylothoraces can be bloody, turbid, or even serous. Furthermore, milky fluid can stain negative for fat and still be chylous.

PL-47. **Answers: d.** Pleural effusions associated with CHF in the subacute or chronic state appear to be due primarily to pulmonary venous hypertension; clinically, there usually is combined systemic venous hypertension. The typical roentgenographic findings are cardiomegaly, pulmonary edema, and bilateral pleural effusions, right larger than left. Ten to 15% of patients will have an isolated left pleural effusion, and 25% will have a pleural effusion isolated to the right hemithorax. The fluid is a serous transudate with a paucity of lymphocytes and mesothelial cells, a glucose level equal to that of serum, and a pH of about 7.50. Acute diuretic therapy usually will raise the pleural fluid protein concentration but only rarely into the exudative range; chronic diuretic therapy may result in an exudative fluid in a higher percentage of cases.

PL-48. **Answer: e.** Only a small percentage (5–6%) of patients with cirrhosis and clinical ascites develop pleural effusions due to either a diaphragmatic defect or diaphragmatic lymphatic transport. Fluid moves from the peritoneal to pleural cavity because of the pressure gradient across the diaphragm. Bilateral effusions are usually due to diaphragmatic lymphatic passage and tend to be small to moderate in size, whereas unilateral large effusions result from a diaphragmatic defect. The pleural fluid is a serous transudate with less than 1000 cells/µl, mostly lymphocytes and mesothelial cells. Pleural and ascitic fluid total proteins are equivalent, but pleural fluid values tend to be slightly greater. The diagnosis can be confirmed by simultaneous peritoneal and pleural taps with equivalent findings; if doubt exists, intraperitoneal radionuclide injection and scanning over the thorax at 20, 40, and 60 minutes or at 12 and 24 hours will be definitive. In a diaphragm defect, radioactive tracer is detected over the thorax within 1 hour, while normal lymphatic transfer may not result in appearance over the thorax until 12–24 hours.

PL-49. **Answers: a, c, e.** Pulmonary embolism is frequent (25%) in nephrotic syndrome whether or not renal vein thrombosis is documented. A possible etiology of this hypercoagulable state is loss of clotting inhibitors in the urine, such as protein S, which has been documented to be deficient in nephrotic syndrome. The transudates, usually with total protein concentrations less than 1.0 gm/dl, tend to be bilateral, small, and subpulmonic. A unilateral effusion, bilateral effusions of disparate size, or a bloody exudate should heighten the suspicion of pulmonary embolism.

PL-50. **Answer: d.** Parapneumonic effusions occur in almost 50% of patients with all types of bacterial pneumonias, 60% of patients with pneumococcal pneumonias, and 40% of patients with anaerobic pneumonias. Anaerobes are responsible for most postpneumonic empyemas because the pneumonia is generally at an advanced stage at presentation. It is not possible to predict accurately from the clinical presentation whether a parapneumonic effusion exists or whether it is complicated or uncomplicated. Pleural fluid analysis is the only method for differentiating between an uncomplicated (resolves with antibiotics only) and complicated effusion (requires chest tube drainage or thoracotomy). An uncomplicated effusion is nonpurulent and free-flowing, with a pH greater than 7.30, LDH <1000 U/L and a glucose >60 mg/dl.

A complicated effusion is either a classic empyema or a turbid fluid with a pH less than 7.10, LDH >1000 U/L, and glucose <40 mg/dl. Fluids with pH between 7.10 and 7.29 are indeterminate, and patients should have serial thoracenteses to decide on therapy. Antibiotic dosage does not need to be increased simply because patients with pneumonia develop an effusion. Continued pleural sepsis despite tube thoracostomy requires empyemectomy or open drainage, depending upon the clinical circumstance.

PL-51. **Answer: e.** Malignant pleural effusions are the most common cause of exudative effusions in patients over the age of 60. Patients with low pH effusions have a shorter survival, higher diagnostic yield on cytology and biopsy, and a poorer response to tetracycline pleurodesis than those with normal pH effusions. Pleural fluid cytology is more sensitive diagnostically than pleural biopsy, as the latter has the problem of sampling error. Malignant effusions are serous or bloody exudates with a predominance of mononuclear cells; 15–20% are transudates due to early lymphatic blockage, endobronchial obstruction with atelectasis, or concomitant CHF. Pleural effusions in lung cancer are ipsilateral due to contiguous spread and pulmonary arterial invasion and embolization. The finding of an effusion in lung cancer is an ominous sign but does not exclude curative resection as the effusion may be due to an endobronchial lesion with atelectasis.

PL-52. **Answer: b.** Malignant mesothelioma, but not benign fibrous mesothelioma, is associated with asbestos exposure. At presentation, patients are almost always symptomatic with chest pain being the most common symptom. Dyspnea, the second most frequent symptom, is due to large pleural effusions, an early occurrence in mesothelioma. As the disease progresses, the effusion resolves and the tumor encases the lung causing ipsilateral mediastinal shift with an apparent large effusion (actually tumor). About 70% of patients present with a low pH, low glucose effusion due to the markedly abnormal pleura inhibiting glucose entry and the efflux of glucose metabolites.

PL-53. **Answer: d.** Pleural effusions occur in 40–50% of patients with PE and are present in almost all patients on admission and certainly within 24 hours. Even though most emboli are bilateral, effusions are unilateral and small to moderate in size. If no radiographic infarction is present, the effusion peaks in size within a day or two and resolves in a week. Effusions associated with chest film consolidation tend to last longer than 7 days. Most effusions are exudates, but up to 25% are transudates presumably owing to atelectasis. Only a third of patients have the classic bloody, PMN-predominant exudate.

PL-54. **Answer: d.** Three weeks (range 3 days to 6 months) following myocardial-pericardial injury, a syndrome characterized by pleuritic chest pain, fever, pericarditis, leukocytosis, and left-sided pleural effusion and infiltrate occurs in up to 5% of patients with myocardial infarction and up to 30% following cardiac surgery. Pleural effusions occur in 80–85% of patients and usually are left-sided or bilateral, and rarely unilateral on the right. The most typical feature of the effusion is that it is bloody (70%); it is an exudate with normal pH and glucose. Postcardiac injury syndrome effusions cannot be distinguished from effusions due to pulmonary embolism by fluid analysis. Patients with postcardiac injury syndrome tend to have higher levels of antimyocardial antibodies than patients with cardiac injury who do not have postcardiac injury syndrome.

PL-55. **Answer: b, e.** Rheumatoid pleurisy is most commonly seen in males (4:1 male:

female ratio) with rheumatoid nodules and active articular disease. The onset usually is within the first 5 years of the disease but may occur prior to and simultaneously with articular manifestations. The pleural fluid often has a yellow-green tint and may appear to contain debris, a result of sloughing of the necrotic rheumatoid nodule into the pleural space. The effusion has the characteristic triad of pH 7.00, glucose less than 30 mg/dl, and LDH more than 1000 U/L. However, 15% of patients will have a glucose higher than 50 mg/dl and a pH greater than 7.30. Rheumatoid effusions usually resolve over several weeks to months but may result in marked pleural thickening, trapped lung, and a cholesterol effusion.

PL-56. **Answer: d.** Lupus pleuritis is the most common pleuropulmonary manifestation of SLE and may be the presenting feature. Patients are almost always symptomatic with pleuritic chest pain, fever, and cough in contrast to those with rheumatoid pleurisy. Bilateral effusions are characteristic, and a pericardial effusion may be present. The effusion is a nonspecific serous exudate with pH and glucose being low in 20% of patients. Finding LE cells in pleural fluid is diagnostic, and an ANA more than 1:160 or greater than the serum ANA is supportive of the diagnosis. Native and lupus pleuritis cannot be distinguished by pleural fluid analysis.

PL-57. **Answer: c.** Malignancy, largely lymphoma, is the most common etiology of chylothorax (content of thoracic duct leaking into pleural space). Chylothorax may appear milky, bloody, serous, or turbid; a turbid or serous fluid occurs in the malnourished individual. The diagnosis is established most simply by measuring the triglyceride concentration of the pleural fluid. If the triglyceride concentration is more than 110 mg/dl, the diagnosis is virtually assured; however, if it is less than

50 mg/dl, chylothorax can be excluded. Levels between 50 and 110 mg/dl, usually seen in malnourished individuals indicate that a lipoprotein electrophoresis should be done to evaluate the presence or absence of chylomicrons. Seventy-five per cent of patients with lymphangioleiomyomatosis will develop a chylothorax during the course of their disease, as these atypical smooth muscle cells involve lymphatics as well as bronchioles and venules. Prolonged tube drainage of the pleural space in patients with dyspnea will result in malnutrition and immunocompromise.

PL-58. **Answer: d.** Spontaneous esophageal rupture frequently results following a severe bout of vomiting or retching and presents as a thoracoabdominal syndrome with pain, fever, and variable degrees of dyspnea. However, patients initially may be asymptomatic. The lower third of the esophagus is the most common site of tear because that portion of the esophagus is devoid of striated muscle and is deficient in extramural support. The time between perforation and radiographic examination, the site of perforation, and the integrity of the mediastinal pleura all determine the chest radiographic findings. Pleural fluid may result from mediastinitis (exudate with normal pH and low amylase) or from an anaerobic empyema when the mediastinal pleura tears (pH 6.00 and high amylase). Early diagnosis and surgical treatment (within 24 hours) result in excellent survival.

PL-59. **Answer: c.** Urinothorax is an ipsilateral pleural effusion due to obstructive uropathy as urine leaks from the obstructed kidney and moves into the pleural space via diaphragmatic defects or lymphatics. It has the triad of transudate, low pH, and pleural fluid/serum creatinine 1.0. Splenic infarction occurs with endocarditis, hemoglobinopathy, and myeloproliferative disorders. It presents as a thoracoabdominal syndrome with a small left pleural effusion that is a serous, PMN-predominant exudate. Subphrenic abscess most commonly follows upper abdominal surgery (biliary tract and gastric) and results in a small, sterile exudate with normal pH and glucose due to diaphragmatic pleural inflammation. Approximately 10% of patients with pancreatitis develop pleural effusions, which are small and left-sided in 60%. The initial pleural fluid amylase may be normal but becomes greater than serum amylase on serial measurement; the fluid is an exudate with pH between 7.30 and 7.35 and a WBC usually 10,000/μl. Amebic liver abscess may produce a "sympathetic" pleural effusion (sterile, PMN-predominant exudate) or a brownish, thick fluid when the abscess ruptures through the diaphragm into the pleural space.

PL-60. **Answer: e.** Yellow nail syndrome consists of the triad of yellow nails, lymphedema, and respiratory tract involvement (pleural effusions, sinusitis, bronchiectasis). The triad rarely occurs simultaneously and may occur in variable combinations; however, the occurence of pleural effusion and yellow nails without lymphedema is rare. In Noonan's syndrome, a Turner's phenotype with a normal karyotype, chylothorax may develop owing to pulmonary lymphangiectasia. Triglyceride concentration of greater than 110 mg/dl in pleural fluid essentially establishes the diagnosis of chylothorax.

PL-61. **Answer: a, b, e.** Approximately one half of the patients who undergo endoscopic variceal sclerotherapy develop pleural effusions and/or paramediastinal densi-

2-7 Infection

I-1. **Answers: a, d.** Herpes simplex virus classically infects squamous epithelium, and so patients at risk for squamous metaplasia (smokers, burn patients) are predisposed. Often, but not always, patients have a defect in cellular immunity or lung injury (ARDS, burns, organ transplant, carcinomas, leukemias most commonly). Histologic confirmation is needed as few symptomatic patients have positive HSV cultures from sputum (5–10%) and lower respiratory tract. Absence of a rise in antibody titer is an ominous sign in HSV infection. Acyclovir is recommended as the treatment of choice, despite several reports of patients improving without therapy.

I-2. **Answer: d.** Histologic findings at autopsy include tissue necrosis, degeneration of cells, ground-glass nuclei, multinucleated giant cells, and eosinophilic intranuclear inclusions.

I-3. **Answer: e.** Oropharyngeal anaerobic bacteria would be the primary etiology in a non-immunosuppressed patient admitted from the community. Penicillin and clindamycin are active against oral anaerobes, but ciprofloxacin is not. Ceftazidime has only marginal activity. Abnormalities in host defense such as alterations in serum complement or reduced PMN chemotaxis play no role in the pathogenesis of pulmonary disease associated with HIV. *Pneumocystis* and *Mycobacterium avium-intracellulare* are the most common pulmonary pathogens in patients with AIDS. Intrathoracic adenopathy is not seen on chest film with *P. carinii* pneumonia. The fluorescein-tagged monoclonal antibody, Giemsa stain, and methenamine silver stain are used to identify *P. carinii*.

I-4. **Answer: b.** Skin tests indicate exposure to histoplasmosis, and results are frequently positive in endemic areas. The complement fixation has sensitivity of 50% and cross-reacts with *Blastomyces*. A positive titer (greater than 1:32) is useful, but only in the context of other clinical findings. Sputum cultures are diagnostic if positive but are often negative in early disease. Sputum cultures may have a sensitivity of 70% in patients with thick wall cavities who are coughing. A Wright's-stained smear showing the organism with an unstained refractile wall will be positive in most patients with a positive culture. Urine cultures have proved to be useful in coccidioidomycosis and in cryptococcosis, but not in histoplasmosis.

I-5. **Answers: a, c, e.** Hilar lymphadenopathy is common in primary histoplasmosis. Pleural effusion is uncommon. Cavitation may be present in postprimary disease, but hilar adenopathy is uncommon in postprimary disease. Calcified foci are very common in postprimary disease.

I-6. **Answers: b, d.** *Legionella* is a gram-negative bacillus of which there are 23 species. There are 12 serogroups of *L. pneumophila*, and serogroup 1 is the most prevalent. The other species that cause diseases in humans are *L. micdadei*, *L. long-beachae*, *L. dumoffii*, and *L. bozemanii*. There are several other bacterial infections that cause a false rise in the serum titers, including *B. fragilis*, *Chlamydia psittaci*, and *Pseudomonas aeruginosa*. The direct fluorescent antibody (DFA) test is only effective for serogroups 1–6. The radioimmunoassay, enzyme-linked immunosorbent assay (ELISA), and latex agglutination tests can detect the *Legionella* antigen in the urine. The test is useful in patients who are not producing sputum so that a DFA or sputum culture cannot be obtained. Unfortunately, it is only specific for *L. pneumophila* serogroup 1. The gold standard test is a culture, and over the past few years a culture medium containing buffered charcoal yeast extract medium, supplemented with alpha-ketoglutarate, has been developed. Normally it takes the *Legionella* 3–4 days to grow on the culture medium.

I-7.   **Answers: b, c, e.** More than 50 outbreaks of nosocomial legionellosis have been described since 1980. In some hospitals it makes up 30% of the nosocomial pneumonias. Superheating water, hyperchlorination, and surveillance culturing reduce the probability of infection. Risk factors include advanced age, cigarettes, COPD, cancer, and general anesthesia. The organism breeds in hot water tanks at less than 140°F and then is distributed around the hospital; it is cultured in showerheads and faucets; 25 50% of all cases of noso comial *Legionella* pneumonia occur is surgical patients, with the highest attack rates in transplant patients. *Legionella* pneumonia occurs at a mean of 9 days after operation.

I-8.   **Answers: c.** Erythromycin, 1.5–3.0 gm per day, as prophylaxis has been shown to prevent *Legionella* pneumonia in renal transplant patients. Erythromycin increases serum cyclosporine levels by competing with the same hepatic enzyme system (one of the cytochrome p450 mixed-function oxidase systems) for its metabolism. When the cyclosporine levels rise, nephrotoxicity and hepatotoxicity can occur. Some patients may develop pulmonary fibrosis, which may lead to functional impairment or death despite prompt antibiotic treatment. The condition is indistinguishable from many other fibrotic pulmonary disorders. Treatment

consists of erythromycin, 4 gm IV per day (watch for ototoxicity) for 10–14 days. Clinical response usually occurs within 72 hours. Rifampin, trimethoprim-sulfamethoxazole (TMP-SMZ), TCN, and perhaps imipenem and ciprofloxacin are other active agents.

I-9.   **Answers: a, b, d.** The clinical features in *L. bozemanii* are similar to those seen in *L. pneumophila*. In cases of *Legionella* unresponsive to erythromycin, an additional antibiotic has been recommended (rifampin, Bactrim). *Legionella* infections can be diagnosed by demonstration of serologic response, by recognition of the bacterial antigen, and by recovery of the pathogen in culture. The CDC criteria for a positive indirect immunofluorescent assay (IFA) is a four-fold increase in titer during convalescence to ≥128. Seroconversion can be detected in many patients within the first week of the illness. Most cultures will be positive in 3–5 days.

I-10.   **Answers: a, c, d.** *Nocardia* is a soil-borne aerobic actinomycete causing suppurative necrosis, nonencapsulated abscess formation, and granulomas. Consolidation is not always clearly confined to lobes or segments. There may be a solitary irregular mass, several masses or large irregular nodules, diffuse tiny nodules, multiple small irregular nodules, an interstitial reticular pattern, or a normal chest roentgenogram. Concomitant therapy with corticosteroids or antineoplastic agents is associated with high mortality. Effective agents include trimethoprim-sulfamethoxazole (TMP-SMX), sulfonamides alone, imipenem, amikacin, minocycline and doxycycline, cycloserine, and cefotaxime. Synergy is apparent with various combinations. There are no good serologic tests.

I-11.   **Answer: d.** The incidence of nocardiosis is thought to be rising because of newer antineoplastic regimens, organ transplantation, and HIV disease. Two thirds of patients are male. *N. brasiliensis* usually causes skin infection (including the classic Madura foot) but can also result in pulmonary disease in as many as 15%. *N. asteroides* produces 80% of pulmonary disease. Sputum cultures are positive in 25–35% of cases, but they may take weeks and require special handling. Organs involved in descending order of frequency include pleura, spleen, kidney, heart, liver, bones and joints, peritoneum, lymph nodes, adrenals, GI tract, meninges, pancreas, thyroid, eye, ear, marrow, endocardium, spinal cord, pituitary, and bladder.

I-12. **Answer: c.** Pneumococcal pneumonia occurs especially in patients with poor defense functions of the respiratory tract. *Streptococcus pneumoniae* initially produces hyperemia and edema and neutrophil mobilization in the alveoli (congestive stage). Resolution results in complete healing, and there is no tissue necrosis. Of the 84 serotypes identified, serotypes 1,2,3,4,7,8,12, and 14 cause the most severe disease, with type 3 being the most virulent. The pneumococcus elaborates hemolysin, or pneumolysin and neuraminidase.

I-13. **Answer: d.** The concentration of organisms in ambient air and the duration of exposure are important determinants of tuberculous infection. Previous infection with tuberculosis may lead to reactivation. End-stage renal disease is a risk factor for TB. Laboratory handling of infected sputum is not a risk factor.

I-14. **Answers: a, b, d, e.** Thirty per cent of individuals who are close contacts of patients with infectious tuberculosis become infected, and about 5% develop active disease immediately; 5% will develop active disease later, whereas in 90% the TB is contained and active infection does not ever develop. INH prophy-

laxis reduces the possibility of TB infection in HIV-positive patients. Obesity is not a risk factor for tuberculosis. Previous BCG vaccination reduces the severity of extrapulmonary TB.

I-15. **Answer: d.** Intravenous drug use, radiographic "old TB," immunosuppression (especially HIV positivity), and endstage renal disease are all risk factors for tuberculosis.

I-16. **Answers: a, c, d, e.** A positive skin test indicates active infection. It is positive in about 80% of asymptomatic HIV-positive patients with TB, which is similar to the rate seen in other groups who have TB. A positive test requires intact cell-mediated immunity, and there is no evidence that IL-3 and IL-5 are involved in a positive response.

I-17. **Answer: c.** People with conversion of their PPD, people who are HIV-positive and have a positive PPD or have been in contact with a new case, and older people with upper lobe scarring on the chest film, especially if they come from the far east, should receive prophylactic INH.

I-18. **Answer: e.** Erythema nodosum is most common in tuberculosis and coccidioidomycosis but can also be seen in histoplasmosis and blastomycosis.

I-19. **Answers: b, c.** Aspergilloma is encountered in patients with sarcoidosis with advanced parenchymal disease (cystic cavitary). Spontaneous resolution can occur as the cavity contracts and disappears. Recurrent hemoptysis does occur, and a patient may die from massive hemoptysis. Surgery may be indicated when there is recurrent life-threatening hemorrhage. Amphotericin has no impact on any aspect of this disease. Prednisone therapy, either before or after the diagnosis of aspergilloma, does not seem to promote occurrence or dissemination.

I-20. **Answer: e.** Signs suggestive of endo-bronchial tuberculosis include lung collapse, air trapping, consolidation, atelectasis, and intrathoracic adenopathy. Pleural effusion is not a consequence of endobronchial tuberculosis.

I-21. **Answers: a, b, c, d, e.** There is a relatively continuous spectrum of macroscopic manifestations in endobronchial tuberculosis: erythema with edema followed by ulceration, "cobblestone" mucosa usually with sterile granuloma, an obstructing mass containing caseous material, inflammatory polyps, and fibrostenosis of the trachea or major bronchi. Early lesions may show caseating granulomas, which are usually free of acid-fast bacillus. Late lesions such as fibrostenosis show chronic inflammation with fibrosis and without granulomas and acid-fast bacilli. The PPD is positive in about 45% of patients.

I-22. **Answer: c.** Pulmonary candidiasis is rare. In the neonate, aspiration may be a common mechanism. In the adult, lung involvement occurs almost exclusively in the immunosuppressed host (especially the neutropenic host) by hematogenous seeding, presumably from the gastrointestinal tract.

I-23. **Answers: b, c, d, e.** Varicella is usually a benign childhood malady. Varicella pneumonia is more common in adults (16 to 50% incidence) and, when it does occur, can be associated with significant morbidity and mortality. Risk factors include the presence of an underlying malignancy, cytotoxic and steroid therapy, pregnancy, and tobacco use. Varicella pneumonia typically presents 1–6 days after the onset of the rash, with cough, dyspnea, and fever. The chest radiograph will typically display a patchy or diffuse bilateral nodular infiltrate with a prominent peribronchial distribution. It is generally recommended that intravenous

acyclovir (500 mg/m^2 BSA IV q8h) be administered to normal hosts with clinically evident varicella pneumonia due to the high mortality associated with this complication.

I-24. **Answers: a, c, d.** The finding of intrathoracic adenopathy or diffuse infiltration on the chest film in patients with HIV infection should trigger suspicion of tuberculosis. Toxic delirium, hypoglycemia, hyperglycemia, and hypotension have all been seen following administration of pentamidine in patients with AIDS. Fever, skin rash with mucositis, hepatitis, and neutropenia have been reported following administration of trimethoprim-sulfamethoxazole in patients with AIDS.

I-25. **Answers: a, b, c.** HIV-positive patients reported as developing primary pulmonary hypertension have all been hemophiliacs and had used lyophilized factor VII. There is a well-recognized form of pulmonary hypertension associated with intravenous drug abusers. Its pathology is granulomatous, and it is believed to be secondary to talc or other foreign body emboli. The anticardiolipin antibody seen in AIDS is an IgG and is apparently not associated with an increased risk of DVT/pulmonary emboli. Although the combination of autoimmunity and severe immunodeficiency seems paradoxical, autoimmune phenomena are common in AIDS, and there is evidence that most of the CD 4 depletion is not on a retroviral cytopathic basis but rather a consequence of immune dysregulation.

I-26. **Answers: a, c, d, e.** Serum protein electrophoresis with a diffuse hypergammaglobulinemia and two or more monoclonal "spikes" is found in only a few diseases: EBV, CMV, and HIV infections; polyclonal B cell lymphomas; SLE; and Sjögren's syndrome. Usually during the course of acute mononucleosis, B cells are infected with the Epstein-Barr virus, causing polyclonal immunoglobulin secretion. By the second or third week of infection, the number of activated Epstein-Barr virus-infected B cells decreases as a result of specific suppressor cell activation. During the acute phase of the infection, patients frequently exhibit depressed cellular immunity. Suppressor cell function gradually returns to normal in 4–8 weeks, correlating with clinical recovery. Antibodies classically associated with collagen vascular diseases have also been reported in patients with Epstein-Barr virus infections. There have been numerous reports of positive rheumatoid factor in Epstein-Barr virus infections. Recently, anticardiolipin antibodies (usually low-titer IgM antibodies rather than IgG) have been described with acute Epstein-Barr virus infections.

I-27. **Answers: a, b, c, d, e.** Patients with SLE have clinically significant anticardiolipin antibodies. The anticardiolipin antibody is one in a family of antiphospholipid antibodies which include the false-positive VDRL and the lupus anticoagulant. All three classes of antiphospholipid antibody are frequently present simultaneously. The antiphospholipid antibodies have been associated with arterial and venous thrombosis, thrombocytopenia, recurrent spontaneous abortions, pulmonary hypertension, and livedo reticularis. In retrospective studies, 25–35% of patients with the lupus anticoagulant and 50% of patients with high levels of IgG anticardiolipin Ab have episodes of thrombosis. There are two leading hypotheses describing the pathogenesis of the phospholipid antibodies: (1) they alter platelet membranes leading to increased platelet adhesion, and/or (2) they affect endothelial membranes leading to a decrease in prostacyclin release.

I-28. **Answer: e.** The lupus anticoagulant is an IgG or IgM antibody known to occur in various immune disorders such as SLE,

myeloproliferative disorders, neoplasms, pregnancy, drug therapies, and most recently in AIDS. In the laboratory they inhibit phospholipid-dependent coagulation tests (PT, PTT, Russell's viper venom time) resulting in higher than normal values for PTT (typically elevated into the 40–55 range) and PT (sometimes). They appear to inhibit coagulation at the level of the prothrombin activator complex (factors Va, Xa, Ca+ , and phospholipid), and therefore both the intrinsic and extrinsic pathways are affected. The earliest reports were in association with hemorrhagic events. However it is now clear that in the absence of thrombocytopenia, hypoprothrombinemia, functional platelet abnormality, or underlying coagulopathy, there is no clinical bleeding, although there is anecdotal evidence of excessive bleeding after transbronchial biopsy.

I-29. **Answers: a, b.** Platelet dysfunction is well documented, and immune-mediated thrombocytopenia and thrombotic thrombocytopenic purpura have been described. Most patients who are HIV-positive with elevated PTTs will have lupus anticoagulant demonstrated in their plasma. As many as 70% of patients who are HIV-positive with ongoing opportunistic infections have the lupus anticoagulant demonstrable. The presence of lupus anticoagulant does not appear to increase the risk of thromboembolic disease in patients who are HIV-positive.

I-30. **Answers: a, c, d.** Pleural effusion is common in *Entamoeba histolytica* infection and in actinomycosis (empyema). Cavitation is common in coccidioidomycosis and actinomycosis, in which chest wall extension is also common.

I-31. **Answer: b.** Cavitation may occur in *Klebsiella* pneumonia, actinomycosis, ankylosing spondylitis, and Wegener's granulomatosis. It is not seen in Löffler's syndrome.

I-32. **Answers: a, b, d, e.** *Cryptococcus neoformans* is a soil saprophyte that can cause infection after inhalation. Despite this portal of entry, cryptococcosis presents most commonly as subacute meningitis (over 80% of those cases reported). Pulmonary involvement may be present in as many as 45% of patients. It is the 4th leading cause of opportunistic infection in the acquired immunodeficiency syndrome. Roentgenographic findings include homogeneous or nodular-appearing infiltrates, solitary nodules often subpleural in location, cavitary lesions, and pleural effusions. Characteristic budding, encapsulated yeast forms can be easily seen after mucicarmine staining.

I-33. **Answers: b, d.** The fetal lung undergoes extensive anatomic and histologic differentiation, which continues through infancy and childhood. Lobar bronchi appear at the sixth week of gestation, and by the sixteenth week of intrauterine life the bronchial tree is almost fully developed. Respiratory bronchioles appear between the sixteenth week and birth, and during this period the acini develop as well. Alveolar multiplication continues through the first decade when the adult complement of alveoli are attained.

I-34. **Answers: a, b, c, d, e.** Bronchopulmonary dysplasia, a clinical-radiologic diagnosis, often occurs in premature infants who require mechanical ventilation or high oxygen concentrations at birth. The lungs of infants with bronchopulmonary dysplasia who have died have histologic evidence of necrotizing bronchiolitis, alveolar fibrosis, emphysema, and arterial changes characteristic of pulmonary hypertension. Long-term follow-up in 26 patients who survived with BPD (at ages 13 to 20 years) revealed that 70% had airway obstruction, and 52% had reactive airway disease as determined by methacholine challenge and bronchodilator response.

I-35. **Answers: a, b, d, e.** Certain strains of adenovirus—especially types 5, 7, and 21—seem to cause more significant disease. Bronchiolar obliteration in infancy with subsequent inhibition of the normal development of one lung or lobe has been proposed as a cause of unilateral radiolucency of the lung (Swyer-James syndrome or Macleod's syndrome). Both pulmonary circulation and alveolar development are inadequate in the damaged lung or lobe. The affected area appears hyperlucent on radiograph with reduced lung volume on inspiration and little change in lung volume on the expiratory film. Although usually asymptomatic, some patients may have cough and chronic pulmonary infections.

I-36. **Answers: a, b, c, d, e.** Bilateral or diffuse radiographic densities of interstitial, alveolar, or mixed patterns are typical of *Pneumocystis carinii* pneumonia, but many atypical presentations have been encountered. The diffuse disease may be asymmetric or predominate in the upper lobes when the patient is on prophylactic inhaled pentamidine. Sometimes the process appears to be unilateral or the chest films may be negative despite impressive clinical pneumonia. Small pleural effusions can occur. Many cases with cyst-like (and bullous) air spaces, with or without complicating pneumothorax, have been reported in AIDS with PCP.

I-37. **Answers: a, b, e.** The incidence of *Pneumocystis carinii* pneumonia in AIDS exceeds 50% (compared to 1% in acute lymphatic leukemia), and recurrence is frequent unless prophylactic treatment is given. The clinical onset is often subtle and slowly progressive over weeks or even months. Organisms are more numerous, more often detected on sputum examination, and more persistent after clearing of the clinical pneumonia. Adverse reactions to drug therapy are greatly increased.

I-38. **Answers: b, c, e.** The clinical tuberculosis of advanced HIV infection has special features. In AIDS the pulmonary infiltrates tend to be randomly distributed, not favoring an apical location, and are nearly always without cavitation. Sputum or bronchial washings are commonly positive for tuberculosis on smear or culture. Extrapulmonary tuberculosis is present in more than half of the patients. A striking feature is mediastinal and/or hilar lymphadenopathy, which is often marked. Somewhat unexpectedly, patients generally respond promptly to antituberculous drug therapy, and they may be cured of the tuberculosis but not of AIDS.

I-39. **Answer: b, c, d.** Impressive intrathoracic adenopathy is uncommon in AIDS except in tuberculosis. The differential diagnosis of the adenopathy includes Kaposi's sarcoma (especially when known to be present in skin or elsewhere) and poorly differentiated lymphomas. Cytomegalovirus (CMV) is the most frequent agent found post mortem in AIDS patients, but its actual significance is often unclear. Evidence of CMV increases as the AIDS patient becomes sicker and the blood helper T cell count drops below 200/mm³. Fungal pneumonia is relatively uncommon in AIDS patients. *Candida* and occasionally *Aspergillus* may colonize the bronchial lumen but rarely cause invasive infections.

I-40. **Answers: a, c, d.** The incidence of disseminated histoplasmosis and coccidioidomycosis in AIDS is directly related to the prevalence of endemic disease in the region. Nonspecific diffuse bilateral reticulonodular or nodular infiltrates are most characteristic of coccidioidomycosis. Bacterial pulmonary infections due particularly to *Streptococcus pneumoniae* and *Haemophilus influenzae* are common. On the other hand *Legionella* and *Nocardia* pneumonias are rare. Lymphoid interstitial pneumonia (LIP) has been a common complication in children and is seen occasionally in adults. Nonspecific interstitial pneumonitis is apparently common.

I-41. **Answer: c.** The granulomatous lesion that typifies the lung lesions seen in tuberculosis is caused by delayed-type hypersensitivity responses to *Mycobacterium tuberculosis*. *Mycobacterium tuberculosis* does not secrete toxins or grow rapidly enough to cause physical damage early in the disease; it is not resisted by cytotoxic T cells, nor does it have an endotoxin.

I-42. **Answer: a.** Several studies have documented an increased risk of INH-related hepatitis in patients over age 50, although all ages are potentially vulnerable. The risk of hepatitis does not vary according to acetylation status. Most cases occur in the first 3 months; however, they are noted as late as the twelfth month. There is no evidence that postpartum women are more vulnerable. The great majority of cases resolve without any sequelae.

I-43. **Answers: a, b, c, d.** Patients with HIV infection are susceptible to opportunistic infections because of defects in T lymphocyte, B lymphocyte, neutrophil, and macrophage function. Although much attention has been focused on pathogens such as *Pneumocystis* and atypical mycobacteria, pyogenic bacteria are the cause of a substantial number of respiratory infections in patients infected with HIV, most commonly *Streptococcus pneumoniae* and *Haemophilus influenzae*. HIV-positive patients are roughly seven times more likely to develop pneumococcal pneumonia than are non–HIV-positive patients and five times as likely as HIV-negative patients to develop any bacterial pneumonia, even when controlling for life style and socioeconomic class. B cells undergo spontaneous activation, producing a nonspecific, polyclonal hypergammaglobulinemia. All states of HIV infection are affected (HIV-positive, ARC, AIDS).

I-44. **Answers: a, d.** B cell differentiation and proliferation in response to specific antigens is markedly reduced in patients with AIDS and is subnormal in patients with other stages of HIV infection. HIV-infected patients with pneumococcal pneumonia show a lack of production of type-specific antibodies following disease, and therefore a high rate of recurrence. Some studies have shown that neutrophil chemotaxis, phagocytosis, and bacterial killing are decreased in advanced HIV infection. In HIV infection, B cells undergo spontaneous activation, producing a nonspecific, polyclonal hypergammaglobulinemia.

I-45. **Answers: a, b, e.** The clinical manifestations of pneumococcal pneumonia in HIV-positive patients are indistinguishable from those in HIV-negative patients. All (90–100%) have cough, fever, and hypoxia; most (50–70%) have purulent sputum, pleuritic chest pain, dyspnea, leukocytosis with left shift, and focal infiltrates; some (20–30%) have an increased LDH. The duration of symptoms in HIV-positive pneumococcal pneumonia is always less than 1 week, and most patients with pneumocystosis are sick for 1 month prior to admission. Approximately 50–80% of HIV-positive pneumococcal pneumonias and 5–25% with *Haemophilus influenzae* have positive blood cultures. Prompt response to therapy is the rule. Over 90% are completely well by the fifth treatment day. The mortality rate for HIV-positive patients with pneumococcal pneumonia may be lower than for HIV-negative patients, but HIV-positive patients have a high rate of recurrence (25–50%).

I-46. **Answers: a, b, d.** The clinical presentation of TB in HIV-infected individuals with CD-4 counts greater than 300–400 is often indistinguishable from classic reactivation TB with upper lobe cavitary infiltrates. The impaired cell-mediated immunity contributes to an inability to kill the intracytoplasmic TB bacilli, poor formation of granulomas, frequent bacteremia, and dissemination of disease. Most cases are secondary to reactivation of latent foci, but primary infection with accelerated features also occurs. If TB occurs early, the diagnosis of TB often precedes the diagnosis of AIDS. Extrapulmonary disease occurs in at least 25% of these patients, and probably in more than 50%.

I-47. **Answers: b, c, d, e.** Approximately one half of patients with pulmonary TB early in the course of HIV infection have positive acid-fast smears. In more severely compromised patients with roentgenograms typical of primary or miliary disease, the sensitivity of smears is lower. INH should be given to any patient with 5 mm or more induration regardless of age or prior skin testing results. It should also be considered for anergic patients who are known contacts of persons with active disease, and for high-risk groups including IV drug abusers, prison inmates, homeless persons, and natives of countries with an increased prevalence of TB. For drug-susceptible infection, INH, rifampin, and PZA should be given for at least 6 months beyond conversion of sputum cultures to negative, or for 9 months, whichever is longer. Prophylaxis should continue for 12 months.

I-48. **Answers: a, b, c, d.** For disseminated TB with CNS involvement, ethambutol should be added to INH, rifampin, and PZA pending susceptibility tests. If drug-resistance is suspected based on epidemiologic data, four-drug therapy is indicated. If drug-resistance is documented, five drugs should probably be employed for at least 12 months after cultures become negative. Interactions between antituberculous drugs and antifungals can result in subtherapeutic levels of rifampin. HIV-positive patients appear to have substantially higher rates of untoward reactions to antituberculous medications (18% versus 4% in normals). Compared with other "opportunistic" infections and other AIDS-defining illnesses, TB tends to occur earlier in the course of HIV infection because of its relative virulence.

I-49. **Answers: a, b, d, e.** Serum protein electrophoresis with a diffuse hypergammaglobulinemia and two or more monoclonal "spikes" is found in only a few diseases: EBV, CMV, HIV, polyclonal B cell lymphomas, SLE, and Sjögren's syndrome.

I-50. **Answers: a, b, c.** Usually during the course of acute mononucleosis, B cells are infected with the Epstein-Barr virus, causing polyclonal immunoglobulin secretion. By the second or third week of infection, the number of activated EBV-infected B cells decreases as a result of specific T suppressor cell activation. During the acute phase of the infection, patients frequently exhibit depressed cellular immunity. T suppressor cell function will gradually return to normal in 4–8 weeks, correlating with clinical recovery. Less commonly, B cell activation can exist from weeks to months without T suppressor cell activation, leading to a polyclonal gammopathy.

I-51. **Answers: a, b, c, e.** Sera from patients with infectious mononucleosis have been shown to contain heterophile antibodies, cold agglutinins to antigen, and a false-positive VDRL. There have been numerous reports of positive rheumatoid factor in EBV infections. Kaplan and Tan reported 14 of 21 young patients with acute mononucleosis who had positive ANAs, usually at low titer with a speckled

pattern. Recently, Misra noted anticardiolipin antibodies (ACA) in 17 of 33 patients with acute EBV infections, usually low-titer IgM antibodies rather than IgG. The ACA is one in a family of antiphospholipid Ab, which include the false-positive VDRL and the lupus anticoagulant. All three classes of antiphospholipid Ab are frequently present simultaneously, but 35% of patients with ACA do not have a lupus anticoagulant, and 50% do not have a false-positive VDRL.

I-52. **Answers: a, c, d.** The antiphospholipid Ab has been associated with arterial and venous thrombosis, thrombocytopenia, recurrent spontaneous abortions, pulmonary hypertension, and livedo reticularis. There is no definite evidence that the antiphospholipid Abs cause thrombosis. However, they may alter platelet membranes leading to increased platelet adhesion and/or affect endothelial membranes leading to a decrease in prostacyclin release. Between 25 and 35% of patients with the lupus anticoagulant and 50% of patients with high levels of IgG anticardiolipin Ab have episodes of thrombosis.

I-53. **Answers: a, b, c, d.** Appropriate therapy for patients with anticardiolipin Ab is controversial. In patients who have a documented thrombotic event and an ACA, the general consensus is to continue anticoagulation as long as the Ab is present regardless of the ACA titer or Ig class. In patients who do not have a disorder attributable to the Ab, no therapy is required. In patients with repeated episodes despite adequate anticoagulation, steroids and/or immunosuppressives should be considered. Corticosteroids have been shown to decrease the titer of ACA, but they have not been shown in a randomized trial to decrease the incidence of thrombosis in the absence of anticoagulation therapy.

I-54. **Answer: a.** An increased incidence of tuberculosis (TB) has been reported in patients with chronic renal failure; TB causes 0.5–1% of all deaths in patients on chronic hemodialysis. Proclivity toward TB infection is mediated by impaired cell-mediated immunity. Lymphocytes from uremic patients have depressed responsiveness to mitogenic stimuli, and serum from uremic patients suppresses the mitogenic response of normal lymphocytes.

I-55. **Answers: a, b, e.** Rifampin is hepatically metabolized and can be administered normally. Isoniazid is acetylated in the liver and its metabolites excreted in the urine; it is, however, dialyzable. Ethambutol is dependent on renal function for excretion.

I-56. **Answers: a, c, d.** Miliary TB accounts for 1% of patients with active tuberculosis. There is an increased incidence in Blacks, males, HIV-positive persons, and pregnant females. Middle lobe syndrome (recurrent atelectasis of the RML) is most commonly due to "benign" poorly characterized inflammatory disease, presumably secondary to bacterial or viral processes (47%); tumors (24%) including primary lung cancer and metastatic endobronchial tumors; bronchiectasis (15%); tuberculosis (9%);benign tumors (2%); aspiration (2%); and a miscellaneous group including isolated cases of endobronchial sarcoid, amyloidosis, esophageal perforation, esophageal diverticula, histoplasmosis, psittacosis, ABPA, and cystic fibrosis. Lower thoracic and thoracolumbar spine are the most common sites (48–67%) of spinal TB. Treatment consists of INH, streptomycin, and PAS, all of which reach therapeutic levels in bone lesions. The proper duration of chemotherapy is unclear: the MRC group found 6 months of INH, rifampin, and streptomycin as effective as 9 months, in conjunction with surgery.

I-57. **Answers: a, c, e.** Paralysis of a vocal cord is rarely caused by infectious disease. The causes are commonly found along the course of the corresponding recurrent or inferior laryngeal branch of the vagus nerve. Carcinoma and trauma are the leading causes of paralysis of the larynx. The cervical or supraclavicular nodes are involved in 90% of cases of tuberculous lymphadenitis. Tuberculous meningitis is usually due to the rupture of a juxtaependymal tubercle (Rich focus) into the subarachnoid space. Cervical nodes are involved in 90% of cases of tuberculous lymphadenitis. There is evidence of other TB in 18% of cases. Meningitis is strongly associated with miliary TB but may occur in the absence of other evidence of extracranial TB. Treatment for tuberculous pericarditis is the same as for pulmonary tuberculosis. Steroids, beginning with 60–80 mg per day of prednisolone with a taper over several weeks, have been advocated to prevent cardiac constriction.

I-58. **Answers: a, e.** About two thirds of patients are male. No age group is unaffected (range 4 months to 87 years), but the majority of cases occur in middle age (mean 45 years). Pulmonary disease alone occurs in 31%, CNS alone in 5%, skin and subcutaneous tissues alone in 14%, and disseminated disease in 30%. Other organs involved in descending order of frequency include pleura, spleen, kidney, heart, liver, bones and joints, peritoneum, lymph nodes, adrenals, GI tract, meninges, pancreas, thyroid, eye, ear, marrow, endocardium, spinal cord, pituitary, and bladder. Disease associations include leukemia, Hodgkin's disease, lupus erythematosus, asthma, pemphigus vulgaris, pulmonary alveolar proteinosis, breast cancer, TB, COPD, bronchiectasis, anthracosilicosis, Paget's disease, dysproteinemia, collagen vascular disease, trauma, and diabetes. Significant associations included pleural effusions, cavitation, and lymphadenopathy occurring as hilar, mediastinal, or both types of involvement.

I-59. **Answers: d, e.** In the majority of cases infection occurs through the respiratory tract (73%); 5% occur through the skin, and almost 20% have an unknown primary site of infection. *N. asteroides* produces 80% of pulmonary disease. *N. brasiliensis* usually causes skin infection (including the classic Madura foot) but can also result in pulmonary disease in as many as 15% of cases. *Nocardia* causes suppurative necrosis, nonencapsulated abscess formation, and granulomas. It disseminates hematogenously with an unexplained predilection for the CNS.

I-60. **Answers: a, b, c, d, e.** Radiographic findings seen in proven cases of nocardial pulmonary infections are consolidation not always clearly confined to lobes or segments, a solitary irregular mass, several masses or large irregular nodules, diffuse tiny nodules, multiple small irregular nodules, an interstitial reticular pattern, and a normal chest roentgenogram. Significant associations included pleural effusions, cavitation, and lymphadenopathy occurring as hilar, mediastinal, or both types of involvement.

I-61. **Answers: b, c, d.** The mainstay of medical therapy of aspergilloma is aggressive pulmonary toilet, along with nutritional supplementation and antibiotic therapy of frequent bacterial superinfection. Systemic amphotericin B is not effective, probably due to inadequate cavity penetration. Chronic necrotizing pulmonary aspergillosis is an indolent, cavitary process caused by the invasion of lung tissue by a species of *Aspergillus*. Organ systems involved with invasive aspergillosis include the skin, nose and paranasal sinuses, eyes, CNS, bone, and the heart. Disseminated disease is the most severe

form of clinical aspergillosis. In the majority of cases, the lung is the predominant organ involved, followed by the CNS, kidney, liver, and the thyroid gland. There is some evidence of synergy between amphotericin B and rifampin.

I-62. **Answers: c, e.** Invasive aspergillosis often presents a dilemma and can only be diagnosed with certainty only by demonstrating fungal elements invading the tissue. In the right clinical picture, isolation of *Aspergillus* from specimens of the lower respiratory tract (sputum or BAL) usually indicates invasive aspergillosis and not contamination. A positive culture alone is not proof of tissue invasion. The "gold standard" remains demonstration of fungal hyphae in tissues. Serum precipitins are positive in 70–80% of patients with invasive aspergillosis, but have low specificity and predictive value. There is an association between invasive pulmonary aspergillosis and influenza A infection, which seems to affect young female smokers predominantly.

I-63. **Answers: a, b, c, d, e.** The lung is involved in about 90% of invasive aspergillosis infections and is the only site in 70%. *Aspergillus fumigatus* accounts for 50–75% of clinical disease, with *Aspergillus flavus* accounting for most of the remainder. Invasive pulmonary aspergillosis occurs almost exclusively in immunosuppressed and myelosuppressed patients. Patients with hematopoietic or lymphoreticular malignancies are at especially high risk, accounting for over 80% of all cases. Other predisposing factors include organ transplantation, cytotoxic drug therapy, corticosteroids, and antibiotic therapy. Approximately 40% of patients will have hemoptysis, which is sometimes massive in association with pulmonary hemorrhage. Recent data (Denning et al) have shown that oral itraconazole has considerable efficacy in treating invasive pulmonary aspergillosis and may in fact be more efficacious than amphotericin B.

I-64. **Answers: b, c, d, e.** *Blastomyces dermatitidis* is a dimorphic soil fungus endemic in the south central and midwestern United States. It presents usually as a flu-like illness that generally resolves with rare reactivation, or occasionally disseminating to the bone, skin, prostate, and lung. Blastomycosis is a rare infection in AIDS. HIV patients often have visceral, cerebral, or meningeal involvement. Nearly all disseminated cases have pulmonary involvement, usually evident on chest roentgenogram.

I-65. **Answers: a, c, d.** The organism takes 2–4 weeks to culture. Biopsies of affected organs or CSF often reveal the characteristic microscopic character of *Blastomyces dermatitidis*. Serology is not helpful. Amphotericin B is the treatment of choice. Thereafter, most authors suggest chronic suppression with either ketoconazole or itraconazole. Unlike classic *Blastomyces* infection, HIV patients have a rash about 20% of the time.

I-66. **Answers: a, c.** Acute epiglottitis or supraglottitis is an acute inflammatory disease of the epiglottis, the aryepiglottic folds, the arytenoid soft tissues, lingular tonsils, the vallecula, and the base of the tongue. Classically, it is nonsuppurative but may be associated with a "cellulitis," with tissue invasion by infecting bacteria and frank abscesses. Systemic illness with fever and bacteremia is also common. Patients have complaints of sore throat, dysphagia/odynophagia, and a muffled but not hoarse voice, because the cords are not involved. Drooling and mild respiratory distress are common.

I-67. **Answers: c, d, e.** The microbiology associated with adult epiglottitis differs from that of pediatric epiglottitis, with only 25% being associated with *Haemophilus*

influenzae (versus 90%). The majority of cases are associated with no identifiable organism and raise suspicion of viral or atypical bacterial infection. In immunocompromised hosts, *Pasteurella* and *Candida* have been described. Diagnosis can be clinical, based on the classic triad of fever, stridor, and drooling. If there is only a high suspicion, confirmation with lateral neck radiographs (enlarged epiglottis, swollen supraglottic structures, and a ballooning hypopharynx) is not critical. When there is airway compromise, a postobstructive pulmonary edema pattern is well described. In addition to securing a patent airway, treatment consists of beta-lactamase–resistant cephalosporins and Unasyn (covers *Haemophilus influenzae* and *Neisseria*). Steroids, humidified O_2 mist, Heliox, and racemic epinephrine also have a role in treatment. Rifampin prophylaxis (600 mg/day for 2 days) is recommended for health care personnel.

I-68. **Answers: a, b, c, d.** Profound suppression of cell-mediated immunity is the hallmark of infection with the HIV virus, and has altered the spectrum and the natural history of neoplasia in certain segments of the population. Kaposi's sarcoma, once a rare and indolent tumor, is now seen in up to 40% of homosexuals with AIDS, and behaves in a much more aggressive fashion. Other tumors frequently associated with AIDS include malignant lymphomas of several histologic types, including Burkitt's lymphoma and Hodgkin's disease, often behaving aggressively and involving the CNS. Nonspecific lymphocytic alveolitis characterized by lymphocytosis in BAL is seen in up to two thirds of patients regardless of concurrent pulmonary infection. Pulmonary Kaposi's sarcoma lesions are less cellular than the cutaneous ones.

I-69. **Answers: b, d, e.** Hospital-acquired lung abscess is often colonized with gram-negative bacilli and *S. aureus*. Broncho-scopy should be performed to rule out obstruction such as foreign body or carcinoma. Most experts believe that penicillin G is the first choice in therapy and that clindamycin is reserved for critically ill patients or true penicillin failures. The mortality rate with prolonged medical therapy and that for surgical management are the same.

I-70. **Answers: a, b, c, d, e.** The characteristic course of a lung abscess is chronic and indolent, with the potential for sudden severe complications such as brain abscess, massive hemoptysis, or rupture of the pleura and development of a pyo-pneumothorax. Other complications include bronchopulmonary fistula, empyema necessitatis and amyloidosis.

I-71. **Answer: b, c, e.** Bronchoalveolar lavage in normal subjects contains macrophages (80–85%), lymphocytes (10–15%), neutrophils (5% or less), and a few eosinophils. Of the lymphocytes, the vast majority are T cells. Approximately 80% of macrophages display surface membrane HLA-DR. All major immunoglobulin isotypes, including IgA, IgG, IgM, and IgE, have been identified in bronchial secretions. Unlike serum, the concentration of IgA usually exceeds that of IgG in bronchial secretions. The ratio of IgG to IgA is lowest in upper airway secretions but rises progressively as sampling proceeds peripherally in the lower respiratory tract. IgG considerably exceeds IgA in samples of bronchoalveolar lavage fluid.

I-72. **Answers: b, c, d, e.** Tuberculosis is particularly common in non-Whites, and is predominantly extrapulmonary. Rifampin can be given in normal doses but, in the pre-dialysis patient, rifampin can, in rare instances, cause nephrotoxicity. The frequency of infection with atypical mycobacteria is increased. Ethambutal hydro-chloride is a toxic drug and can cause ophthalmic damage.

I-73. **Answer: d.** Pulmonary conditions associated with an increased incidence of anaerobic infections in the lung are those characterized by stasis or tissue necrosis, such as pulmonary infarction, bronchial carcinomas or other obstructing lesions, or bronchiectasis.

I-74. **Answer: c.** In general, anaerobic bacterial infections do not occur with increased frequency in the immunocompromised host. The usual pathophysiologic mechanism underlying anaerobic bacterial infection is a breach in the mucocutaneous defense barrier. In the lung, the usual mechanism is drainage from periodontal disease, such as gingivitis.

I-75. **Answers: a, b, c, d, e.** The frequency distribution of anaerobic bacteria in lung abscess or aspiration pneumonia ranges from 6% to 100%. In empyema, the recovery rate ranges from 25%–76%. The incidence of anaerobic bacteria is second to *Streptococcus* pneumonia in community-acquired pneumonia (21–33%), and in hospital-acquired pneumonia the incidence is around 35%.

I-76. **Answers: a, d, e.** Histoplasmosis in AIDS is virtually always disseminated. It is the first AIDS-defining illness in about 80% of all reported cases. There are no apparent risk factors within the HIV-positive population (IVDA versus homosexual). Physical examination is generally nonspecific, the most common findings being hepatosplenomegaly and adenopathy. Skin lesions have been reported in less than 10% of cases. Most cases will show some CNS involvement (encephalitis, meningitis, or focal lesion) at autopsy. The complement fixation assay using yeast or mycelial antigen is greater than 1:8 in 70% of cases, but specificity of this test is limited by cross-reaction with *Cryptococcus*.

I-77. **Answer: e.** Once it has been determined that there is alveolar filling on the chest roentgenogram and symptoms are of short duration, suspicion should focus on atypical pneumonias giving rise to diffuse alveolar filling such as mycoplasmal pneumonia, *Legionella* pneumonia, and viral pneumonias. If the patient is immunosuppressed, infection with *Pneumocystis carinii* or cytomegalic inclusion virus is possible. Other causes include smoke, hydrocarbon or toxic gas inhalation, aspiration, high-altitude pulmonary edema, and the adult respiratory distress syndrome due to sepsis, burns, or fat embolization.

I-78. **Answers: a, c, e.** The histoplasma polysaccharide antigen by RIA is found in urine with 97% sensitivity, blood with 85%, and even CSF with 67%. Response to amphotericin is generally good—around 80%—if it is started in time (i.e., if patients live long enough to receive 2 gm). Therapy consists of induction with amphotericin 1–2 gm (1 mg/kg/day), followed by maintenance with 50–80 mg/week. Ketaconazole is no good. Lifelong therapy is necessary.

I-79. **Answers: a, b, c, d.** Nonspecific laboratory findings in legionnaires' disease include elevated CPK and liver function tests, and myoglobinuria. Hyponatremia and hypophosphatemia are common in this disorder.

I-80. **Answers: a, c, e.** With new improvements, *L. pneumophila* can be readily isolated from the sputum. Bronchoscopy can be useful in obtaining adequate specimens; bronchial washing gives a higher yield than bronchoalveolar lavage. Saline and lidocaine used in the procedure may inhibit *Legionella* growth. Indirect immunofluorescent antibody determination is the most widely used method, but obtaining a four-fold rise in titer may take up to 6–9 weeks. Urinary antigen detection is highly accurate, low in cost, easy to perform, and easy to obtain. Although it detects only serogroup 1 of *L. pneumophila*, 90% of *Legionella* infections are due to this serogroup.

I-81. **Answers: a, b, c, d.** The retropharyngeal space is bounded anteriorly by pharyngeal constrictions, posteriorly by the prevertebral fascia, and laterally by the carotid sheaths. The space extends inferiorly to the superior mediastinum (T1–T2). Extension below T1–T2 indicates involvement of the prevertebral space, which is posterior to the retropharyngeal space. Studies from the Mayo Clinic suggest that prevertebral tissues measuring more than 7 mm at C2 or 22 mm at C6 indicate a pathologic process. Mediastinal extension is characterized by a widening of the mediastinum on chest film. Diagnosis is confirmed by CT scan.

I-82. **Answers: a, b, d, e.** Retropharyngeal abscesses are usually caused by a contiguous infection of the ears, nose, or throat with lymph nodes lying within the retropharyngeal space. Less common causes include penetrating foreign bodies, dental procedures, and complications of endoscopy or oroendotracheal intubation. Clinically, retropharyngeal abscess presents initially with symptoms of acute pharyngitis. Symptoms heralding a more serious infection include sialorrhea, dysphonia, odynophagia, dysphagia, dyspnea, and shoulder/back pain made worse with swallowing. The incidence is rare in adults due to atrophy of the retropharyngeal lymph nodes, which occurs during childhood. The most frequent complication is dissection of the abscess to the posterior mediastinum with resultant mediastinitis, pleuritis, and pericarditis. Spontaneous rupture of the abscess results in pneumonia, empyema, or asphyxiation. Treatment centers around the mandatory surgical drainage of the abscess and intravenous antibiotics.

I-83. **Answers: c, e.** The respiratory system is the most frequent site of infection, followed by the skin, bones and joints, genitourinary tract, and central nervous system. The fungus exists in mycelial form in moist soil. When the soil is disturbed, fungal spores are aerosolized and may be inhaled. Once in the lung, the spores convert to yeast form. In acute infections most immunocompetent persons are asymptomatic or have flu-like symptoms. The chest roentgenogram is frequently abnormal even in asymptomatic patients, with consolidation the most common finding. Hilar and mediastinal adenopathy are uncommon. For reasons that are not well understood, blastomycosis is not a frequent opportunistic pathogen in the immunocompromised, and there are few reports of blastomycosis in the transplant population or in AIDS patients.

I-84. **Answer: c, e.** The radiographic finding of single or multiple pulmonary nodules is relatively unusual in advanced HIV disease. In general, focal lung nodules or distinctly nodular infiltrates are seen most frequently in patients with AIDS-related neoplasms. *Pneumocystis carinii* can present radiologically as a solitary pulmonary nodule, as reported in a few patients with AIDS. However, in one series of 150 microscopically proven cases of *P. carinii* pneumonia, only two patients (1.3%) presented with a solitary pulmonary nodule. Other infectious causes of focal lung nodules in AIDS include septic emboli, mycobacterial infections (*M. tuberculosis* more frequently than *M. avium-intracellulare*), and fungal disease (most commonly *Cryptococcus neoformans* and *Histoplasma capsulatum*).

I-85. **Answers: d, e.** Pulmonary non-Hodgkin's lymphoma in AIDS presents as both multiple nodules and as a diffuse infiltrate. AIDS-related pulmonary non-Hodgkin's lymphoma virtually always presents with extranodal involvement, but pulmonary involvement is relatively uncommon, occurring in less than 10% of reported cases. Along with pulmonary non-Hodgkin's lymphoma, Kaposi's sarcoma is the most frequently reported malignancy in AIDS. Although it can have a wide range of radiographic appearances, the most common finding is a bilateral interstitial and/or alveolar infiltrate, frequently with pleural effusions. Well-defined pulmonary nodules are an uncommon radiographic finding, occurring in approximately 15% of cases. It is becoming evident that patients with AIDS are at higher risk to develop other malignancies, and adenocarcinoma of the lung occurs frequently.

I-86. **Answers: a, b, c, d, e.** Individuals who lived in the early part of the 20th century were exposed to epidemic TB and have harbored latent infection for decades. The appearance of active TB in them is most likely due to diminished cell-mediated immunity with aging. The incidence in nursing homes, is much higher than in the general population, presumably owing to intercurrent illness and a variety of stresses. Mini-epidemics have been noted in nursing homes, with high rates of contact infection and the rapid appearance of disease. INH prevention, while associated with a somewhat higher risk of hepatitis, has been effective in limiting disease in those recently infected.

I-87. **Answers: b, c, d.** Extrapulmonary TB now constitutes one in seven new cases of TB in America. Rarely is there simultaneous active pulmonary disease. Except in AIDS patients, virtually all forms of extrapulmonary TB can be treated with short-course chemotherapy (adjuncts such as surgery or steroids may be useful). As with pulmonary disease, there is a higher prevalence of all forms of extrapulmonary TB among non-Whites. Most patients have intact immunity.

I-88. **Answers: a, b, c.** The antiphospholipid Ab has been associated with arterial and venous thrombosis, thrombocytopenia, recurrent spontaneous abortions, pulmonary hypertension, and livedo reticularis. The antiphospholipid Ab may alter platelet membranes, leading to increased platelet adhesion, and/or they may affect endothelial membranes, leading to a decrease in prostacyclin release. There is no evidence of an alteration in BAL lymphocytes.

I-89. **Answers: a, b, c, d, e.** Varicella is usually a benign childhood malady infrequently associated with serious complications. Varicella pneumonia is the most common complication; it is more common in adults (16 to 50% incidence). It occurs 1 to 6 days after the onset of the rash, and can be associated with significant morbidity and mortality. Pregnancy and tobacco use are risk factors. Intravenous acyclovir should be administered to normal hosts with clinically evident pneumonia.

I-90. **Answers: children, a; adults, b.** In children, respiratory syncytial virus, and in adults, influenza A are the most common causes of viral pneumonia.

I-91. **Answers: a, b.** Secondary bacterial pneumonia is a serious complication of influenza pneumonia. The patients have "classic" influenza followed by a period of improvement of 1–4 days. Fever and signs of purulent pneumonia then ensue. The most common etiologies are (in order): *S. pneumoniae*, *S. aureus* (the classic association), and *Haemophilus influenzae*.

I-92. **Answers: a, b.** During outbreaks of influenza, amantadine hydrochloride can be administered as short-term (weeks) prophylaxis for high-risk individuals who did not receive the vaccine. It may also be given for 2 weeks only, if the vaccine is given simultaneously. Rimantadin hydro-

chloride is a newly released structural analog of amantadine hydrochloride, which appears to be comparable to amantadine hydrochloride in terms of efficacy and safety.

I-93. **Answers: a, b, c, e.** Pneumococcal vaccine has been recommended for all of the groups, except children with leukemia.

I-94. **Answers: d, e.** *Pneumococcus* and *Haemophilus* should be readily diagnosed by examination of blood, pleural fluid, and sputum. The sensitivity of bronchoscopy specimens seems to be comparable to that of sputum for *Legionella*. There are studies showing that the yield from bronchoscopy for *M. tuberculosis* is slightly better than that for sputum. Bronchoscopy with BAL is the current procedure of choice for detecting *Pneumocystis*, although yield with sputum has been respectable in some centers.

I-95. **Answers: a, b, c, d.** Streptococci produce three erythrogenic toxins called exotoxins A, B, and C. There has been a gradual increase in the virulence of group A streptococci, and emergence of the streptococcal "toxic shock" syndrome. The suspected portals of entry are primarily the skin, the mucous membranes, and the lungs. Localized swelling and erythema appear, as well as thin yellow bullae on the skin. There is mild leukocytosis with a striking left shift and eventually thrombocytopenia and hypoprothrombinemia. Progressive azotemia requiring dialysis, hypocalcemia out of proportion to hypoalbuminemia, and hematuria are frequent. The clinical course is one of multi-organ failure with ARDS in more than 50% of the patients (as compared with 8% in routine gram-positive sepsis) and mortality of 30–100%. The majority of patients require surgical debridement and/or amputation for control of sepsis. The treatment of choice is still penicillin G, to which streptococci are exquisitely sensitive. In penicillin-allergic patients, vancomycin, a first- or second-generation cephalosporin, or erythromycin can be used.

I-96. **Answers: a, b, d.** Staphylococci can produce several toxins: (1) alpha toxin, which is dermonecrotic and lyses erythrocytes and leukocytes; (2) beta toxin, which degrades sphingomyelin in erythrocytes, leukocytes, and fibroblasts; (3) gamma toxin, which causes acute diarrhea by inhibiting water absorption and stimulating cAMP in gut; (4) leukocidin, which causes potent lysis of leukocytes; (5) exfoliatin, responsible for staphylococcal scalded skin syndrome (SSSS); (6) TSST-1, responsible for the systemic and cutaneous symptoms of TSS; (7) enterotoxin A–E, responsible for the systemic symptoms of staphylococcal sepsis. In toxic shock syndrome, the toxin can be demonstrated in serum using a monoclonal antibody assay. TSST-1 antibody is present in plasma of 90% of the general population.

I-97. **Answers: b, c, d, e.** Although cooling towers were implicated in early studies, newer information shows that potable water distribution systems are, by far, the most common reservoir. In addition, evaporative condensors and whirlpools have been implicated in Pontiac fever.

I-98. **Answer: e.** The clinical presentation of legionnaires' disease is varied and non-specific. Although all of the symptoms given have been reported as occurring more often in legionnaires' disease, only hyponatremia (Na less than 131 mEq/L) has emerged as statistically significant in comparative studies.

I-99. **Answer: b.** *Legionella bozemanii*, a species of the genus *Legionella* whose origin can be in soil, accounts for 3.5% (range 0.6–4.8%) of sporadic cases, with *L. pneumophila* accounting for 85% and *L. micdadei* for 6.2% The clinical features in *L. bozemanii* are similar to those seen in *L. pneumophila*. *Legionella* infec-

tions can be diagnosed by the indirect immunofluorescence assay (IFA). Direct immunofluorescence (DFA) has a sensitivity of 25–50%, but it is highly specific and is rapidly available. The yield of DFA staining is directly related to the number of organisms recoverable from the sputum. Culture of the organism has been possible since 1978.

I-100. **Answers: a, c, d, e.** The only one not associated is eosinophilic granuloma.

I-101. **Answers: a, b.** Oropharyngeal anaerobic bacteria would be the primary etiology in a non-immunosuppressed patient admitted from the community. Penicillin and clindamycin are active against oral anaerobes, while ciprofloxacin and ceftazidime are not. Cefotaxime has only marginal activity. Broader-spectrum coverage would be acceptable if the patient were immunosuppressed or hospitalized, or came from a nursing home.

I-102. **Answers: d, e.** *Mycobacterium avium-intracellulare* and *Cytomegalovirus* are most common of these pulmonary pathogens in patients with AIDS.

I-103. **Answers: a, c, d.** The fluorescein-tagged monoclonal antibody, Giemsa stain, and the methenamine silver stain can be used to identify *P. carinii*.

I-104. **Answers: b, d, e.** The incidence of nocardiosis is thought to be rising because of newer antineoplastic regimens, organ transplantation, and HIV disease. Two thirds of patients are male. Pulmonary disease alone occurs in about 31%, CNS alone in 5%, skin and subcutaneous tissues alone in 30%, and disseminated disease in about 30%. Sputum cultures are positive in 25–35% of cases, but they may take weeks and require special handling. Organs involved in descending order of frequency include pleura, spleen, kidney, heart, liver, bones and joints, peritoneum, lymph nodes, adrenals, GI tract, meninges, pancreas, thyroid, eye, ear, marrow, endocardium, spinal cord, pituitary, and bladder. *N. asteroides* produces 80% of pulmonary disease. *N. brasiliensis* usually causes skin infection (including the classic Madura foot) but can also result in pulmonary disease in as many as 15%.

I-105. **Answer: b.** TWAR is a new chlamydial species that has been implicated in pneumonia. TW refers to Taiwan, one of the sources for the original isolate. The syndrome includes pharyngitis, fever, and nonproductive cough, and the disease is self-limiting. Erythromycin and tetracycline are treatment options. The CDC code name for *Legionella pneumophila* is OLDA.

I-106. **Answers: b, d, e.** Abnormalities in host defense such as alterations in serum complement or reduced PMN chemotaxis play no role in the pathogenesis of pulmonary disease associated with HIV.

I-107. **Answer: c.** All of the radiologic patterns may be seen in *Pneumocystis* infection except adenopathy.

I-108. **Answers: b, d.** The major infectious agents to worry about are mycobacteria and *Pneumocystis carinii*.

I-109. **Answers: a, b, c, d, e.** All of these, especially the finding of intrathoracic adenopathy or diffuse infiltration on the chest film, should trigger suspicion of tuberculosis.

I-110. **Answer: d.** Amphotericin B is the antibiotic of choice. Ketoconazole and miconazole have proven efficacy for mucocutaneous candidiasis, but are not therapies of choice for deep-seated infection. Flucytosine and rifampin have activity *in vitro* against *Candida*, but cannot be given as monotherapy because of the rapid emergence of resistance.

I-111. **Answers: b, c, d, e.** Toxic delirium, hypoglycemia, hyperglycemia, and hypo-

tension have all been seen following pentamidine administration.

I-112. **Answers: a, b, c, d.** Fever, skin rash with mucositis, hepatitis, and neutropenia have all been reported with trimethoprim-sulfamethoxazole.

I-113. **Answer: b.** Aspergillomas are masses of fungi that colonize a preexisting cavity, such as in tuberculosis. Tissue invasion is rare. Aspergillomas complicating asthma or other fungal infections are rare. Instillation of amphotericin B directly into the cavity via catheter or percutaneous injection has been successful in anecdotal reports.

I-114. **Answer: d.** *Aspergillus* may colonize the oropharynx of patients who are smokers or have preexisting lung disease. Its presence in the neutropenic host, with pulmonary infiltrates, however, is virtually diagnostic of invasive disease. Visualization of hyphae within lung tissue (but not sputum) is diagnostic of disease. The organism is rarely isolated from blood even in endocarditis.

I-115. **Answers: a, b, c, e.** Any individuals living in, or visitors to, endemic regions are at high risk for disseminated coccidioidomycosis. As with most superimposed infection, immunosuppressed individuals are at particular risk. However, there is no particular predilection for alcoholics.

I-116. **Answer: c.** Of the agents listed, only ketoconazole and amphotericin B have activity against *H. capsulatum*. Ketoconazole has been used in selected patients with chronic pulmonary histoplasmosis, but is not the therapy of choice for disseminated histoplasmosis.

I-117. **Answers: a, b.** As far as is known, standard precautions against infection (i.e., gloves, mask, eyewear, and gown) and good air hygiene (i.e., a well-ventilated room) are the only important ingredients of good infection control.

I-118. **Answer: e.** Although the portal of entry is the lung, the most common clinical manifestation is meningitis.

I-119. **Answers: a, b, c, d, e.** Direct immunofluorescence assay (DFA) is specific and is rapidly available. The yield of DFA staining is directly related to the number of organisms recoverable from the sputum. Indirect immunofluorescence assay (IFA) is the most commonly employed serologic test. The CDC criteria for a positive result is a four-fold increase in titer during convalescence. A presumptive diagnosis is made with a single titer >256. Culture media have been significantly improved over the past 10 years, and the medium currently in use is a buffered charcoal yeast extract agar with the addition of various antibiotics and dyes to increase its sensitivity. Most cultures will be positive in 3–5 days.

I-120. **Answers: a, b, c, d, e.** All five drugs have bactericidal activity when used in the correct dose. INH and RIF are the most active, followed by EMB, SM, and PZA. PZA's power in reducing the duration of therapy may not be related to its antimycobacterial effect.

I-121. **Answers: a, b, c, d.** Choice a, the Arkansas regimen, has been reported to work well in that state, where there is a low prevalence of INH resistance and there is a superb system to monitor patients on therapy and sustaining compliance. In other areas, such a regimen might well result in unacceptable rates of treatment failure/relapses and progressive drug resistance. The other 6- or 9-month regimens have been shown to be effective. The 4-month regimen has an unacceptably high (15–20%) risk of relapse.

I-122. **Answers: a, b, c.** There are roughly 3000 cases of pulmonary *M. avium-intracellulare* complex in AIDS. Up to 50% of AIDS victims die with evidence of disseminated infection. Most pulmonary cases are seen among those with underlying COPD, bronchiectasis, or fibrosis. However, pulmonary disease is also seen among those with no discernible disturbance of immunity or abnormalities of the lung. Cases are found in large numbers throughout the entire United States. Best estimates indicate that only 30% of patients with MAC in sputum cultures have invasive disease.

I-123. **Answers: a, b, c, d.** Although there have been no controlled clinical trials with placebo to prove the merit of therapy, there are abundant data that indicate untreated or poorly treated pulmonary MAC infection has a poor prognosis. Recently, experts have recommended initial INH, RIF, EMB with 2–4 months of SM for the usual case. If, however, the patient does not respond, a retreatment regimen based on *in vitro* susceptibility studies should be employed. For patients with localized disease, resectional surgery may enhance the outcome; however, there have been no controlled trials.

I-124. **Answers: a, b, c, d, e.** *M. fortuitum-chelonei* was nearly as prevalent as *M. kansasii* in a recent CDC survey. Some pulmonary disease is due to reflux from dilated esophagus (e.g., achalasia). It is seen in a variety of iatrogenic/nosocomial conditions (dialysis, cardiac surgery, breast implants). *M. fortuitum-chelonei* is almost universally resistant to anti-TB drugs. Regular antibiotics such as cefoxitin, amikacin, erythromycin, sulfamethoxasole, and the tetracyclines may be active against individual strains.

I-125. **Answers: a, c, e.** Virtually any mycobacterial species can be pathogenic in certain clinical settings. However, *M. gordonae* and *M. terrae* are rarely associated with disease. *M. gordonae* is, in the great majority of cases, a laboratory contaminant, not a saprophyte, in patients.

I-126. **Answers: b, c, e.** In contrast to *M. avium-intracellulare* complex, *M. kansasii* occurs among younger patients, many of whom have no underlying lung or immunologic disturbances. In the great majority of cases, chemotherapy alone is sufficient to cure. There usually is partial resistance to INH with lower levels of resistance to the other drugs. In spite of this, a regimen of INH, RIF, and EMB for 18 months results in 95% cure rates. Regimens less than 12 months in duration result in grossly unacceptable relapse rates. Patients with *M. kansasii* disease who receive an inadequate regimen (e.g., INH and RIF) may develop clinically significant higher levels of drug resistance in a relatively short period of time.

I-127. **Answer: d.** Although the incidence of TB is higher among non-Whites, the majority of cases are in white Americans. Presumably due to AIDS, the excess morbidity of TB has been among men 25 to 44 years old. This, not immigration, is believed to be responsible for the upturn. Evidence for spread of new infection is common in nursing homes. There has been a slow upward drift of resistance rates.

I-128. **Answer: e.** The AIDS virus infects CD 4+ helper T cells, which secrete lymphokines. These cause increased phagocyte-mediated antibacterial activity, which is involved in resistance to facultative intracellular bacteria, such as *Mycobacterium* sp. The AIDS virus does not infect CD 8+ cells.

2-8 Critical Care

C-1. **Answers: b, c, d.** Amyotrophic lateral sclerosis mainly affects men over 40 years old. It involves the loss of both upper and lower motor neurons in the spinal cord and/or brain stem. Anal and bladder sphincters are usually spared. Muscle weakness, atrophy, and fasciculations are common, as are bulbar deficits with difficulty in swallowing or speaking. Respiratory failure is a common but not ordinarily early feature of ALS. Mechanisms include impaired intercostal and diaphragmatic muscle function as well as paresis of glottic and pharyngeal function, culminating in atelectasis, aspiration, and pneumonia. Hypoventilation ultimately

occurs, and pulmonary emboli occasionally complicate a patient's course.

C-2. **Answers: a, b, c, d.** Paresis of the glottic and pharyngeal function can lead to aspiration, atelectasis, and pneumonia. These patients are vulnerable to upper airway closure when sleeping. These events may result in severe hypoxemia or hypercapnia, are usually associated with periods of REM sleep, and are exacerbated by the use of negative pressure ventilators. If muscle relaxation is required for intubation, depolarizing agents such as succinylcholine should be avoided since massive release of potassium is occasionally induced by this drug in patients with ALS. Low-dose heparin or pneumatic leg compression devices are indicated to prevent DVT and pulmonary embolism.

C-3. **Answers: a, b, c, e.** Colchicine overdose often results in progressive multi-organ failure and death. The drug interferes with microtubule assembly and function, thus having effects in all tissues to various extents. Its value in gout is believed to be due to interference with neutrophil granule release. Death from colchicine overdose has been described from as little as 6 mg in someone with normal physiology. Doses over 50 mg are usually fatal. The diagnosis is made usually from the history. Routine toxicology screens do not detect colchicine. The Pelger-Huët anomaly on peripheral smear (arrested mitotic figures in PMNs) is suggestive.

C-4. **Answers: a, c, d, e.** Early signs of colchicine overdose are the well-known GI side effects: nausea, vomiting, abdominal pain, and diarrhea. Dehydration follows. In the first 12 hours marked leukocytosis, fever, tachycardia, and hypotension are often seen. The next 12–72 hours bring multi-organ failure with ARDS, acute respiratory failure, metabolic acidosis, shock due to both vasodilation and heart failure, seizures and ascending paralysis, and thrombocytopenia. Late effects are pancytopenia, aplasia, skin rash, and alopecia.

C-5. **Answers: b, c, d.** There is no antidote. Treatment is supportive of the various organ failures. Aggressive fluid resuscitation, hemodynamic monitoring, blood product replacement, bicarbonate, and early mechanical ventilation are often required, as are pressors. Most of the drug is cleared in >72 hours; however, few patients survive to this point, succumbing to multi-organ failure and refractory hypotension. Iatrogenic overdose can be prevented by limiting IV dose to 3 mg, by

giving no more than 5 mg per gout attack, by decreasing doses in hepatic disease, and by forgoing its use in cases of combined hepatorenal disease (owing to dual paths of metabolism).

C-6. **Answers: a, b, c.** Pulmonary emboli occur almost solely from deep venous thrombosis, but cases associated with right heart thrombi have been increasingly described. Right heart thrombi form by two mechanisms: *in situ* or as emboli from systemic veins. *In situ* emboli occur in association with RA enlargement, pacer wires, PA or venous catheters, infarction of the right ventricle, and CHF. Right atrial clot is more common than right ventricular clot, and biventricular clot is unusual. Both sessile and serpiginous (or "worm-like") types of thrombi are seen on echocardiography.

C-7. **Answers: c, d, e.** Sessile thrombi occur usually in the setting of right ventricular failure or the non-DVT associations; serpiginous thrombi are seen mostly related to DVTs. Left-sided thromboemboli can occur with a patent foramen ovale. Treatment with heparin/coumadin is nearly always successful with sessile thrombi. Catheter-related thrombi are treated with thrombolysis, successfully in most cases.

C-8. **Answers: b, c, d, e.** One or more segmental or larger unmatched perfusion defects are not specific. Similar findings occur in fibrosing mediastinitis, pulmonary artery agenesis, primary tumors of the pulmonary artery, congenital branch stenosis, and extrinsic compression. This test can help to distinguish between chronic embolism and primary pulmonary hypertension.

C-9. **Answers: a, c, d.** ARDS patients suffer from diffuse injury of the pulmonary microvasculature with increased permeability to plasma proteins. The disease is characterized by an increased venous admixture (e.g., Qs/Qt > 30 or $PaO_2/FiO_2 < 250$), acute bilateral diffuse radiographic infiltrates, and a pulmonary capillary wedge pressure of less than 18 mm Hg. In late-stage ARDS the PAP may be greater than 40 mm Hg, and the patient can exhibit a low cardiac output, high PCWP and right ventricular end diastolic pressure, and an enlarged poorly contracting right ventricle with a small, hyperdynamic left ventricle.

C-10. **Answers: a, c, e.** The pulmonary artery pressure and vascular resistance can be elevated within a few hours after acute lung injury despite a normal PaO_2. Late in ARDS the PVR cannot be reduced by infusing vasodilators (nitroprusside, phentolamine, ibuprofen), but early in ARDS, infusing nitroprusside reduces the PAP and pulmonary capillary wedge pressure (PCWP), while increasing cardiac output, suggesting vasodilation or vascular recruitment. Recently, it has been reported that inhaling nitrous oxide, an endothelium-derived relaxing factor, can cause marked and selective pulmonary vasodilation without any decrease of the systemic vascular resistance and a fall in Qva/Qt level, probably because inhaled nitrous oxide selectively dilates ventilated alveoli. A reduction of PVR and increased right ventricular ejection fraction has been reported following inhaled nitrous oxide.

C-11. **Answers: a, b, d, e.** Balloon occlusion pulmonary arteriography has demonstrated multiple PA filling defects in some patients, associated with DIC, and a death rate of approximately 85%. At least two studies reported thromboemboli in most ARDS lungs at autopsy. In addition, there is major remodeling of the pulmonary arteries with marked medial muscular thickening and growth of smooth muscle into distal regions of the pulmonary artery where muscle is not normally present. There is a general finding that as PAP

increases the right ventricular ejection fraction decreases. ARDS can follow severe trauma (thoracic or extrathoracic), fat embolization, bacteremia, aspiration of gastrointestinal contents, smoke or toxic gas inhalation, surface burns, hydrocarbon ingestion, toxic drugs (heroin, paraquat), neurogenic pulmonary edema, viral, mycoplasma, or bacterial pneumonia, legionnaires' disease, Pittsburgh pneumonia agent, acute vasculitis, Goodpasture's syndrome, anaphylactic reaction to drugs and blood, radiation of thorax, immunosuppression and infection (*Pneumocystis*), thrombus, amniotic fluid, or tumor embolism to the lung. In late-stage ARDS with the PAP greater than 40 mm Hg, the patient can exhibit a low cardiac output, high PCWP and right ventricular end diastolic pressure, and an enlarged poorly contracting right ventricle with a small, hyperdynamic left ventricle.

C-12. **Answers: a, b, c, e.** Perhaps the most common cause of ARDS is sepsis, whether the primary focus is within the lung or elsewhere. Mediators of lung injury are directly and indirectly stimulated by exposure to gram-negative bacterial lipopolysaccharide (LPS). LPS given intravenously to sheep causes leukopenia, fever, and an increased transpulmonary flux of protein-rich edema fluid. LPS causes the release of a host of secondary mediators of injury including thromboxane and the endoperoxide metabolites of arachidonic acid. Thromboxane is a profound pulmonary vasoconstrictor. Tumor necrosis factor alpha is a polypeptide hormone produced by macrophages and monocytes. Tumor necrosis factor alpha, infused intravenously into rats and dogs after endotoxin injection, causes hypotension, metabolic acidosis, hemoconcentration, and death within a few hours.

C-13. **Answers: a, c, e.** Auto-PEEP can be measured by occluding the expiratory port, thereby equalizing the pressure in the system which, in turn, is measured on the pressure dial. The incidence of auto-PEEP is very high in COPD when ventilation is great, and increases with patient age. Increasing inspiratory flow (thereby allowing more time on the ventilatory cycle for exhalation) and use of a circuit with low compressible volume reduce auto-PEEP.

C-14. **Answers: a, c, e.** Auto-PEEP rises with smaller endotracheal tubes. Auto-PEEP causes the static pressure determination to be measured at a falsely elevated value, thereby underestimating the static compliance. Auto-PEEP is reduced by lowering frequency and tidal volume (increasing expiratory time which may decrease ventilation). Addition of PEEP up to a level equal to the auto-PEEP decreases auto-PEEP. Intrinsic PEEP acts as an additional inspiratory load, i.e., as a threshold load to the inspiratory muscles. The magnitude of intrinsic PEEP depends on the time available for expiration (T_e) and on the forces governing expiration.

C-15. **Answers: a, b, c, d, e.** When normal individuals breathe at rest, the inspiratory muscles must overcome the elastance and flow resistance of the total respiratory system. Expiratory muscle activity is usually absent, and hence the pressure driving expiration is due entirely to the elastic recoil pressure stored in the lung and chest wall during the preceding inspiration. This pressure is used in part to overcome the flow resistance offered by the total respiratory system during expiration, and part of it is normally dissipated against the postinspiration activity of the inspiratory muscles. Normal subjects exhibit substantial braking due to activity of inspiratory muscles early in expiration.

C-16. **Answers: a, b, c.** In patients with chronic airflow limitation, the rate of lung emptying is unduly slowed by the increased airway resistance and, by necessity, they develop auto-PEEP. Tachypnea promotes dynamic hyperinflation. One can reduce substantially the breathing efforts in acutely ill patients by application of CPAP or continuous negative pressure around the thorax (CNTP). This is valid only in expiratory flow limitation, so that the application of CPAP does not result in a further increase in the end expiratory lung volume. Here, a decrease in transthoracic driving pressure due to an increase in airway pressure (CPAP) or a decrease in pressure around the thorax (CNTP) should not affect the rate of lung emptying so that end expiratory lung volume should not change. If so, inspiratory muscle pressure required to initiate lung inflation should be reduced by an amount approximately equal to end expiratory elastic recoil pressure before application CPAP or end expiratory elastic recoil pressure before application +CNTP, and thus should reduce the inspiratory threshold load due to auto-PEEP, without affecting the FRC and hence the effectiveness of the inspiratory muscles as pressure generators.

C-17. **Answers: a, b, c, d, e.** Amyotrophic lateral sclerosis (ALS) is an idiopathic degenerative disease of the upper and lower motor neurons and is characterized by anterior horn cell degeneration. Male predominance is 2:1. Clinically, ALS presents with insidious onset of focal muscle weakness (100%), although occasionally as atrophy and fasciculations (90%) or spasticity (47%). Typical bulbar signs include tongue weakness and fasciculations, dysarthria, pharyngeal weakness, swallowing difficulties, and symmetric facial weakness. ALS can also present with subtle signs of respiratory insufficiency, such as altered sleep patterns, headache, or polycythemia.

C-18. **Answer: c.** Disseminated intravascular coagulation (DIC) results from the simultaneous activation of the coagulation and fibrinolytic systems as a consequence of a severe underlying disorder, such as sepsis, malignancy, trauma, shock, or serious obstetric complications. Platelets and clotting factors are consumed, and fibrin split products are released. Clinically, there is widespread hemorrhage. The consumptive coagulopathy of DIC cannot be interrupted until the underlying pathologic process that precipitated the disorder has been controlled. Until this is accomplished, administration of platelets, fresh frozen plasma, and cryoprecipitate are helpful adjuncts. Heparin administration, although advocated by some, probably is inadvisable in the profusely bleeding patient with DIC.

C-19. **Answers: a, b, c, d, e.** "Freebasing," the intravenous use of cocaine, results in immediate and direct absorption of the drug and produces a quicker and intense euphoria. These routes also result in pulmonary complications: a decreased diffusing capacity, which is postulated to be due to cocaine-induced pulmonary vasoconstriction eventually causing pulmonary hypertension; pneumothorax, pneumomediastinum, and pneumopericardium, which is believed to be due to a sudden rise in intraalveolar pressure secondary to the forced and prolonged inspiratory effort and Valsalva maneuver; cardiogenic and noncardiogenic pulmonary edema; acute pneumonitis, characterized by fever, dyspnea, hypoxemia, diffuse alveolar infiltrates, and respiratory failure; an acute, self-limited pulmonary syndrome with dyspnea and hypoxemia but no fever; symptoms usually resolve spontaneously within 36 hours of discontinuing cocaine and (usually with freebase cocaine) include alveolar hemorrhage and organizing pneumonitis/BOOP.

C-20. **Answers: a, b, d, e.** Methemoglobin (metHb) is formed by the oxidation of the iron moieties in deoxyhemoglobin to the ferric (Fe^{3+}) states. It is incapable of binding and transporting oxygen. It causes a shift to the left of the oxygen dissociation curve in the remaining hemoglobin, thereby further impairing oxygen delivery to tissues. Small amounts of metHb are continuously formed under normal circumstances, but these are readily reduced by the enzyme NADH-dependent metHb reductase, keeping normal levels less than 1% of total hemoglobin.

C-21. **Answers: a, c, d, e.** Methemoglobinemia may be hereditary or acquired. Hereditary forms are uncommon and include hemoglobin variants, which stabilize the ferric state and deficiencies of NADH-dependent metHb reductase. The hereditary methemoglobinemias generally have no clinical manifestations other than cyanosis, unless patients are exposed to oxidant stresses. Acquired methemoglobinemias are caused by exposure to oxidant agents. These include nitrites and nitrates, which may be environmental (e.g., from well water) or pharmacologic; they also include sulfonamides (e.g., dapsone), aniline derivatives, topical anesthetic agents (e.g., benzocaine), and Pyridium. Most elevations in metHb are asymptomatic; the earliest sign is the bluish-brown cyanosis.

C-22. **Answers: b, c, e.** Most elevations in metHb are asymptomatic. When metHb levels approach 30% of total Hb, symptoms of hypoxia such as dyspnea, headache, and malaise may be seen. Levels of 50–70% are associated with acidosis, arrhythmias, and coma. Higher levels are frequently fatal. Patients with underlying problems with O_2 delivery may have symptoms with lower levels. Diagnosis is suggested by otherwise unexplained cyanosis and dark brown blood that fails to brighten with exposure to oxygen. Accurate diagnosis is usually made with a spectrophotometric heme oximeter (CO-oximeter) during blood gas analysis. Since most cases are associated with few or no symptoms, treatment usually consists of withdrawing the offending agent. For significant symptoms or levels greater than 30%, IV methylene blue (1–2 mg/kg of 1% solution) may be given. In severe cases of methemoglobinemia, exchange transfusion or hyperbaric oxygen may be tried.

C-23. **Answers: a.** Pulse oximetry estimates oxygen saturation based on the absorption of light at two wavelengths (oxyhemoglobin absorbing primarily at 940 nm and deoxyhemoglobin absorbing mainly at 660 nm). The ratio between these absorbencies is compared to experimentally derived standards to provide oxygen saturation. This method is accurate as long as only oxyHb and deoxyHb are present. When additional hemoglobins are present, however, erroneous pulse oximetry results may occur. MetHb absorbs reasonably well at both wavelengths, so that the ratio of the two wavelengths approaches unity. In the experimentally designed standard, the ratio at unity gives a saturation of approximately 85%. In practice, low levels of metHb cause relatively small overestimations of true Hb saturation. At larger concentrations, as the overall ratio approaches unity, saturation by pulse oximetry remains near 85% even in the face of markedly reduced oxyHb. Thus, assessing oxygen delivery is best accomplished by means of arterial blood gas analysis with CO-oximetry.

C-24. **Answers: a, b, d, e.** In hypothyroidism or its extreme, myxedema, one can encounter alveolar hypoventilation, sleep apnea, exudative pleural effusions, and pulmonary edema, which, along with cardiomegaly and EKG abnormalities, may mimic CHF clinically.

C-25. **Answers: a, d, e.** Patients with myxedema and obesity demonstrate reductions in lung volumes, maximum breathing capacity, and D_LCO, and most subjects manifest alveolar hypoventilation and a reduced ventilatory response to carbon dioxide.

C-26. **Answers: a, b, c.** In myxedema without obesity, lung volumes and ABGs are normal, but MBC and D_LCO are reduced, as is hypercapnic ventilatory responsiveness. Other studies have reported reduced hypoxic drives in patients with either myxedema or hypothyroidism, but only those patients with myxedema also had reduced hypercapnic drives.

C-27. **Answer: b.** Reported associations are with *Campylobacter* infections, Hodgkin's disease, trauma, and following epidural and general surgery.

C-28. **Answer: b.** The classic presentation is progressive symmetric muscle weakness, which spreads proximally and is associated with areflexia. One third of these patients have associated sensory symptoms (paresthesias, pain, numbness), and cranial nerves are affected in half. Patients commonly have transient autonomic dysfunction characterized by flushing and sweating.

C-29. **Answer: a.** Patients commonly have transient autonomic dysfunction characterized by flushing, sweating, hypo- and hypertension, tachy- and bradycardia. The CSF is acellular with a striking increase in protein; glucose is normal. The typical findings on nerve conduction studies and EMG are slowed conduction (a consequence of the demyelination), prolonged distal latencies, small amounts of axonal dropout, and, much later, mild denervation.

C-30. **Answers: b, c.** The direct mechanism of organ toxicity is not well understood. It had been thought that most damage was due to deposition of calcium oxalate crystals in blood vessel walls, but it is now known that such deposition is neither a necessary nor a sufficient condition for organ damage to occur. Oxalate is produced by sequential oxidation of ethylene glycol and is in itself a highly toxic compound capable of causing renal damage, acidosis, or death if ingested directly. Hypocalcemia is a common finding, and is probably due to formation of calcium oxalate. The "classic" crystals are needle-shaped calcium oxalate monohydrate crystals, which are often erroneously reported as hippuric acid crystals. Ethanol has a 100-fold greater affinity for alcohol dehydrogenase than ethylene glycol has.

C-31. **Answers: a. 1, b. 1, c. 2, d. 1, e. 3.** Three stages of ethylene glycol poisoning have been described:

Stage 1, predominantly CNS effects: inebriation, nausea and vomiting, seizures, stupor, coma, cranial nerve abnormalities (VII, IX, X), decreased visual acuity, optic atrophy, ophthalmoplegia, metabolic acidosis, and calcium oxaluria.

Stage 2, predominantly cardiopulmonary effects: tachycardia, tachypnea, hypertension, pulmonary edema, cardiac dilatation, hypoxia, and dysrhythmias.

Stage 3, predominantly renal effects: proteinuria, hematuria, flank pain, and acute tubular necrosis.

C-32. **Answer: b.** Since the metabolites of ethylene glycol are much more toxic than the ethylene glycol itself, blocking the metabolism of ethylene glycol is one mainstay of therapy. Ethanol has a 100-fold greater affinity for alcohol dehydrogenase than ethylene glycol has, and so a loading dose of 8 ml/kg of 10% ethanol is given with a maintenance infusion of 1–1.5 ml/kg/hour, maintaining ETOH levels at 100–150 mg% until ethylene glycol levels are zero. Both ethylene glycol and its toxic metabolites are readily dialyzable, and hemodialysis is another mainstay of therapy. Bicarbonate and alkaline diuresis are also useful.

C-33. **Answers: a, b, c, d, e.** High-dose chemotherapy followed by autologous bone marrow transplant has been increasingly utilized in patients with Hodgkin's and non-Hodgkin's lymphoma, breast and ovarian carcinoma, small cell carcinoma of the lung, malignant melanoma, and nonseminomatous germ cell tumors.

C-34. **Answers: a. V, b. V, c. V, d. V, e. P.** The potential advantages of volume-controlled inverse-ratio ventilation include the delivery of a guaranteed tidal volume and precise manipulation of the inspiratory flow pattern. However, peak alveolar pressures can vary with changes in respiratory mechanics. Sedation is mandatory during volume-controlled inverse-ratio ventilation because of the danger that the patient will inadvertently cause increases in frequency and associated gas trapping. As with any pressure-limited mode of ventilation, the volume delivered with pressure-controlled inverse-ratio ventilation varies with respiratory system compliance and resistance.

C-35. **Answer: b.** The predominant causes of an anion gap are salicylate intoxication, lactic acidosis, uremia, methanol toxicity, paraldehyde toxicity, ethylene glycol toxicity, and ketoacidosis.

C-36. **Answer: e.** Tracheoesophageal fistula may result from a cervical Zenker's diverticulum, infectious organisms such as *Candida*, tracheal or esophageal infection, blunt chest trauma, vasculitis (i.e., Wegener's granulomatosis), as well as malignant disorders such as lymphoma.

C-37. **Answers: b, c, e.** Allopurinol is often incorrectly prescribed for asymptomatic hyperuricemia, for which no data supports the contention that treating asymptomatic high serum urate levels reduces the incidence of urate nephropathy. At standard doses of allopurinol (i.e., 300 mg/day), a patient with renal insufficiency will accumulate high levels of oxypurinol and be more at risk of developing the syndrome. In a patient for whom allopurinol is clearly indicated, the dosage must be adjusted for renal function and the patient cautioned to be aware of the first signs of toxicity (usually a rash). Complications of the syndrome include worsened renal function, infection, and GI, neurologic, dermatologic, and ocular sequelae. There is no effective treatment except for early recognition of the syndrome, withdrawal of the drug, and supportive care. Steroids have been used but have no proven benefit. The likely mechanism of toxicity is a hypersensitivity reaction to allopurinol or its metabolite, oxypurinol, leading to immune-complex deposition and vasculitis.

C-38. **Answers: a, e.** Like allogeneic bone marrow transplant recipients, patients with autologous bone marrow transplant have a high incidence of pulmonary complications (40–60%). However, the spectrum of disease appears to be significantly different. Diffuse alveolar hemorrhage has been described in "immunocompromised" hosts, but it is usually a "secondary" phenomenon, often seen in association with thrombocytopenia and/or invasive fungal infection. In contrast, autologous bone marrow transplant recipients appear to be at risk for developing a "primary" or idiopathic form of diffuse alveolar hemorrhage, which may in fact be the most common pulmonary complication. The frequency of diffuse alveolar hemorrhage appears to be associated with age over 40, treatment of solid malignancies (especially melanoma), mucositis, WBC recovery, and renal insufficiency. There appears to be little correlation with thrombocytopenia or type of chemotherapy. Diffuse alveolar hemorrhage most commonly occurs

within 40 days of transplantation, although there have been case reports of diffuse alveolar hemorrhage occurring 1 to 2 years following autologous bone marrow transplant.

C-39. **Answers: b, d, e.** Inverse-ratio ventilation extends the inspiratory time. Although there are many anecdotal reports, there are no controlled studies comparing outcome in ARDS patients treated with inverse-ratio ventilation and with conventional ventilation. There are two methods for administering inverse-ratio ventilation: (1) volume-cycled ventilation with an end inspiratory pause or with a slow or decelerating inspiratory flow rate; or (2) pressure-controlled ventilation applied with a long inspiratory time.

C-40. **Answers: b, c, d.** When performed within the first 10 days of disease onset, computed tomographic scans demonstrate marked heterogeneity in the roentgenographic density of the lung with areas that have the density of normally aerated tissue, as well as areas that appear poorly aerated or consolidated. There is often a striking gravitational distribution of the infiltrates. Areas of consolidation appear more extensively in dependent portions of the lung. With ventilatory support, most patients with the adult respiratory distress syndrome (ARDS) do not die of respiratory insufficiency; they die of sepsis and multiple organ failure. The incidence of these complications rises with the duration of mechanical ventilation. Recent evidence suggests that conventional ventilatory support of patients with ARDS (i.e., volume-cycled ventilation with applied positive end expiratory pressure) may perpetuate or extend lung damage by injuring delicate alveolar tissues with high pressures. The use of inverse-ratio ventilation, which extends the percentage of inspiratory time to the point of inverting the conventional I:E ratio of 1:4, may improve gas exchange while limiting or decreasing the peak airway pressures.

C-41. **Answers: a, c, e.** Analyses of gas exchange using inert gas techniques suggest that ARDS alters lung function in a nonhomogeneous pattern. The proportion of venous admixture correlates with the proportion of nonaerated lung. A significant fraction of lung units appears to have normal V/Q ratios despite the marked increases in shunt and dead space. The surface tension of alveoli may be higher than normal at low lung volumes owing to depleted or dysfunctional surfactant. Using gas dilution methods, aerated lung volume at FRC is significantly less in patients with ARDS than in other patients requiring mechanical ventilation, perhaps because flooding of alveoli with edema fluid and inflammatory debris forces gas out of the lung. Early in the disease process, the inflation portion of the P-V curve is typically flat, and significant hysteresis tends to be present, i.e., the volume of aerated lung is greater during deflation than during inflation at the same transpulmonary pressure.

C-42. **Answers: a, e.** Gas extravasated from alveoli during ventilatory support for ARDS is visible roentgenographically as pneumothoraces, pulmonary interstitial emphysema, pneumomediastinum, pneumoperitoneum, and tension air cysts. Early animal investigations demonstrated that alveolar disruption appeared to occur in alveoli that bordered the bronchovascular sheath, particularly when an excessive pressure gradient exists across this boundary. Peak airway pressure over 40–50 cm H_2O is thought to be associated with an increased risk of alveolar rupture during mechanical ventilation. The incidence of barotrauma exceeds 40% in patients exposed to a peak airway pressure above 70 cm H_2O. It has been

suggested that ventilator-induced alveolar edema may occur at relatively low levels of peak airway pressure. In animal models of ARDS, large tidal volumes contributed to increased lung edema, even if peak airway pressure, end inspiratory lung volume, and pulmonary capillary wedge pressures were held constant.

C-43. **Answers: b, d.** During positive ventilation of a passive subject, mean airway pressure over the entire respiratory cycle reflects the average pressure applied by the ventilator, and mean alveolar pressure is the average pressure acting to distend the alveoli against the combined recoil of lung and chest wall. During volume-controlled ventilation, the peak airway pressure always exceeds the peak alveolar pressure. In contrast, during pressure-controlled inverse-ratio ventilation, the "peak" or set airway pressure and the peak alveolar pressure will equilibrate. A potential problem with inverse-ratio ventilation is that cardiac output may fall as mean airway pressure increases. Most patients do not tolerate inverted I:E ratios without sedation, and paralytic medications in some cases. This is particularly important in volume-controlled inverse-ratio ventilation. If the patient is allowed to trigger the ventilator during volume-controlled inverse-ratio ventilation, dyssynchrony is almost inevitable, and alveolar pressures will increase dangerously because of gas trapping. Increasing the frequency during pressure-controlled inverse-ratio ventilation may actually reduce the alveolar ventilation.

C-44. **Answers: a, b, c, d.** The aspartate aminotransferase has been found to be elevated in 88% of cases of the allopurinol hypersensitivity syndrome. Leukocytosis may be accompanied not only by eosinophilia but also by a left shift, without clear evidence of infection. Many patients have underlying chronic diseases, the most common being chronic renal failure, hypertension, diabetes mellitus, and congestive heart failure. The onset of the syndrome on the average, follows 6 weeks of therapy, but the range is large (1-728 days).

C-45. **Answers: c, e.** In addition to thyroid replacement, management of myxedema involves avoidance of CNS depressants, avoidance of hypotonic fluids, meticulous search for a precipitating event or infection, and passive rewarming to avoid peripheral vasodilation. Corticosteroids should be given initially to cover for possible coexistent adrenal insufficiency.

C-46. **Answers: d, e.** Myxedema may be associated with obstructive sleep apnea, which is reversible and may not be related to obesity. Hypoglycemia may occur and suggests coexistent primary or secondary adrenal insufficiency. Renal impairment with hyponatremia is often associated with myxedema and is due to a decrease in free-water clearance. The etiology is unclear, but is associated with inappropriate ADH secretion or inability to suppress ADH with a water load and altered renal hemodynamics with reduced delivery of water to the distal nephron causing a dilutional hyponatremia.

C-47. **Answers: a, b, c, d, e.** Hypothyroidism exists when the amount of thyroid hormone reaching the peripheral tissues is insufficient for normal metabolic requirements. Decompensation is usually caused by a precipitating event or illness. The skin is characteristically dry, pale, and scaly, and may have a yellow tinge due to deposits of carotene. Important causes of hypothyroidism in the United States include chronic autoimmune (Hashimoto's) thyroiditis, nongoitrous variants, and ablative hypothyroidism. The pulmonary manifestations are myriad but culminate in alveolar hypoventilation with

progressive CO_2 retention due to decreased ventilatory responses to both hypercarbia and hypoxia. Important drugs that cause hypothyroidism are iodide and lithium carbonate in susceptible individuals (those with preexistent Hashimoto's thyroiditis or Graves' disease).

C-48. **Answers: a, d.** In the "toxic strep" syndrome, the suspected portals of entry are primarily skin, the mucous membranes, and the lungs. There is localized swelling and erythema, as well as thin yellow bullae on the skin. There is mild leukocytosis with a striking left shift, and eventually thrombocytopenia and hypoprothrombinemia. Progressive azotemia requiring dialysis, hypocalcemia out of proportion to hypoalbuminemia, and hematuria are frequent. The clinical course is one of multi-organ failure with ARDS in more than 50% of the patients (as compared with 8% in routine gram-positive sepsis); the mortality rate is 30–100%. The majority of patients require surgical debridement and/or amputation for control of sepsis. The treatment of choice is still penicillin G, to which streptococci are exquisitely sensitive. In penicillin-allergic patients, vancomycin, a first- or second-generation cephalosporin, or erythromycin can be used.

C-49. **Answers: a, b, e.** Staphylococcal alpha toxin is dermonecrotic and lyses erythrocytes/leukocytes. Beta toxin degrades sphingomyelin in erythrocytes, leukocytes, and fibroblasts. Gamma toxin causes acute diarrhea by inhibiting water absorption and stimulating cAMP in gut. TSST-1 antibody is present in plasma of 90% of the general population. The toxin can be demonstrated in serum using a monoclonal antibody assay in toxic shock syndrome.

C-50. **Answer: d.** Major physical signs of respiratory distress include tachypnea, tachycardia, arrhythmias, hypotension, diaphoresis, nasal flaring, and recession of the suprasternal/supraclavicular space.

C-51. **Answers: a, b, d, e.** The increased intracranial pressure often seen in patients with bacterial meningitis is most probably multifactorial. The cerebral edema that occurs may be vasogenic, cytotoxic, or interstitial in origin. In addition, the secretion of antidiuretic hormone contributes to the pathogenesis of edema. The inflammatory response in CSF is reduced by inhibiting the cyclooxygenase pathway of arachidonic acid metabolism. When tested after the intracisternal inoculation of live pneumococci, administration of cyclooxygenase inhibitors in conjunction with beta-lactum antibiotics markedly reduce inflammation. Preliminary evidence suggests that the combination of dexamethasone and antibiotics decreases CSF tumor necrosis factor and interleukin-1 more rapidly than antibiotics alone.

C-52. **Answers: b, c, e.** The three most common causative agents of bacterial meningitis are *Haemophilus influenzae*, *Neisseria meningitidis*, and *Streptococcus pneumoniae*. A critical step in the initiation of meningitis is the host acquisition of a new organism by nasopharyngeal colonization. The mechanism underlying bacterial traversal across a presumably intact blood-brain barrier is largely unknown, but once bacteria enter the subarachnoid space, host defense mechanisms are inadequate to control the infection. Also, specific antibody formation and complement levels are essential for opsonization of the encapsulated meningeal pathogens and efficient phagocytosis; however, their relative absence in CSF has been well documented. The presence of tumor necrosis factor in CSF may be specific for bacterial meningitis.

C-53. **Answers: a, b, e.** Phospholipase A and the complement cascade are thought to be involved in mediating increased permeability. Diabetic ketoacidosis can cause ARDS and it can be unilateral. It is common to see an elevated serum amylase in diabetic ketoacidosis, and thus it has been suggested that acute pancreatitis is common during diabetic ketoacidosis and may in fact precipitate it. There is no correlation between degree of elevation of amylase and severity of diabetic ketoacidosis. Acute pancreatitis has been established as a cause of ARDS. Most studies indicate that fulminant ARDS is seen almost exclusively with hemorrhagic pancreatitis or ongoing pancreatic inflammation.

C-54. **Answer: e.** Pressure-support ventilation is triggered by the patient (or by a time lapse back-up in some systems) and continues until the patient's inspiratory flow decreases to a system-specific minimal level (usually 5 L/min or 25% of peak inspiratory flow), at which time exhalation ensues. Every breath must be triggered by the patient (unless the ventilator is equipped with a back-up mode). Delivered tidal volume will decrease if patient effort decreases or lung mechanics deteriorate. In patients receiving in-line continuous nebulizers, the flow rate of the nebulizer may exceed the patient's mean inspiratory flow, so that the negative pressure necessary to trigger pressure-support ventilation will not be generated. The low minute ventilation alarm may fail because the ventilator monitoring system falsely interprets the nebulizer flow as coming from the patient. There is no evidence that the work of breathing is reduced particularly in those with heightened respiratory drive and high minute ventilation.

C-55. **Answers: c, d.** The optimal amount of ventilator support in a patient requiring prolonged mechanical ventilation is unknown. Too much support may produce disuse atrophy and weakness of the respiratory muscles, whereas insufficient support predisposes to respiratory muscle fatigue and may produce or aggravate respiratory distress. Recent studies of respiratory muscle suggest that negative-pressure ventilation yields improvement in respiratory performance for 3 days in some patients with COPD. Several investigators have shown that intermittent mandatory ventilation leads to a two-fold or greater increase in work of breathing. During the breaths being delivered by the ventilator, a patient's work of breathing is about 80% of that during an unassisted breath.

C-56. **Answer: a.** Abdominal distension resulting from gastric distension, ascites, peritoneal dialysis, or bowel perforation may cause elevation of the diaphragm, basilar atelectasis, and deterioration in ventilation-perfusion relationships. Gastric distension may result from elevation of airway pressure above lower esophageal sphincter pressure during the delivery of manual ventilation, from elevation of tracheal pressure above cuff and lower esophageal sphincter pressure, during mechanical ventilation (with mouth closed), or during a prolonged or difficult attempt at intubation. Massive distension (i.e., meteorism) can result in gastric rupture.

C-57. **Answer: a.** An increased respiratory drive may result from pain, anxiety, hypoxic stimulation, hypercapnic stimulation, peripheral sensory-receptor stimulation, medications, increased ventilatory demands, or improper ventilatory settings. An alteration in body posture can cause significant hypoxemia, especially in patients with unilateral lung disease because of gravity, as blood is shunted through the diseased dependent lung. Agitation or seizures may result from use of theophylline. Aminoglycoside antibiotics can provoke or aggravate neuromuscular blockade and produce respiratory embarrassment. Hypoxemia may result

from worsening of ventilation-perfusion relationships secondary to bronchodilators.

C-58. **Answer: e.** Fighting the ventilator may be due to either a patient-related or a ventilator-related cause. If the latter is suspected, one should vary (one setting at a time) the trigger sensitivity, inspiratory flow, delivered tidal volume, mode of mechanical ventilation, and even consider the use of PEEP (to minimize the effect of auto-PEEP). If medical and mechanical problems have been excluded and distress persists, a sedative agent with or without a neuromuscular blocking agent can be administered, but these should only be given as a last resort because of the dangers associated with neuromuscular blockade and the inability to carry out spontaneous ventilation should a disconnection of the ventilator circuit occur.

C-59. **Answers: b, c, e.** Controlling intracranial pressure is beneficial in neurologic recovery of patients with head injuries. Mechanical ventilation-induced hypocapnia is effective in acutely and chronically lowering elevated intracranial pressure. IPPV in excess of 12 bpm may result in an increase in intrathoracic pressure and in intracranial pressure. With a rapid ventilator rate, the intracranial pressure may never return to baseline, and the positive effects of hypocapnia may thus be negated. High-frequency jet ventilation is characterized by low tidal volumes, high respiratory rates, and low peak airway pressures, and this may reduce any elevation in intracranial pressure that occurs with IPPV.

C-60. **Answer: b.** IPPV in excess of 12 bpm may result in an increase in intrathoracic pressure and a rise in intracranial pressure. If the ventilator rate is rapid, intracranial pressure may never return to baseline levels, thus negating the positive effects of hypocarbia. High-frequency jet ventilation is characterized by low tidal volumes, high respiratory rates, and low peak airway pressures. Low volumes and low peak airway pressures reduce the elevations of intracranial pressure with IPPV. The addition of CPAP and IMV breaths to high-frequency jet ventilation allows hyperventilation and adequate oxygenation in most patients.

C-61. **Answers: c, d, e.** Auto-PEEP is the development of hyperinflation and positive end expiratory pressure within the alveoli during mechanical or spontaneous ventilation due to insufficient expiratory time. The complications of auto-PEEP are similar to those of applied extrinsic PEEP: diminished cardiac output due to decreased venous return, increased cranial pressure, increased risk of barotrauma, especially pneumothorax due to hyperinflation, and inaccurate pulmonary artery catheter measurements of intrathoracic vascular pressures. Patients at risk include those with airflow limitation, a high respiratory frequency, or minute ventilation, and a small-diameter endotracheal tube.

C-62. **Answers: a, b.** Auto-PEEP (also termed occult PEEP, inadvertent PEEP, or intrinsic PEEP) is the development of hyperinflation and positive end expiratory pressure within the alveoli during mechanical or spontaneous ventilation. It develops because there is insufficient expiratory time. Patients with airflow limitation such as asthma, emphysema, or chronic bronchitis are at risk for auto-PEEP, as are patients on ventilators set to deliver a high respiratory frequency or a high minute ventilation. One can measure the amount of auto-PEEP by occlusion of the exhalation port at end expiration.

C-63. **Answers: c, d, e.** Treatment of auto-PEEP consists of inserting a larger endotracheal tube if possible, increasing the inspiratory flow rates and lengthening the expiratory time, or decreasing the respiratory frequency and/or minute ventilation,

using a circuit with low compressible volume, and/or adding positive end expiratory pressure to a level that equals the auto-PEEP.

C-64. **Answers: b, e.** The level of auto-PEEP does not register on the ventilator pressure manometer because it is open to the atmosphere. Auto-PEEP predisposes to barotrauma and hemodynamic embarrassment, increases the work of breathing, and decreases the efficiency of force generation of the respiratory muscles. It imposes a significant inspiratory threshold load, so that a patient with auto-PEEP who is triggering a ventilator must generate a negative pressure equal to the level of auto-PEEP in addition to the minimum circuit-pressure drop to initiate an assisted breath.

C-65. **Answers: a, c, d.** In normal subjects, lung volume at end expiration approximates the relaxation volume of the respiratory system (static balance between the elastic forces of the lung and the chest wall). In some critically ill patients, end expiratory lung volume exceeds the predicted FRC as a result of dynamic airway collapse in patients with airflow limitation and inadequate expiratory time. The relaxation pressure of the respiratory system is zero at end expiration in normal individuals. The end expiratory volume rises when expiratory resistance is increased.

C-66. **Answers: a, b, e.** Anticholinergic agents primarily antagonize acetylcholine competitively at the neuroreceptor site. The "anticholinergic syndrome" consists of both central (anxiety, delirium, disorientation, hallucinations, hyperactivity, seizures, coma) and peripheral (tachycardia, hypertension, fever, mydriasis, warm dry skin, diminished Gl motility, urinary retention) signs and symptoms. Toxicity may be due to, or potentiated by, drugs with anticholinergic profiles such as antihistamines, phenothiazines, and tricyclic antidepressants. Benzodiazepines may be useful for mild or moderate agitation and hyperactivity. Severe CNS toxicity generally warrants reversal of the syndrome with an anticholinesterase. Physostigmine, unlike other anticholinesterases, has excellent CNS penetration, and reversal of central toxicity is rapid and dramatic. Too-rapid IV administration of physostigmine may result in hypotension and seizures. Cholinergic toxicity (bradycardia, bronchoconstriction, excessive salivation, vomiting) may occur, especially in the patient who has been misdiagnosed as having anticholinergic toxicity.

C-67. **Answer: e.** The patient who is failing a weaning trial is characterized as being tachypneic, with an increased ventilation and respiratory rate, usually with a reduced tidal volume. This results in a reduced alveolar ventilation and an increased dead space/tidal volume ratio.

C-68. **Answers: a, b, d, e.** Endoscopic variceal sclerotherapy (EVS) is often the treatment of choice for managing esophageal varices acutely and prophylactically. Pleural effusions are common after EVS and may occur in as many as 50% of the patients; most are asymptomatic. The effusion is typically an exudate with normal pH, glucose, and amylase, and it may occur unilaterally or bilaterally. Another common roentgenographic finding after EVS is the development of a retrocardiac or mediastinal density believed to be due to paraesophageal and contiguous mediastinal inflammation; this is often mistaken for a left lower lobe infiltrate or collapse. Late perforations and esophago-bronchopleural fistulas develop from ulceration and subsequent transmural necrosis of the esophagus in 1–2% of patients, typically 7–14 days after EVS.

C-69. **Answers: a, b, c, d, e.** Pathologically, two responses are seen: an acute alveolitis, which peaks at 3 days and disappears by 10 days, and a chronic proliferative process, which peaks at 10 days and resolves over several weeks. Autopsy findings of fatal cases demonstrate bronchospasm, atelectasis, emphysema, signs of inflammation such as edema, hyperemia, and infiltration of PMNs, vascular thrombosis, hemorrhage, and necrosis of bronchial, bronchiolar, and alveolar tissues.

C-70. **Answers: e.** There is conclusive evidence to suggest that the pulmonary lesions are caused by aspiration and not by gastrointestinal absorption of the hydrocarbon. The management of hydrocarbon ingestion and pneumonitis is fairly straightforward. Acutely, large volumes of hydrocarbons in the gut can generally be tolerated without severe systemic effects, and vomiting should not be induced, as aspiration is the principal hazard. Corticosteroid therapy to prevent the development of fibrosis and to decrease the amount of hemorrhage and edema has been proposed, but does not appear to be effective and is not recommended. Antibiotics are frequently used for prevention of bacterial superinfection, but the majority of patients do not develop a bacterial superinfection, and the empiric use of antibiotics on all patients is controversial. Bronchodilators may be of benefit in patients with symptoms of bronchospasm.

C-71. **Answers: b, c, d, e.** Hypophosphatemia is a relatively common in-hospital condition. Serious hypophosphatemia (<1 mg/dl or 0.33 mmol/L) develops in nearly 1% of patients admitted to a medical service and up to 5% of patients in the medical intensive care unit. It is particularly associated with certain conditions including alcoholism and alcohol withdrawal, diabetic ketoacidosis, sepsis, and malnutrition.

C-72. **Answers: a, b, d, e.** Although significant phosphate deficiency may result from decreased input (particularly with the use of phosphate-binding antacids or with malabsorption) or increased renal excretion, which may be due to drugs (e.g., diuretics), the most common cause of hypophosphatemia seen in hospitalized patients is transcellular shifts from the extra- to the intracellular space. This is most frequently due to (1) respiratory alkalosis (CO_2 moves out of cells, raising intracellular pH and activating glycolysis, in which phosphates is incorporated into intermediate metabolites); (2) glucose and/or insulin administration, which results in movement of glucose and phosphorus into cells; and (3) aggressive nutrition, which also leads to the incorporation of phosphates into intracellular molecules.

C-73. **Answers: a, b, c, e.** The serum phosphate level is an inexact indicator of total phosphate stores, and a low level does not necessarily indicate phosphate deficiency, and vice versa. Nevertheless, clinical symptoms rarely occur in the absence of markedly reduced levels. Although detectable diaphragmatic dysfunction may be present with levels <2 mg/dl, significant problems generally occur with levels <1 mg/dl. A reduction in red cell 2,3 DPG and ATP leads to a left shift in the oxygen dissociation curve of hemoglobin, which decreases oxygen transport. Central nervous system manifestations of hypophosphatemia range from irritability and paresthesias to a Guillain-Barré like ascending paralysis to seizures and coma.

C-74. **Answers: b, c, d.** There is probably no need for intravenous supplementation in diabetic patients unless levels fall to <1 mg/dl. Moderate hypophosphatemia (1–2.5 mg/dl) can be treated enterally, with skim milk or sodium phosphate salts. Intravenous replacement is indicated for levels <1 mg/dl (usually sodium or potassium phosphate, 10 mmol/L over 8–12 hours, repeating as necessary until

levels approach 1.5–2 mg/day) with the remainder repleted enterally. Potassium and magnesium are frequently also low and should be repleted. Potential complications of IV phosphate therapy include hyperphosphatemia and precipitation of calcium phosphate crystals if the Ca/P product is >60, and symptomatic hypocalcemia if the phosphate is administered too quickly.

C-75. **Answers: a, b, d, e.** The epidemiologic data in Reye's syndrome seem to indicate that both genetic susceptibility and environmental factors are involved. The association of aspirin use and the increased risk of Reye's syndrome was initially controversial, but numerous sound epidemiologic studies now implicate aspirin ingestion with an increased risk, albeit small, of Reye's syndrome. There have been 23 previous reports of adult Reye's syndrome in the English literature, patients ranging in age from 16 to 62. URI/influenza B is the antecedent illness in many cases, as is varicella infection. Reye's syndrome is often divided into an infectious phase followed by an encephalitic phase.

C-76. **Answers: d, e.** There is overwhelming metabolic and histopathologic evidence that there is a universal mitochondrial injury in Reye's syndrome, and this so-called "mitochondrial phase" is equivalent to the "encephalitic phase" noted clinically. The activities of nearly all mitochondrial enzymes are decreased, including those involved in the urea cycle, oxidative phosphorylation, and the Krebs cycle. In contrast, the cytosolic enzyme activities are normal. These biochemical differences parallel the EM evidence of widespread mitochondrial degeneration in almost all tissues studied. The clinical severity and recovery seem to parallel the morphologic distortion and recovery of the mitochondria themselves.

C-77. **Answers: a, b, c, d, e.** Lactic acidosis is generally believed to be a reliable indicator of oxygen debt. When oxygen delivery is inadequate to meet cellular energy needs, anaerobic generation of ATP is favored with shifting of glucose metabolism to pyruvate production and subsequent formation of lactate and excess hydrogen ions.

C-78. **Answers: d, e.** In normals, Vo_2 is independent of O_2 delivery above about 350 ml/min/m². Below this, O_2 consumption is dependent on O_2 delivery. The normal relationship between O_2 supply and demand fails to hold in the septic state. In septic patients O_2 consumption depends on O_2 delivery at levels well above normal threshold for anaerobic metabolism. When oxygen delivery is inadequate to meet cellular energy needs, there is formation of lactate and excess hydrogen ions. Despite apparently optimal O_2 delivery, the presence of ongoing lactic acidosis should raise concern regarding ongoing tissue hypoxia and inadequate resuscitation at a cellular level, which are a prognostic indicator of a bad outcome.

C-79. **Answers: b, c, d, e.** Given that some 2 million prescriptions for allopurinol are written each year, the incidence of life-threatening reactions is low. Approximately 100 cases have been reported in the literature. In one large series, 3% of patients developed some reaction to the drug. The syndrome is defined by: (1) a clear history of allopurinol use, (2) lack of exposure to another drug, (3) a clinical picture consisting of two major criteria: (a) rash (diffuse maculopapular or exfoliative dermatitis, erythema multiforme, or toxic epidermal necrolysis) and (b) worsening renal function or acute hepatotoxicity; or by one major criterion and one minor criterion (fever, eosinophilia, leukocytosis).

C-80. **Answers: a, b.** The occurrence of this syndrome has been reported to be 67.3 % males and 32.7 % females. Aspartate aminotransferase is elevated in 88% and renal failure develops in 84%. No effective treatment exists except for early recognition of the syndrome, withdrawal of the drug, and supportive care. Steroids have been used but are of no proven benefit. The overall mortality in the reported cases is 26%, and many complications related to allopurinol hypersensitivity syndrome occur. Allopurinol is often incorrectly prescribed for asymptomatic hyperuricemia, but there are no data supporting the contention that treating asymptomatic high serum urate levels reduces the incidence of urate nephropathy.

C-81. **Answers: a, b, c, d.** The likely mechanism of toxicity is a hypersensitivity reaction to allopurinol or its metabolite, oxypurinol, leading to immune-complex deposition and vasculitis. Almost all organs have been involved. The accumulation of oxypurinol correlates with development of the syndrome, and is directly related to renal function, thus explaining the high association of AHS with renal insufficiency. The half-life of oxypurinol (approximately 20 hours with normal renal function) is extended to 250 hours in anuria. Mortality is more likely among patients with toxic epidermal necrolysis, hepatitis, or sepsis, but not with acute or acute-on-chronic renal failure.

C-82. **Answers: a, b, c, d.** The first report of pulmonary complications from the drug appeared in 1962 when a man developed fever and chills, eosinophilia, and pulmonary infiltrates over a 5-week course of intermittent nitrofurantoin therapy for a urinary tract infection. Patients with acute reactions present with fever (always), dyspnea, and eosinophilia (usually) a mean of 5 days after therapy was started. Although interstitial disease is usually associated with this drug, acute pulmonary reactions are much more common. Of 921 adverse reactions reported in Sweden between 1966 and 1976, 40% involved acute pulmonary reactions, 42% allergic reactions (mainly hives), and only 5% of patients had chronic interstitial pneumonitis.

C-83. **Answers: b, c, d, e.** The pathogenesis of pulmonary reactions is not known. Acute manifestations are likely to be a hypersensitivity reaction, with a previous history of exposure, rapid onset of symptoms, rapid disappearance after drug cessation, high incidence of eosinophilia, and some cases of anaphylactoid reactions. Chronic nitrofurantoin complications, however, are thought to involve some type of cumulative toxicity caused by the drug or one of its metabolites. Rat pulmonary endothelial cells incubated with nitrofurantoin are stimulated to produce the toxic oxygen radicals superoxide anion and hydrogen peroxide. Some postulate that direct oxidant injury of the lung represents one mechanism of pulmonary toxicity of nitrofurantoin. Cases of circulatory collapse have been reported. Resolution occurs quickly after the drug is discontinued, but re-exposure invariably leads to recurrence of symptoms. Chronic pulmonary toxicity rarely occurs in less than 6 months, but can be seen after years of seemingly uncomplicated therapy.

C-84. **Answer: e.** Women predominate and make up 80% of cases. Bibasilar interstitial infiltrates are the most common radiographic appearance, and pleural effusions are infrequently seen. Eosinophilia and leukocytosis are uncommon in patients with chronic pneumonitis. Lung biopsy often shows a nonspecific interstitial pneumonitis difficult to distinguish from other causes of interstitial pneumonitis. No specific pathologic finding can distinguish nitrofurantoin-induced fibrosis from other causes of fibrosis. Desquamative interstitial pneumonia has been reported in some patients.

C-85. **Answers: a.** Nitric oxide (NO) is a potent endogenous mediator previously known as endothelium-derived relaxing factor (EDRF). NO was first reported in the vascular endothelium, where it serves as a potent determinant of basal and induced vasodilator tone. NO is a labile, diffusable factor released from endothelium under basal conditions and in response to a wide variety of endogenous hormones and chemicals that increase intracellular calcium. Once produced, NO directly stimulates cyclic GMP in vascular smooth muscle causing relaxation. NO production is inhibited by hypoxia and may play a role in hypoxic pulmonary vasoconstriction.

C-86. **Answers: a.** Nitric oxide is avidly bound to hemoglobin and inactivated, thereby decreasing its availability for causing systemic vasodilatation and allowing selective pulmonary vasodilatations, mostly those associated with the best ventilated areas, and thus enhancing ventilation/perfusion matching. Nitric oxide causes inactivation of enzymes, as in the cytochrome system required for electron transport. Inhaled nitric oxide has been shown to decrease pulmonary vascular resistance (PVR) in patients with primary pulmonary hypertension.

C-87. **Answers: b.** It appears that steroidal neuromuscular blocking agents (e.g., pan- and vecuronium bromide) are more likely to be involved with this syndrome than the nonsteroid type agents (e.g., atracurium besylate), but this has not been confirmed by prospective studies. Pancuronium and vecuronium bromide and their active 3-hydroxy metabolites accumulate in patients with renal failure (and to some extent liver failure) and lead to prolonged neuromuscular blockade. Other factors associated with prolonged neuromuscular blockade include metabolic acidosis, female sex, and hypermagnesemia. Atracurium besylate is metabolized nonenzymatically and does not accumulate in renal or hepatic dysfunction, and therefore is likely to be less of a problem.

C-88. **Answers: a, c, d.** Patients treated concomitantly with high-dose corticosteroids and neuromuscular blocking agents seem to be particularly at risk. The resulting myopathy differs from chronic steroid myopathy in that the acute myopathy has distal as well as proximal weakness and is frequently associated with an elevated CPK. Other cases of prolonged paralysis have shown electrophysiologic evidence of neuropathy, either alone or with myopathy. The deficits are typically reversible, but may resolve slowly over weeks to months. There is no specific treatment, but physical therapy is essential to facilitate rehabilitation.

C-89. **Answers: c, d, e.** Critical illness polyneuropathy syndrome is characterized by weakness (with occasional respiratory muscle failure), decreased deep tendon reflexes, variable sensory deficits, and electrophysiologic evidence of axonal degeneration involving both motor and sensory fibers. The neuropathy is generally seen in patients with the multiple organ dysfunction syndrome after 2–4 weeks in the ICU. It is believed to represent another organ system involvement in multiple organ dysfunction syndrome (MODS).

C-90. **Answers: b, e.** Therapeutic levels needed for the anti-inflammatory effects of salicylates range from 15–30 mg/dl, with toxic effects occurring with levels greater than 30 mg/dl. Chronic intoxication is seen less frequently, but generally has a poorer outcome because of a low index of suspicion and delay in proper treatment. Hepatocellular necrosis can occur when levels exceed 20 mg/dl, but it is usually mild. Forced alkaline diuresis can be achieved with intravenous sodium bicar-

bonate and should be considered for all patients with salicylate level greater than 35 mg/dl.

C-91. **Answers: a, c.** Noncardiogenic pulmonary edema is a frequent complication of salicylate intoxication and is believed to be an increased alveolar capillary permeability as a result of platelet or prostaglandin interaction, a direct salicylate pulmonary microvascular injury, or a direct CNS toxic effect. The primary pathophysiologic effects include stimulation of the CNS respiratory center, uncoupling of oxidative phosphorylation, inhibition of the Krebs cycle, and interference with hemostatic mechanisms. An inhibition of the extrinsic coagulation cascade results in interference with the synthesis of factor VIII, but an increase of prothrombin is usually not clinically significant The respiratory stimulation leads to respiratory alkalosis, with a compensatory increase in renal excretion of bicarbonate. Concurrently with inhibition of the Krebs cycle enzymes, metabolic acidosis is generated from lactate and ketoacids. Salicylate excess can also interfere with carbohydrate metabolism, causing hyperglycemia followed by hypoglycemia as glucose stores are depleted in chronic or severe cases.

C-92. **Answers: a, b, c, d.** Therapy is directed toward treating the metabolic and electrolyte derangements, decreasing further absorption, and enhancing elimination. Gastric lavage, followed by multiple doses of activated charcoal, should be performed. Hydration along with electrolyte replacement and alkalinization are the primary therapy. Therapy is directed at maintaining a urinary pH of 8.0–8.5. The effect of bicarbonate therapy includes correcting the metabolic acidosis and alkalinizing the urine to promote excretion and prevent passage into the CNS and other tissues by increasing the ionized or nonabsorbable fraction. For patients with respiratory compromise or mental status changes, intubation and mechanical ventilation should be performed for airway protection, for alkalinization by hyperventilation, and for assistance in decreasing intracranial pressure from cerebral edema.

C-93.   **Answers: c, d.** In general, hemodialysis is indicated for severe toxicity that is not responsive to alkaline diuresis. Specific indications for hemodialysis include levels greater than 100 mg/dl in acute ingestion and greater than 70 mg/dl in chronic toxicity, rising levels, CNS abnormalities, and pulmonary edema.

C-94.   **Answers: a, b.** Inhalation injuries occur in approximately one third of all major burns and have a mortality of 45–78%. Inhalation of air heated to 150°C or higher usually results in burns confined to the face, oropharynx, and upper airway. Heat damage to pulmonary parenchyma is rarely seen and is generally prevented by laryngeal reflexes and the efficiency of heat dissipation of the oropharynx. At levels of CO between 0–10%, the patient is asymptomatic; 15–25% results in nausea and headache; 30% causes confusion and weakness; and 40–60% unconsciousness and death.

C-95.   **Answers: a, b, d, e.** The half-life is 4 hours but is reduced to 45–60 minutes with 100% FiO_2. CO not only causes hypoxia and anoxia by shifting the oxyhemoglobin desaturation curve to the left, but also binds to myoglobin, causing decreased O_2 transport to cardiac muscle as well, and interferes with the cytochrome oxidase system of cellular respiration.

C-96.   **Answers: b, e.** The course of ALS is relentlessly progressive, with mean survival of 4 years. There is a trend toward decreased survival for progressive bulbar palsy. Survival is further shortened for males and the elderly. Pulmonary function in ALS is impaired at diagnosis in the majority of patients. At onset, PFTs reveal decreased ERV, increased RV, and a normal TLC, while MVV is the most abnormal test of function.

C-97.   **Answer: a, b, c, e.** Many individuals aspirate to some degree during the night, and aspiration per se is not a major problem for the lungs as the pH is rapidly neutralized. The critical factors are the pH of the aspirate (pH of gastric aspirate <2.5), the volume of aspirate, and particulate matter/bacterial content. If any one of these occurs, there is lung damage.

C-98.   **Answer: b.** The first rule is to ensure an adequate ventilation. The patient should be disconnected from the ventilator and manually ventilated with 100% oxygen using an anesthesia bag, while a systematic effort is made to determine the cause of the distress. Relief by ventilating with the bag suggests that the distress was ventilator related. The source of the malfunction should then be determined by evaluating each component of the defective ventilator.

C-99.   **Answers: a, c, e.** Botulism is a disease resulting from a neurotoxin produced by the organism *Clostridium botulinum*. These are gram-positive, rod-shaped, spore-forming anaerobic bacteria that are widely distributed in the soil and water. The spores are capable of surviving at 100°C for up to 6 hours. The killing temperature is at least 120°C for 5–10 minutes. The formed toxin is more heat-labile and is denatured at 80°C. Food-borne, infantile, wound, and adult enteric infections are the four diseases caused by the toxin. In food-borne disease the toxin is ingested from contaminated food products, whereas in the other disease types the organism is allowed to grow in a wound or within the GI tract, producing toxin.

C-100. **Answer: d.** Most cases of human disease are the result of toxin types A, B, E, and F. Types C and D cause botulism in birds and mammals. Type A disease is found west of the Mississippi river, type B east, and type E is associated with marine products and is usually reported from the northwest and Alaska. Type A disease tends to be more severe, with more cases resulting in mechanical ventilation, whereas type E has the shortest latency between ingestion and symptoms. The toxin is absorbed from its source (GI tract or wound) into the blood stream and lymphatics, and targets the presynaptic terminal of neuromotor end plates in the peripheral nervous system. Endocytic vesicular uptake into the presynaptic terminal results in the prevention of acetylcholine release from the nerve terminal by a mechanism that is still unclear. The effects of the toxin can last for months.

C-101. **Answers: a, b, c, d, e.** The toxin is absorbed from its source (GI tract or wound) into the blood stream and lymphatics and targets the presynaptic terminal of neuromotor end plates in the peripheral nervous system. Endocytic vesicular uptake into the presynaptic terminal results in the prevention of acetylcholine release from the nerve terminal by a mechanism that is still unclear. Interruption of the cholinergic autonomic system results in diminished saliva and dryness of the mouth, which can lead to a sore throat. The effects of the toxin can last for months.

C-102. **Answers: c, e.** The Tensilon test is negative in botulism. The CSF fluid is frequently normal, although the fluid may have mildly elevated protein. The EMG has characteristic alterations implicating the neuromuscular junctions. The culture of stool or gastric aspirate is usually positive.

C-103. **Answers: a, c, d, e.** The clinical manifestations of botulism usually begin within 12–36 hours of toxin ingestion. Nausea and vomiting occur in only a third of types A and B, but are more common in type E. Early symptoms include weakness, lassitude, and dizziness. Most cases of food-borne botulism are from improper canning of fruits and vegetables in the home; however, restaurant outbreaks account for large numbers of patients because of the numbers of people affected prior to identification of the source. The autonomic dysfunction can lead to an ileus, constipation, and urinary retention.

C-104. **Answers: a, c, d, e.** Cranial nerve motor end plates are a common target as reflected in such symptoms as diplopia, blurred vision, photophobia, dysphonia, dysarthria, and dysphagia. Symmetric weakness of the extremities usually occurs in a descending fashion. Sensation is classically not affected. Respiratory arrest can occur, and ventilatory support may be necessary for months. Symptoms can persist for as long as a year, with persistent fatigue and dyspnea on exertion.

C-105. **Answers: b, c.** Antimicrobial therapy has no impact. An equine trivalent antitoxin has been shown to shorten the course of the disease and to decrease mortality. The antitoxin has a significantly greater effect on morbidity and mortality if given within 24 hours of the onset of symptoms. Guanidine was thought to be efficacious, as reported in the early 70s, but is no longer thought to be beneficial.

C-106. **Answers: a, b, c.** Paralysis occurs as a result of the toxin binding irreversibly to calcium channels at the motor neuron end plate. Acetylcholine release, a calcium dependent process, is subsequently inhibited. Symptoms begin within 12–36 hours of ingestion. The proximal muscles are more involved than the distal. Generally, sensory function is intact.

C-107. **Answers: a, b, c.** High-altitude pulmonary edema is a form of noncardiogenic pulmonary edema that develops in people who ascend to over 8000–9000 feet of elevation. Symptoms usually occur within 24–96 hours and include dyspnea, cough and fatigue, cyanosis, fever, and leukocytosis in the majority of patients.

C-108. **Answer: e.** Hemodialysis may result in hypoxemia and an increased $P(A-a)O_2$ as well as a reduced D_LCO. Complement activation has been implicated in the gas exchange impairment. Bicarbonate dialysate decreases the incidence of pulmonary complications.

C-109. **Answer: e.** In sickle cell disease the hemoglobin O_2 saturation curve is shifted to the right, and the PaO_2 at 50% Hb saturation (P50) is increased. The 2–3 DPG is increased, and the pulmonary capillary blood volume is increased. Reducing the percentage of Hb S cells improves blood viscosity, increases the Hb concentration, and increases the oxygen-carrying capacity.

C-110. **Answer: b.** Lower esophageal sphincter pressure is decreased by theophylline, beta agonists, smoking, and alcohol. The FVC and FEV_1 are reduced with gastric but not duodenal ulcer, regardless of smoking history. Theophylline increases gastric acid secretion.

C-111. **Answers: a, b, c, d, e.** Injuries causing ARDS include severe trauma (thoracic or extrathoracic), fat embolization, bacteremia, aspiration of gastrointestinal contents, smoke or toxic gas inhalation, surface burns, hydrocarbon ingestion, toxic drugs (heroin, paraquat), neurogenic pulmonary edema, viral, mycoplasmal, or bacterial pneumonia, legionnaires' disease, Pittsburgh agent, acute vasculitis, Goodpasture's syndrome, anaphylactic reaction to drugs and blood, radiation of thorax, immunosuppression and infection

(pneumocystis), thrombus, amniotic fluid, and tumor embolism to the lung.

C-112. **Answers: b, d.** During positive-pressure ventilation of a passive subject, mean airway pressure over the entire respiratory cycle reflects the average pressure applied by the ventilator, and mean alveolar pressure is the average pressure acting to distend the alveoli against the combined recoil of lung and chest wall. During volume-controlled ventilation, the peak airway pressure always exceeds the peak alveolar pressure. In contrast, during pressure-controlled inverse-ratio ventilation, the "peak" or set airway pressure and the peak alveolar pressure will equilibrate. A potential problem with inverse-ratio ventilation is that cardiac output may fall as mean airway pressure increases. Alveolar ventilation will decrease.

C-113. **Answers: a, b, c.** The three requirements for ARDS are diffuse chest roentgenographic infiltrates (interstitial or alveolar, usually involving all four quadrants), hypoxemia refractory to modest amounts of supplemental oxygen (the need for mechanical ventilation with positive end expiratory pressure is cited by some investigators), and normal left ventricular filling pressures (either estimated clinically, or quantitated by a pulmonary artery occlusion pressure of 18 mm Hg or less).

C-114. **Answer: d.** Normal hemoglobin is 50% saturated at a pO_2 of 27 mm Hg. At a PaO_2 of 40, the oxyhemoglobin saturation is approximately 75%. Therefore the oxygen content of this blood sample is

$$(CO_2 = 15 \times 1.34 \times 0.75) + (40 \times .003) = 15.3 \text{ ml/100 ml}$$

Patients with severe congestive heart failure have increased extraction of oxygen and the mixed venous PO_2 generally is lower than 40 mm Hg. However, this could be a sample from the right atrium of a normal person. Since oxygen extraction has been reported to be low in ARDS, this could also be a mixed venous sample from a patient with ARDS. This pO_2 is too low for an arterial sample from a normal person residing at 10,000 feet.

C-115. **Answer: b.** In primary pulmonary hypertension, plexogenic pulmonary arteriopathy is the most common vascular pathology. It is most often seen in middle-aged females with the clinical correlates or normal-appearing lung fields on chest roentgenogram and normal distribution or radionuclide on pulmonary perfusion lung scan. A male teenager with dyspnea and increased bronchovascular markings on chest film could represent pulmonary veno-occlusive disease or some other cause or parenchymal change on the chest film. An elderly female with increased bronchovascular markings on the chest film and subsegmental perfusion defects on perfusion lung scans would be more likely to have pulmonary veno-occlusive diseases, bronchiectasis, or some other cause of parenchymal disease. A middle-aged female with a normal chest film but patchy distribution or radionuclide on lung scan would be more likely to have thromboembolic pulmonary hypertension. An elderly male with normal chest film and lung scan, but a pulmonary arteriogram that shows widespread segmental and subsegmental filling defects and occlusions, is internally contradictory. This individual should have an abnormal lung scan as well and would be more likely to have thromboembolic disease.

C-116. **Answer: b.** If the pulmonary vascular bed is severely compromised and is incapable of vasodilatation, cardiac output may fall because of decreased right ventricular filling from peripheral vasodilatation and from bradycardia, resulting from decreased blood supply to the right ventricle and nodal area. Pulmonary arterial blood pressure may rise in response to vasodilator therapy because systemic vasodilata-

tion may necessitate an increase in cardiac output if the pulmonary vascular bed is relatively fixed and is not capable of vasodilatation. Then the pulmonary arterial blood pressure will rise with the increasing cardiac output. Generally, with vasodilator therapy the fall in systemic vascular resistance is greater than the fall in pulmonary vascular resistance because the systemic vascular bed is more amenable to vasodilatation. Morphologic abnormalities in the pulmonary resistance vessels do not correlate well with increases in pulmonary arterial blood pressure. This finding has helped to make a strong argument for the role of vasoconstriction in the pathogenesis of pulmonary hypertension. However, as noted above, vasodilators tend to dilate the systemic bed more efficiently than the pulmonary vascular bed.

C-117. **Answer: c.** All major studies of the epidemiology of ARDS stress that sepsis is the major risk factor for development of the syndrome. Sepsis should not be thought of as bacteremia in this regard; the incidence of ARDS with bacteremia varies between 5 and 20% in most series. Rather, systemic responses to sepsis (such as hypotension, low systemic vascular resistance, diminished urine output, and altered mentation), if present, increase the incidence of ARDS to 40–60%. Sepsis with systemic responses has been called the sepsis syndrome.

C-118. **Answer: e.** The pathologic picture of ARDS is also called diffuse alveolar damage. It includes interstitial and alveolar edema (by definition, because ARDS is a capillary leak syndrome), neutrophil and platelet aggregation (unless patients are neutropenic or thrombocytopenic, as has been reported), *in situ* thrombosis, hyaline membranes, and fibrosis.

C-119. **Answer: e.** Immune deficiency is not required for ARDS to occur although immunodeficient patients may manifest the syndrome. Intrapulmonary inflammation involving complement, neutrophils, and other effector cells is implicated by many authors. Vascular obstruction, atelectasis, and fibrosis also may occur.

C-120. **Answer: a.** Decreased lung volume due to alveolar edema and atelectasis are common in patients with ARDS and are responsible for severe hypoxemia. The diffusing capacity is likely to be reduced (if it was measured) due to vascular obstruction. Hypocapnia occurs early in the syndrome.

C-121. **Answers: a, b, c, d, e.** Controlling intracranial pressure is beneficial for neurologic recovery of patients with head injuries. Mechanical ventilation inducing hypocapnia is effective in acutely and chronically lowering elevated intracranial pressure. If the ventilator rate is rapid, intracranial pressure may never return to baseline levels, thus negating the positive effects of hypocarbia. On the other hand, high-frequency jet ventilation is characterized by low tidal volumes, high respiratory rates, and low peak airway pressures, thus avoiding the elevation of intracranial pressure with IPPV that occurs clinically with large volumes of fluid sequestration and severe hypocalcemia. It is common to see an elevated serum amylase in diabetic ketoacidosis, and thus it has been suggested that acute pancreatitis is common during diabetic ketoacidosis and may in fact precipitate it. Since the true severity of pancreatitis requires pathologic evaluation, it is difficult to know "how much" pancreatitis it takes to cause ARDS. Most studies indicate that fulminant ARDS is seen almost exclusively with hemorrhagic pancreatitis or ongoing pancreatic inflammation.

C-122. **Answer: c.** ARDS can only be diagnosed clinically because there are no biochemi-

cal or physiologic markers that are specific for the syndrome. Thus, although an increased white blood cell count, intrapulmonary shunt, dead space, and circulating immune complexes may be seen, they are not diagnostic.

C-123. **Answer: e.** No therapy has been shown to prevent ARDS, and some may hamper its resolution.

C-124. **Answer: d.** Although they are used in ARDS patients with known infections, antibiotics have not been shown to improve outcome. Heparin is of no proven value, nor are corticosteroids. PEEP improves oxygenation and is therefore therapeutic, but it is merely supportive therapy. Acetylcysteine is of no benefit.

C-125. **Answer: b.** PEEP is known to increase lung volume, which prevents atelectasis, opens airways, and redistributes lung water (either within the alveoli, where it creates a smaller meniscus for respiratory gases to traverse or by pushing fluid from the alveolar to the interstitial space of the lung). PEEP does not diminish lung water and actually may increase it. Positive end expiratory pressure fails to decrease lung water in alloxan-induced pulmonary edema.

C-126. **Answer: c.** The ventilation-perfusion lung pattern most likely to be associated with an angiographically proven pulmonary embolism consists of segmental and lobar perfusion defects associated with a normal ventilation scan. This pattern is also often associated with a normal or mildly abnormal chest roentgenogram, which only shows minimal volume loss or small pleural effusion, subsegmental defects, whether associated with a normal ventilation scan or with ventilation defects, and infiltrates in the corresponding position on chest film are less likely to be associated with pulmonary embolism. These abnormalities are seen in a number of lung diseases including pneumonia, COPD, and similar problems. The pattern of segmental perfusion defects, associated with a matched ventilation defect and a normal chest film, is also less likely to be associated with pulmonary embolism. However, segmental and larger defects, in general, do raise the possibility of pulmonary embolism in the mind of the clinician and many times will warrant the subsequent performance of a pulmonary angiogram to be certain of the diagnosis, or to effectively exclude it. A single lobar perfusion defect associated with a matched ventilation defect and corresponding evidence on the chest film for lobar atelectasis is unlikely to be associated with pulmonary embolism. Such a defect is more likely to be associated with intrabronchial obstruction on the basis of carcinoma, mucus plug, or foreign body. It is important to realize that although the segmental and lobar perfusion defect with a normal ventilation scan is the most specific ventilation/perfusion pattern, this pattern only accounts for some 30–40% of patients with angiographically proven pulmonary embolism. Any of the other patterns can also be associated with pulmonary embolism, When the diagnosis is still in doubt, an angiogram is indicated to ascertain or effectively exclude the diagnosis.

C-127. **Answer: d.** The oxygen tension of systemic arterial blood primarily reflects lung function. The pulmonary artery occlusion (wedge) pressure is a rough guide to left ventricular end diastolic volume. Cardiac output reflects cardiac function only. The systemic oxygen transport is the product of cardiac output and the oxygen content of systemic arterial blood; it therefore is determined by heart, lung, and hematopoietic function and is a better monitoring tool than the aforementioned parameters. Tissue oxygen extraction, as reflected in the mixed venous oxygen tension, or the systemic arterial to mixed venous oxygen tension, saturation or content difference, does not correlate well with oxygen transport in patients with ARDS.

C-128. **Answer: b.** Several recent studies have shown that patients with ARDS (especially that associated with sepsis) and perhaps other critically ill patients, manifest an oxygen delivery dependence in that their oxygen consumption is determined by oxygen delivery and not vice-versa. The clinical implication of this phenomenon is that measures to increase oxygen delivery (e.g., increasing intravascular volume, hemoglobin concentration, and cardiac output) may increase oxygen consumption and perhaps improve survival.

C-129. **Answers: a, b.** Positive pressure ventilation is known to decrease cardiac output primarily by reducing venous return (preload) to the right (and then left) ventricle. However, the high pulmonary artery pressure (afterload) faced by the right ventricle may cause the interventricular septum to bulge into the left ventricle and decrease its filling. Systemic arterial pressure, roughly equivalent to left ventricular afterload, is actually decreased by positive pressure ventilation.

C-130. **Answers: a, b, c, d, e.** Phospholipase A and the complement cascade are thought to be involved in mediating increased permeability. Diabetic ketoacidosis can cause ARDS. ARDS can be unilateral. Controlling intracranial pressure is beneficial in neurologic recovery of patients with a head injury. Mechanical ventilation inducing hypocapnia is effective in acutely and chronically lowering elevated intracranial pressure.

C-131. **Answer: e.** A recent study has demonstrated that a minority of patients with ARDS die within 3 days of hospital admission due to respiratory or cardiovascular failure, or such problems as pulmonary embolism, viral infection, or disseminated intravascular coagulation. Of the conditions associated with ARDS on admission, sepsis is the most lethal. Three days and more after admission, sepsis remains the most lethal associated condition; in this situation, the sepsis may be a complication of prolonged stay in the intensive care unit. Many patients with sepsis develop multi-organ system failure, which is the leading cause of mortality.

C-132. **Answer: a.** Although residual deficits may be seen in some survivors of ARDS, most return to relatively normal lung function after one year despite previously extensive alveolar damage. If deficits do persist beyond one year they are likely to last.

C-133. **Answer: b.** A well-designed controlled clinical trial of warfarin treatment of deep venous thrombosis has shown that prolongation of the prothrombin time, measured with rabbit brain thromboplastin between 1.3 and 1.5 times control, is sufficient to significantly reduce recurrent venous thromboembolism. Furthermore, prolongation of the prothrombin time beyond 1.5 times control only resulted in a greater number of major bleeding complications. The 1-mg daily regimen is under investigation for prophylaxis, but it is not adequate therapy for venous thrombosis in most patients.

C-134. **Answer: e.** Most neurosurgeons consider any anticoagulant or antiplatelet regimen to be contraindicated in neurosurgical procedures because of the low but real risk for intracerebral bleeding. TED stockings and early ambulation are not adequate prophylaxes in an older patient undergoing major surgery. Pneumatic compression of the legs is noninvasive, does not induce a hemostatic defect, and is effective in nearly every instance in which it has been tested for prevention of deep venous thrombosis.

C-135. **Answer: e.** Retrospective clinical data and animal studies suggest that the therapeutic range of the activated partial thromboplastin time for heparin therapy of deep venous thrombosis is 1.5–2.0 times control. Further prolongation of the APTT is no more efficacious. Since patients with an APTT below 1.5 seem to be at high risk to suffer recurrent thromboembolism, laboratory monitoring is indicated. Heparin can be given subcutaneously, but sufficient drug must be given to prolong the APTT beyond 1.5 times control.

C-136. **Answer: b.** Generally, factor II takes longer than 2 days to fall to therapeutic levels after warfarin therapy is begun. Protein C, a naturally occurring anticoagulant, is cleared almost as rapidly as factor VII. Consequently, in the first 2 or 3 days of warfarin therapy, it is possible that blood could become more procoagulant even though the prothrombin time might be prolonged. A large loading dose of warfarin does not significantly shorten the time to achievement of therapeutic levels of all the vitamin K-dependent coagulation factors. Heparin in doses to prolong the activated partial thromboplastin time to 1.5–2.0 times control usually does not greatly prolong the prothrombin time and need not be stopped prior to beginning warfarin. Hemorrhagic necrosis of skin occurs rarely following initiation of warfarin therapy. It has been associated with deficiency of protein C and large loading doses of warfarin (30–40 mg).

C-137. **Answer: d.** Airway obstruction obviously needs to be rectified first. Open pneumothorax or tension pneumothorax results in a situation in which the mechanics of breathing are severely impaired. Cardiac tamponade can result in rapid circulatory collapse. Bronchial disruption, on the other hand, usually does not require immediate intervention unless it leads to airway obstruction or a tension pneumothorax. Often bronchial disruption causes no immediate problem and is only recognized when the patient returns weeks or months later with a bronchial stenosis.

C-138. **Answer: e.** In a patient presenting with seemingly isolated chest trauma, the contiguous body areas, mainly the head and neck and the abdomen, always need to be evaluated for associated injuries. Because the diaphragm constitutes a mobile anatomic boundary between the chest and the abdomen, and the dome of the diaphragm can reach to the level of the nipple line on forced expiration, the possibility of abdominal visceral injury must always be entertained. Also, injuries to the diaphragm itself may lead to herniation of abdominal contents and respiratory embarrassment. In a flail chest a tremendous force must be exerted to sustain an abdominal injury. Because of the configuration of the steering wheel, any time there is a significant chest injury with sternal fracture or myocardial contusion, an abdominal injury, especially a liver or splenic tear, must be strongly considered. An abdominal injury should be suspected in any type of penetrating injury below the nipple line, or a gunshot wound to the chest with no evidence of an exit sight. As a general rule, any injury that penetrates the intercostal musculature below the 4th interspace requires peritoneal lavage to rule out an abdominal injury. The isolated stab wound above the 4th interspace, especially when the offending weapon is known to be of short length, does not require peritoneal lavage unless there are associated abdominal findings on physical examination.

C-139. **Answer: c.** A major distinction between the two conditions is the status of the neck veins. Typically in tension pneumothorax, the neck veins are distended because of the increase in intrathoracic pressure, whereas in hemothorax the neck veins are flat due to the loss of intravascu-

lar volume. Although deviation of the trachea is common in both conditions, actual compression may occur with tension pneumothorax, but rarely occurs with massive hemothorax. Although both conditions can be seen with either blunt or penetrating chest trauma, hemothorax is much more likely with a blunt injury, whereas a tension pneumothorax would be more likely with a penetrating injury. Therapeutic maneuvers often need to be instituted prior to obtaining a diagnostic chest roentgenogram. If a tension pneumothorax is present, it must be decompressed immediately. On the other hand, it may be prudent to replace intravascular volume and obtain blood products prior to decompressing a massive hemothorax that may be providing tamponade of a disrupted intrathoracic vessel.

C-140. **Answer: d.** Relief of unilateral increase in intrathoracic pressure and deviation of the mediastinal structures is essential. Because of the rapid onset of this condition and the progressive hemodynamic instability, the quickest and simplest maneuver to relieve the pressure constitutes the most appropriate therapy. Waiting for a diagnostic study such as a chest film or taking the time to insert a large-bore chest tube are both inappropriate. Positive-pressure ventilation will not only be ineffective but will probably aggravate the situation. One can quickly ascertain on clinical grounds the side of the tension pneumothorax and then insert an open-ended needle into the chest cavity. A correct diagnosis is greeted by a loud rush of air through the needle and a return of circulatory function.

C-141. **Answer: a.** The disruption of any air-containing structure—be it lung, tracheobronchial tree, or esophagus—can lead to subcutaneous emphysema. Obstruction of an air-filled structure without disruption, such as an obstructed bronchus, however, cannot in itself cause the development of subcutaneous emphysema.

C-142. **Answer: b.** The necessity of evacuating blood from the pleural space is controversial, as the blood will often be reabsorbed. There are situations, however, in which the chest tube is required not only for the evacuation of the hemothorax, but also in the context of the total management of the trauma patient, such as the patient entering the Emergency Room in shock in whom a hemothorax is suspected. The chest tube should be inserted as part of the initial resuscitation measures. A traumatic hemothorax may not require a chest tube, except in patients who require a general anesthetic in the immediate post-injury period for other indications. A traumatic pneumothorax always requires a chest tube, not only to monitor blood loss but also to evacuate a pneumothorax that may develop if the patient is placed on positive-pressure ventilation. A chest tube is never indicated to monitor blood loss from a suspected disrupted aorta. Such a patient is in imminent danger of exsanguination and should undergo an immediate diagnostic aortogram followed by surgical repair if the diagnosis is confirmed.

C-143. **Answer: b.** Documenting the exact site of the fracture is not necessary, and a physical examination is all that is necessary to diagnose a rib fracture. Anteroposterior compression of the thorax with one hand on the sternum and the other on the vertebral column will invariably elicit pain at or near the fracture site if the fracture is present. Direct palpation of the individual ribs often gives misleading information since a broad area of the chest wall may be contused.

C-144. **Answer: c.** The major reason for obtaining a chest film in patients with suspected rib fractures is to evaluate the status of the underlying pleura and lung. In the initial evaluation, a chest film is obtained to check for a possible pneumothorax or hemothorax since these conditions may require immediate treatment. Usually a pulmonary contusion is not evident radiographically in the immediate post-traumatic period, although it may become apparent 12–24 hours after injury.

C-145. **Answer: a.** A number of easily recognized problems underlie the development of respiratory failure in a flail chest. These include extreme pain, the splinting and resultant ineffective cough that leads to retention of bronchial secretions, and the associated pulmonary contusion. It is assumed that air exchange is hampered to some degree because of loss of the normal bellows function. However, pendelluft (i.e., the exchange of air back and forth across the carina from one lung to the other) was once thought to be a major component of physiologic dysfunction in flail chest, but it is no longer considered a significant factor in the development of respiratory failure.

C-146. **Answer: d.** External traction is no longer used to treat flail chest except in some emergency situations, but internal fixation, along with continuous positive-pressure ventilation, is often used when there are large flail segments. At the present time, the literature would support conservative management for flail segments of 5 or less ribs, with treatment consisting of day and night physical supplemental therapy, oxygen, and the liberal use of analgesics and local rib blocks. If patients fail to maintain certain hemodynamic and pulmonary physiologic parameters, they are electively intubated and placed on continuous positive-pressure ventilation, in which case, a 10-day to 2-week course is usually required before the chest wall becomes adequately stabilized.

C-147. **Answer: c.** Esophageal injuries are uncommon in both blunt and penetrating chest trauma, and they are usually related to either the ingestion of a foreign body or instrumentation. Mostly the perforation occurs at areas of either natural or pathologic narrowing of the esophagus. The three naturally occurring narrowings are at the upper and lower sphincters and at the level of the aortic arch. A cricopharyngeal perforation presents mostly with pain, swelling, and crepitus in the mid-neck region. Perforation in the mid-esophagus often presents with chest pain and subcutaneous emphysema at the thoracic inlet. Perforation at the lower esophageal sphincter is more likely to present with abdominal pain, shortness of breath, and a hydropneumothorax.

C-148. **Answer: e.** Post-traumatic myocardial contusion is a diagnosis considered primarily because of a strong clinical suspicion, based on knowledge of the mechanism of injury and signs and symptoms such as chest pain and arrhythmias. Ischemic changes on an electrocardiogram, a rise in the CPK levels, or an abnormal thallium scan can all substantiate the diagnosis, but none are, in themselves, diagnostic. Patients suspected of sustaining a myocardial contusion should be carefully monitored for the development of arrhythmias, valvular dysfunction, or, rarely, septal defects.

C-149. **Answer: d.** An acute bleed into the pericardium differs substantially from the slow accumulation of pericardial fluid in chronic diseases, in that many of the compensatory mechanisms and classic signs of pericardial tamponade, such as distended neck veins, muffled heart sounds, or a large pulsus paradoxus, may not be present. The chest film will not show an enlarged cardiac silhouette although it may reveal a hemothorax or hemopneumothorax. Insertion of a central venous pressure line and direct measurement of right atrial pressure constitute the best means of diagnosing this condition. In a patient who is hypovolemic, the CVP may be low initially, and a CVP measurement that is rising with fluid resuscitation

in the face of continued systemic hypotension is diagnostic for either a pericardial tamponade or a tension pneumothorax.

C-150. **Answer: a.** Autopsy series have shown that approximately 30% of people who die of blunt injuries exsanguinate from disruption of the thoracic aorta. When the adventitial layer of the aortic wall remains intact, the victim may survive the injury initially but is still at high risk for late disruption or dissection. All of the possibilities can occur with disruption of the thoracic aorta, but the most sensitive indicator is a widening of the mediastinum on chest film. Although the sign is nonspecific, the majority of these injuries can be recognized so that a diagnostic aortogram and emergent surgical repair can be rapidly accomplished.

C-151. **Answer: d.** Disruptions of the thoracic aorta following blunt trauma occur at sites where the aorta is tethered to surrounding tissue: the aortic valve, the isthmus of the aorta, which is just distal to the takeoff of the left subclavian artery, and at the diaphragmatic hiatus. Most disruptions at the aortic valve are immediately fatal. Of patients reaching the hospital with a disrupted thoracic aorta, 70–80% will have disruptions at or close to the isthmus.

C-152. **Answers: a, b, c.** The allopurinol hypersensitivity syndrome is defined by three criteria: (1) a clear history of allopurinol use, (2) a clinical picture consisting of two of the major criteria, or one major and one minor criterion, and (3) lack of exposure to another drug that may have caused a similar clinical picture. The major criteria consist of rash (diffuse maculopapular or exfoliative dermatitis, erythema multiforme, toxic epidermal necrolysis), worsening renal function or acute hepatotoxicity. The minor criteria are fever, eosinophilia, and leukocytosis.

2-9 Case Problems

P-1. **Answer: a.** Estimation of the alveolo-arterial oxygen tension gradient is relatively simple and merely requires knowledge of the partial pressure of the moist inspired air (P_{IO_2}), which equals F_{IO_2} (B.P.-47), the $PaCO_2$, and the respiratory quotient:

Then
$$PAO_2 = P_{IO_2} - (PaCO_2/R)$$
and, in this patient:
$$PAO_2 - PaO_2 = (21 \times (747-47))$$
$$-(70/0.7) - 35$$
$$= (147-100) - 35$$
$$= 12 \text{ mm Hg.}$$

P-2. **Answer: d.** The physiologic dead space (V_D) is that portion of the tidal volume (V_T) that does not take part in gas exchange. The portion that takes part in ventilation is the alveolar component (V_A). V_D can be calculated from the Bohr equation, using carbon dioxide as the reference gas, and analysis of the source and fraction of CO_2 (FCO_2) or pressure of CO_2 (pCO_2) in the expired tidal volume.
$$V_D = ((PACO_2 - PECO_2) / PACO_2) \times V_T$$
$$V_D / V_T = (PACO_2 - PECO_2) / PACO_2$$
Since the alveolar and arterial pCO_2 are the same, and
$$PECO_2 = .05 \times (747-47) = 35$$
then $V_D = (70-35)/70 = 0.5 \times 600 = 300 \text{ ml}$
and $V_A = (600-300) \times 30 = 9.0 \text{ L/min.}$

P-3. **Answer: b, d.** While breathing room air the PaO_2 is 55 mm Hg and the $PaCO_2$ is 55 mm Hg, indicating alveolar hypoventilation. The A-a gradient is 17 mm Hg, indicating the presence of either true venous admixture or ventilation-perfusion imbalance. The gradient between the alveoli and the pulmonary-end capillary is only 1 mm Hg, ruling out a diffusion defect. Similarly, the rise in PaO_2 to greater than 500 mm Hg on 100% O_2 rules out a significant shunt (true venous admixture).

P-4. **Answer: b.** This patient has a reduced exercise tolerance, but has not reached the maximum ventilation possible (MVV), and the respiratory frequency is recruited appropriately. Cardiac rate is excessive, and there is an inordinate rise in systolic and diastolic blood pressure. As a consequence, despite the hyperventilation and lowering of the pCO_2, the respiratory quotient ($\mathring{V}CO_2/\mathring{V}O_2$ rises, and there is an early anaerobic threshold, indicating that the supply of energy (oxygen) to the exercising muscles is not meeting their demands.

P-5. **Answer: b.** When first seen, the patient was suffering from alveolar hypoventilation (elevated $PaCO_2$) and the
$$P(A-a)O_2 = \frac{(21 \times 700) - 80}{0.8} = 47 - 40 = 7 \text{ mm Hg.}$$
While on the ventilator the $PaCO_2$ has been restored to normal, but the
$$P(A-a)O_2 = \frac{(21 \times 700) - 40}{0.8} = 97 - 70 = 27 \text{ mm Hg.}$$
Therefore, something has led to increased mismatching of ventilation and perfusion—such as atelectasis, edema, airway obstruction—and the patient has deteriorated.

P-6. **Answers: a. 2, b. 3, c. 4, d. 1.** In asthma (a), hypoxemia and perhaps the bronchial narrowing, leads to hypoxemia and hyperventilation and hypocapnia. In acute anxiety (b), hyperventilation results in hypocapnia and alkalemia, and there is no hypoxemia. In chronic hyperventilation (c), the hypocapnia persists, but the kidneys have eliminated bicarbonate so that no alkalemia is present. In COPD (d), hypoxemia and hypercapnia, along with mild acidemia often develops in acute exacerbations.

P-7. **Answer: b.** During acute asthma, inhaled beta agonists will effectively cause bronchodilation even if the patient has been using, or abusing, this agent prior to presentation for treatment. High doses of intravenous aminophylline have not been shown to be effective in acute asthma, especially in people who have been receiving aminophylline. Although corticosteroids are effective in severe asthma, their onset of action is delayed for hours. Finally, inhaled anticholinergics are only beneficial when given in large doses and in combination with a beta agonist.

P-8. **Answer: a.** The baseline tests demonstrate overdistension (increased lung volumes) and airflow limitation (low FEV_1 and FEV_1/FVC ratio).

P-9. **Answer: a.** Following inhaled bronchodilator the FEV_1 and maximal expiratory flow rates are not changed, but there is a significant decrease in FRC and TLC, indicating reduction in overdistension, and the maximal expiratory flow rates if examined at equivalent lung volumes (isovolume) are significantly improved.

P-10. **Answer: a.** The clinical features of this case illustrate several difficulties. Wegener's is supported by an absent allergic history or peripheral blood eosinophilia, the location of disease, and the radiographic abnormalities of bilateral noncavitating nodules. Churg-Strauss syndrome would be likely if the histology indicated an eosinophilic vasculitis involving sinuses and lungs. In the absence of pathognomonic clinical signs and diagnostic laboratory tests, recognition of the different disorders relies heavily on the correct interpretation of the morphologic features of the disease. Only an open lung biopsy, and not a transbronchial or needle biopsy, should be relied on for the histologic diagnosis.

P-11. **Answer: b.** This is desquamative interstitial pneumonitis. Note the markedly increased numbers of alveolar macrophages with associated chronic inflammatory infiltrate in the alveolar walls, and minimal fibrosis.

P-12. **Answer: c.** Ventilation is excessively increased and has reached the maximum ventilation possible (MVV). The respiratory frequency is recruited disproportionately. There is alveolar hypoventilation with hypoxemia and hypercapnia. The exercise is limited by a ventilatory problem.

P-13. **Answer: a.** There is recent evidence that treatment with a single dose of corticosteroids in the emergency room reduces the likelihood that patients will require readmission to the emergency ward and hospitalization. The mechanism by which corticosteroids are efficacious in acute asthma is not known. However, unless the patient has severe underlying diabetes or other such complications, this high dose in a single bolus will not be associated with significant side effects. Although beta-adrenergic function does recover in the face of corticosteroid treatment, the importance of this to the efficacy of steroids in asthma is not known. Steroids do not act that quickly.

P-14. **Answer: b.** During severe asthma that has been present for an extended time and associated with fatigue, the arterial blood gas determinations often show severe hypoxia with the carbon dioxide and pH in the "normal range." What this indicates is a transition from hypocapnia to hypercapnia and alkalosis to acidosis. In acute mild asthma, the patient usually has hypoxia, hypocapnia, and alkalosis. In patients with chronic obstructive pulmonary disease who have had severe obstructive disease for an extended period of time, the picture may indicate hypoxia and mild hypercapnia, but the pH has compensated and is in the normal range. Patients who retain carbon dioxide and are severely acidotic have altered levels of consciousness. It would be unusual to find normal levels of oxygen when the patient enters into CO_2 retention. Therefore, the finding of normal levels of pH and pCO_2 is not compatible with severe asthma as described in the above case history.

P-15. **Answer: a.** The physical finding of the tracheal shift to the right indicates either a reduction in volume on the right or an increase on the left. A left pleural effusion would cause dullness on that side, and a pneumothorax would be hyperresonant. A right pleural effusion would cause dullness on that side and tracheal shift to the left. Atelectasis on the left would shift the trachea to the same side. The physical findings on the right could also represent some associated consolidation.

P-16. **Answer: c.** This is the typical history of the Churg-Strauss syndrome, which is also called allergic angiitis and granulomatosis. It is a disorder characterized by hypereosinophilia and systemic vasculitis in patients with asthma and allergic rhinitis. The age of onset is usually in the late 20s or 30s. A history of allergic rhinitis is found in 70% of the patients. Asthma can precede the diagnosis by up to 30 years. Neurologic complications, especially mononeuritis multiplex, abdominal pain, skin rash, musculoskeletal complaints, and cardiac involvement are seen. The chest film may be normal in up to 30% of these cases. The clinical phases are a prodromal phase in which allergic or atopic complaints (asthma, allergic rhinitis) are present; a second phase in which peripheral blood eosinophilia and tissue infiltrates are noted; and then a life-threatening vasculitic phase.

P-17. **Answer: e.** This patient has a reduced exercise tolerance, and the ventilation is excessive, but the respiratory frequency is recruited appropriately. Cardiac rate is not excessive and there is only a modest rise in systolic and diastolic blood pressures. There is the expected amount of hyperventilation, and minimal lowering of the pCO_2 and pH. The anaerobic threshold is normal, indicating that the supply of energy (oxygen) to the exercising muscles is meeting their demands. However, the dead space/tidal volume ratio fails to fall, suggesting that the expected redistribution of blood flow has not taken place and that there may be a pulmonary vascular abnormality.

P-18. **Answer: b.** Although most of the possibilities listed might be considered, this is carcinoma until proved otherwise.

P-19. **Answer: c.** Generally, the first step in an organized work-up of a suspicious lung lesion is to establish a tissue diagnosis. Sometimes this can be accomplished by biopsy of a lesion in the liver, skin, or a lymph node, at the same time establishing the presence of metastatic disease. Because small cell lung cancer is not usually treated surgically, tissue diagnosis of a lesion should precede determination of resectability.

P-20. **Answer: a.** This patient has a reduced exercise tolerance and has not reached the maximum ventilation possible (MVV). The respiratory frequency is recruited appropriately. Cardiac rate is excessive, but systolic and diastolic blood pressures are not abnormal. There is some hyperventilation and lowering of the pCO_2 and there is an early anaerobic threshold indicating that the supply of energy (oxygen) to the exercising muscles is not meeting their demands.

P-21. **Answer: e.** The CT scan is virtually diagnostic of lymphangioleiomyomatosis, which is a rare disease that occurs only in women. The roentgenographic features of lymphangioleiomyomatosis are variable and depend on the time the patient is seen, beginning with some small irregular opacities and progressing to pleural effusions, septal lines, and a cystic honeycomb-like pattern.

P-22. **Answer: a.** This is cryptogenic organizing pneumonia or bronchiolitis obliterans with organizing pneumonia. Note the polyps of immature connective tissue in alveolar ducts and more distal air spaces.

P-23. **Answer: b.** This is the radiograph of a 60-year-old man with pain in the right shoulder radiating to the back, swelling of the right arm, and weakness of the right hand. On physical examination the right pupil is constricted, and there is ptosis of the right eyelid and facial anhydrosis. This is a Pancoast's tumor.

P-24. **Answer: b.** Barring localized disease, 60% of pulmonary function is on the right and 40% on the left. Residual FEV_1 is approximately proportional to residual lung. Thus, provided the tumor itself has not contributed to the FEV_1 present, the patient will have a post-section FEV_1 of $2.4 L \times 0.40 = .960 L$.

P-25. **Answer: d.** The history and chest roentgenogram are consistent with diffuse alveolar hemorrhage.

P-26. **Answer: c.** The low lung volume and FEV_1/FVC ratio is consistent with a restrictive defect. The pCO_2 is normal, thereby ruling out alveolar hypoventilation.

P-27. **Answer: a.** This is an obstructive defect with overdistension of the lungs.

P-28. **Answer: d, e.** The patient clearly has rheumatoid arthritis and has developed a pulmonary complication as well as Sjögren's syndrome. The obstructive pattern and hyperinflation are suggestive of bronchiolitis obliterans.

P-29. **Answer: c.** There is a symmetric enlargement of the hilar nodes and no parenchymal disease. This is sarcoidosis; 50–90 % of patients with sarcoidosis show mediastinal and hilar lymph node enlargement, and approximately 40% of these show diffuse parenchymal disease as well. Hilar adenopathy is rare in hypersensitivity pneumonitis. This is not the picture of eosinophilic granuloma, which is virtually always seen in smokers. Pulmonary non-Hodgkin's lymphoma is relatively uncommon in AIDS; it presents both as multiple nodules and as a diffuse infiltrate, and there is virtually always extranodal involvement. Kaposi's sarcoma can have a wide range of radiographic appearances, but the most common finding consists of bilateral interstitial and/or alveolar infiltrates, frequently with pleural effusions.

P-30. **Answer: a.** This is miliary tuberculosis, which is characterized by the millet-like nodules uniform in size.

P-31. **Answer: a.** Current recommended therapy in this type of case consists of INH, RF, and PZA for 2 months with the addition of EMB or SM if there is CNS involvement or disseminated disease. This is followed by INH and RF for 7 months. Therapy is carried out for at least 9 months, and at least 6 months after culture conversion.

P-32. **Answer: c.** Although there have been no controlled trials, rifampin is probably as effective as INH. While option b may be a good alternative, the use of more than one drug increases the possibility of toxicity. Arguing against simple observation is the fact that the patient may become very ill and infectious to others by the time the TB is recognized. The PPD may never yield a positive result if the HIV infection is far advanced.

P-33. **Answer: e.** This is Wegener's granulomatosis. Note the widely distributed sharply defined nodules. Cavitation may occur in about one third to one half of patients.

P-34. **Answer: a.** It is clearly important to establish the basis of the upper lobe atelectasis and persistent localized wheeze. Although the reduced volume could be due to fibrosis, an endobronchial lesion such as a carcinoma, fibrostenosis, or even a foreign body should be ruled out.

P-35. **Answer: c.** Although almost all of the antibiotics are active against *Pneumococcus*, penicillin is the clear-cut drug of choice.

P-36. **Answer: a.** The drug of choice is ampicillin if beta-lactamase–producing strains are rare in the particular community. Alternative therapy ending culture and beta-lactamase testing include the cephalosporins (cefonicid sodium, cefuroxime, cefamandole, and ceftriaxone sodium) and beta-lactamase inhibitor combinations (Unasyn).

P-37. **Answer: d.** The presence of many epithelial cells indicates the presence of oropharyngeal contamination. The streptococci are part of normal flora; therefore a transtracheal aspirate is indicated.

P-38. **Answer: c, d, e.** *Mycoplasma pneumoniae*, *Legionella pneumophila*, and influenza A are the likely organisms in this case.

P-39. **Answer: a.** This is hypersensitivity pneumonitis, or extrinsic allergic alveolitis. The CT scan shows innumerable fine nodules and some haze in the periphery.

P-40. **Answer: d.** Coccidioides is a dimorphic fungus with its mycelial phase in soil. Airborne spores (arthroconidia) infect the mammalian host and cause coccidioidomycosis. In the tissue phase, the spores swell, become spherical, and develop a thick wall. This spherule reproduces with formation of internal spores called endospores. When it ruptures, the endospores are released and can form new spherules. The spherule is not capable of infecting man. If the spherule returns to the soil, the organism reverts back to the mycelial phase. In the mycelial phase, the infectious spores are produced, re-initiating the cycle.

P-41. **Answer: b.** Enlarged lymph nodes are not necessarily due to tumor; tissue diagnosis is mandatory before discarding the only potentially curative therapy, i.e. surgery.

P-42. **Answer: d.** This is a case of multiple pulmonary arteriovenous fistulas. Note the round, well-defined nodules in the lower lung zones.

P-43. **Answer: e.** Primary tuberculosis must be strongly considered. Pleural effusion may antedate signs and symptoms of rheumatoid arthritis. The combination of pneumonia, pleural fluid, and chest wall involvement would strongly suggest actinomycosis. Nitrofurantoin is one of several drugs that can induce a pleural effusion. Cyclophosphamide can induce a diffuse reticulonodular pattern and is not associated with pleural effusion.

P-44. **Answer: c, d.** This is a Langerhans' cell, which demonstrates the boomerang-shaped X body or Birbeck granule .These cells are characteristically increased in eosinophilic granuloma, but since these cells are present in normal lung, they are not specific for eosinophilic granuloma, and increased numbers can be found in smokers and in patients with bronchoalveolar carcinoma.

P-45. **Answer: c.** This is most likely to be a case of auto-PEEP. In a patient with severe chronic airway obstruction, the end expiratory lung volume often exceeds the relaxation volume of the respiratory system (the volume at which the elastic recoil pressure of the total respiratory system is zero, i.e., the elastic forces of the lungs and thorax are equal and pulling in opposite directions). In this condition, referred to as dynamic hyperinflation, the elastic recoil pressure of the respiratory system is positive, i.e., there is auto-PEEP or intrinsic PEEP (PEEPi). The magnitude of PEEPi depends on the time available for expiration (T_e) and on the forces governing expiration. Although normal subjects exhibit substantial braking due to activity of inspiratory muscles early in expiration, they are still capable of reaching the relaxation volume of the respiratory system before the onset of the next inspiration because the resistance to flow is normally relatively low. In patients with airflow limitation, the rate of lung emptying is unduly slowed by the increased airway resistance and, of necessity, they develop PEEPi. The cardiac output falls due to a continuously elevated intrathoracic pressure and impeded venous return. In this patient, the preload was likely to be diminished, but this was not initially recognized since the wedge pressure was falsely high.

P-46. **Answer: c.** The classic presentation of ethylene glycol poisoning is that of a patient who is inebriated or comatose but who lacks the smell of ethanol on the breath. Classically, there is a metabolic acidosis that is not accounted for by ketones, lactate, or salicylate, along with an elevated anion gap and an elevated osmolar gap not explained by ethanol. Direct measurements indicate that the characteristic metabolic acidosis is due largely to glycolic acid. The finding of calcium-oxalate crystals in the urine completes the picture.

P-47. **Answer: d.** Patients with traumatic tracheoesophageal fistula usually present with hemoptysis after an automobile accident in which a chest injury from a steering wheel has occurred. The majority experience an asymptomatic interval of 3 to 5 days before an episode occurs after ingestion of liquid.

P-48. **Answer: a.** Once a fistula is suspected, a contrast study should be performed, and if suggestive of a fistula, bronchoscopic and endoscopic evaluation are indicated.

P-49. **Answer: d.** This is very suspicious of botulism and should be of prime concern.

P-50. **Answer: c.** The diagnosis is made on clinical grounds; symptoms are associated with ingestion of a contaminated food source. EMG can be helpful by enhancing muscular response after rapid large repetitive stimuli, much like Eaton-Lambert syndrome. Detection of the toxin in the stool, blood, and food is diagnostic but becomes less sensitive as time passes. A negative Tensilon test makes myasthenia less likely, and a normal lumbar puncture (lack of protein) decreases the likelihood of Guillain-Barré syndrome.

P-51. **Answer: c.** Approximately 50% of the positive end expiratory pressure (PEEP) applied to the airway is transmitted to the juxtacardiac regions. Pulmonary arterial wedge pressures reflect intracavitary pressures (assuming they are properly positioned in zone 3). Left ventricular preload is related to the transmural left ventricular pressure or the intracavitary pressure minus the juxtacardiac pressure. His low cardiac output can be accounted for by reduced preload. Dopamine administered in the dose suggested will increase left ventricular afterload and would be an appropriate medication to use if an afterload problem is the cause of the low cardiac output. In this patient, the problem is a reduced preload which will not respond to administration of dopamine. Reducing his PEEP will allow for more venous return and may raise cardiac output sufficiently to render additional fluid volume unnecessary. At an FIO_2 of 0.50 with adequate oxygenation, a PEEP of 20 cm H_2O is not needed. The patient could have sepsis, since this is a common complication in patients with the adult respiratory distress syndrome. If reduction of PEEP does not restore his blood pressure to normal, this should be considered. Wedge pressures measured with the patient removed from PEEP will be meaningless with regard to the hemodynamic status, since removal of PEEP will alter both right and left ventricular preload and afterload.

P-52. **Answer: c.** All the options listed could be correct. However, because the hypotension and tachycardia were temporally related to institution of mechanical ventilation, the most likely possibility is that the patient was experiencing the effects of intrinsic positive end expiratory pressure (PEEPi). When severe airflow limitation is present, the interval between respiratory cycles is insufficient to allow alveoli to empty completely, and the alveolar pressure remains positive at the end of exhalation. In addition, patients may forcefully contract their respiratory muscles, further increasing intrathoracic pressure. Intrinsic PEEP is measured by transiently occluding the expiratory tube of the ventilator immediately before inspiration. The pressure generated by this maneuver is read on the airway pressure manometer and can be taken as the level of intrinsic PEEP.

P-53. **Answer: c.** The acute symptoms with the findings of a widened A-a oxygen gradient and a clear chest film in this postpartum female strongly suggests pulmonary embolism. Since she would be presumed to have normal lungs, the correct response is to give her a bolus of heparin and order a lung scan. If one chooses to begin the diagnostic work-up with a pulmonary angiogram, the bolus of heparin should still be given first.

P-54. **Answer: c.** This is idiopathic pulmonary fibrosis. The diffuse infiltration bilaterally involving the lower lobes predominantly and, more significantly, the HRCT demonstrating extensive subpleural honeycombing with cystic regions of lung destruction with visible walls is characteristic of advanced disease.

P-55. **Answer: b.** This is eosinophilic granuloma. Note the fine reticulonodular opacities in the routine chest film, particularly in the lower zones. This is not usual as the upper lobes are generally more involved. The HRCT is particularly abnormal and reveals the multiple nodules and cystic spaces characteristic of this disorder.

P-56. **Answer: a.** The patient has a history of working as a coal miner and a foundry worker. His chest roentgenogram has the appearance of silicosis, which has a predilection for the upper lobes. As seen in this case, there is incorporation of nodular lesions into massive consolidation, and cavitation may occur. The presence of a cavity in the right upper zone, the cough productive of yellow sputum, and night sweats as well as increasing dyspnea on exertion suggest infection and, in this susceptible individual, tuberculosis.

P-57. **Answer: d.** Multiple well-controlled clinical trials showed that the best therapy for venous thromboembolic disease is 10–14 days of intravenous heparin followed by warfarin in a dose to prolong the prothrombin time to 1.3–1.5 times the control value (using rabbit brain thromboplastin) for 3–4 months. However, the major exception to this is pregnant patients. Warfarin is fetopathic and results in a characteristic embryopathy in the 6th to 12th week of pregnancy. It must not be used at any time during pregnancy, and all women of childbearing potential who take warfarin must avoid pregnancy. Consequently, for a pregnant patient, adjusted-dose heparin given subcutaneously in a dose to prolong the activated partial thromboplastin time to 1.5 times the control value at the mid-dosing intervals is appropriate. Aspirin, 325 mg per day, is not an acceptable regimen for the treatment of established venous thromboembolic disease. Subcutaneous heparin, 5000 units every 12 hours, is unacceptable because it results in an unacceptably high rate of recurrent thromboembolism.

P-58. **Answer: b.** In differentiation of pericardial tamponade from right ventricular infarction, echocardiography would be the simplest most effective test. A pulsatile liver, jugular venous distension, and pulsus paradoxus can be associated with either process. Equalization of right-sided diastolic pressures is characteristic of pericardial tamponade, but can also occur in right ventricular infarction. A technetium pyrophosphate scan would not differentiate myocardial infarction, which is already evident in this patient, from pericardial tamponade. The material might, however, accumulate in the pericardial space. However, the complexity of this test would make it less acceptable than echocardiography.

P-59. **Answer: c.** Shock associated with evidence of clear lungs and elevated right-sided pressure suggests right ventricular dysfunction. An echocardiogram and a right precordial electrocardiogram should be ordered to confirm the diagnosis of right ventricular infarction and rule out pericardial tamponade. The correct treatment is volume loading with saline. Diuretic therapy, vasodilators, and intra-aortic balloon pumping are likely to make the hemodynamic state worse. Digoxin will have little acute effect.

P-60. **Answer: c.** This is a lung abscess. They generally have a predilection for the posterior portions of the upper or lower lobes. Note the round, sharply defined border and the fluid level.

P-61. **Answer: c.** This is lymphangioleiomyomatosis. The biopsy shows proliferating primitive smooth muscle cells, which take the form of nodules and thicken the walls of air spaces and protrude into their lumen. Smooth muscle of the pulmonary lymphatic, perivascular, and peribronchiolar tissues is involved in this disorder. The terminal and respiratory bronchioles are particularly involved and lead to check valve–like obstruction with dilatation of the distal air spaces and cyst formation.

P-62. **Answer: c.** This is active tuberculosis with infiltrates in the right lower and upper lobe and loss of volume in the right upper lobe.

P-63. **Answer: c.** This is sarcoidosis. Note noncaseating granulomas consisting of pale-staining endothelioid cells, some of which have fused to become giant cells. These in turn are surrounded by a ring of lymphocytes and form a sharply defined whorl.

P-64. **Answer: b.** This is a restrictive disorder with reduction in lung volume and little or no airflow limitation.

P-65. **Answer: b.** This is a pleural effusion with an underlying mesothelioma. The impact of this condition has resulted in loss of lung volume function.

P-66. **Answer: d.** This is chronic eosinophilic pneumonia. Note the peripheral ground-glass pattern that almost completely surrounds the lung, suggesting a photographic negative of the opacity seen in pulmonary edema.

P-67. **Answer: e.** This is allergic bronchopulmonary aspergillosis. Note the central bronchiectasis, which is characteristic of this disorder.

P-68. **Answer: b.** This is cystic fibrosis. Note the multiple nodules and rounded opacities or lucencies probably representing small bronchiectatic cavities, prominent hila, and diffuse hyperaeration.

P-69. **Answer: d.** The central pulmonary vessels are markedly enlarged. Note tapered peripheral vessels and oligemia of the lungs.

P-70. **Answer: b.** This is alveolar proteinosis. Note the bilateral symmetric pattern, with a typical batwing or butterfly groundglass pattern identical to that of pulmonary edema. There are no Kerley's B lines and there is no cardiomegaly.

P-71. **Answer: d.** This is a pulmonary embolus. Note the peripheral wedge-shaped infiltrate pointing toward the hilum.

P-72. **Answer: c.** While the patient breathes room air the PaO_2 is 55 mm Hg and the $PaCO_2$ is 30 mm Hg, indicating alveolar hyperventilation. The A-a gradient is 45 mm Hg, indicating true venous admixture, or ventilation-perfusion imbalance, or a diffusion deficit. However, the gradient between the alveoli and the end pulmonary capillary is only 1 mm Hg, ruling out a diffusion defect. The failure of the PaO_2 to rise above 500 mm Hg on 100% O_2 indicates a significant shunt (true venous admixture).

P-73. **Answer: c.** The hemoglobin is 18 gm and so the oxygen-carrying capacity is $18 \times 1.34 = 24.12$ ml. Since there is .03 ml O_2 dissolved in plasma for every 100 mm Hg partial pressure, and the end capillary pO_2 was 700 mm Hg, the amount dissolved in the plasma was 2.1 ml. Thus the O_2 content of the blood leaving the alveoli was 26.22 ml while the arterial O_2 content was $24.12 + (200 \times .03) = 24.72$ ml. Since the O_2 consumption was 300 ml and the cardiac output was 5l/min, the arterial–mixed venous O_2 difference was 6 ml, and mixed venous O_2 content was 18.72 ml.
If the % shunt = X, then:
$(X \times 18.72) + ((100–X) \times 26.22) = (100 \times 24.72)$
and $18.72X + 2622–26.22X = 2472$
or $7.5 X = 150$
and % shunt = 20.

P-74. **Answer: b.** This anterior mediastinal tumor is a thymoma. Note the smooth well-defined borders.

P A R T   3
SELECTED REFERENCES

ADENOCARCINOMA

Greco FA, Hainsworth JD. Tumors of unknown origin. CA Cancer J Clin 1992; 42:96–115.

ADULT RESPIRATORY DISTRESS SYNDROME

Ashbaugh DG, Maier RV. Idiopathic pulmonary fibrosis in adult respiratory distress syndrome. Arch Surg 1985; 120:530.

Basran GS, et al. The effect of methylprednisolone on the pulmonary accumulation of transferrin in the adult respiratory distress syndrome. Eur J Respir Dis 1986; 68:336

DuToit HJ, et al. Methylprednisolone and the adult respiratory distress syndrome. S Afr Med J 1984; 65:1049.

Griffith BP, et al. Selected lobar injury after infusion of oleic acid. J Appl Physiol 1979; 47:706.

James PM. Treatment of shock lung. Ann Surg 1975; 41:451.

Montgomery BA, Stager MA, Carrico CJ, Hudson LD. Causes of mortality in patients with the adult respiratory distress syndrome. Am Rev Respir Dis 1985; 132:485–489.

Radermacher P, Huet Y, Lemaire F. Comparison of ketanserin and sodium nitroprusside in patients with severe ARDS. Anesthesiology 1988; 68:152–157.

Sibbald WJ, et al. Alveolo-capillary permeability in human septic ARDS. Chest 1981; 79:133.

Tomashefski JF, Zapol WM, Reid LM. The pulmonary vascular lesions of the adult respiratory distress syndrome. Am J Pathol 1983; 112:112–126.

Weigelt JA, et al. Early steroid therapy for respiratory failure. Arch Surg 1985; 120:536.

Williams AJ, et al. Pulmonary embolism presenting as adult respiratory distress syndrome—support for a hypothesis. Postgrad Med J 1982; 58:290.

Zapol WM, Snider MT. Pulmonary hypertension in severe acute respiratory failure. N Engl J Med 1977; 296:476–480.

Zapol WM, K Falke K (eds). Acute Respiratory Failure. Lung Biology in Health and Disease series. New York, Marcel Dekker, 1985, pp 241–273.

AIDS

Amorosa JK, Nahass RG, Nosher J, Goeke W. Radiologic distinction of pyogenic pulmonary infection from *Pneumocystis carinii* pneumonia in AIDS patients. Radiology 1990; 175:721–724.

Barrio JL, et al. *Pneumocystis carinii* pneumonia presenting as cavitating and noncavitating solitary pulmonary nodules in patients with AIDS. Am Rev Respir Dis 1986; 134: 1094–1096.

Beers MF, Sahn M, Schwarz M. Recurrent pneumothorax in AIDS patients with *Pneumocystis* pneumonia. Chest 1990; 98:266–270.

Bergin CJ, Wirth RL, Berry GJ, Castellino RA. *Pneumocystis carinii* pneumonia: CT and HRCT observations. J Comput Assist Tomogr 1990; 14:756–759.

Bronnimann DA, Adam RD, Galgiani JN, et al. Coccidioidomycosis in the acquired immunodeficiency syndrome. Ann Intern Med 1987; 106:372–379.

Chaisson RE. Bacterial pneumonia in patients with HIV infection. Semin Respir Infect 1989; 4:133–138.

Chechani V, Kamholz SL. Pulmonary manifestations of disseminated cryptococcosis in patients with AIDS. Chest 1990; 98:1060–1066.

Ellner JJ. Tuberculosis in the time of AIDS. Chest 1990; 98:1051–1052.

Garay SM, et al. Pulmonary manifestations of Kaposi's sarcoma. Chest 1987; 91:39–43.

Glatt AE, et al. Treatment of infections associated with HIV. N Engl J Med 1988; 318:1439–1448.

Guillon JM, Autran B, et al. Human immunodeficiency virus related lymphocytic alveolitis. Chest 1988; 94:1264–1270.

Heitzman ER. Pulmonary neoplastic and lymphoproliferative disease in AIDS: a review. Radiology 1990; 177:347–357.

Hopewell PC. TB and HIV infection. Semin Respir Infect 1989; 2:11.

Horsburgh CR, Selik RM. The epidemiology of disseminated nontuberculous mycobacterial infection in the acquired immunodeficiency syndrome (AIDS). Am Rev Respir Dis 1989; 139:4–7.

Johnson PC, Hamil RJ, Sarosi GA. Clinical review: progressive disseminated histoplasmosis in the AIDS patients. Semin Respir Infect 1989; 4:139–146.

Karp J, et al. Lung cancer in patients with AIDS. Chest 1993; 103:410–413.

Kramer F, et al. Delayed diagnosis of tuberculosis in patients with HIV infection. Am J Med 1990; 89:451.

Naidich DP, et al. Pulmonary manifestations of AIDS: CT and radiographic correlations. Radiol Clin North Am 1991; 29:999–1017.

Klein JS, Warnock M, Webb WR, Gamsu G. Cavitating and noncavitating granulomas in AIDS patients with pneumocystis. AJR 1989; 152:753–754.

Miller WT Jr, Edelman JM, Miller WT. Cryptococcal pulmonary infection in patients with AIDS. Radiographic appearance. Radiology 1990; 175:725–728.

Murray JF, et al. NHLBI workshop summary: pulmonary complications of AIDS: an update. Am Rev Respir Dis l987; 135:504–509.

Murray JF, Mills J. Pulmonary infectious complications of human immuno deficiency viral infections. Am Rev Respir Dis 1990; 141:1356–1372 (Part I), 141:1582–1598 (Part II).

Naidich DP, Garay SM, Goodman PC, et al. Pulmonary manifestations of AIDS. *In* Federle MP, et al (eds): Radiology of Acquired Immune Deficiency. New York, Raven Press, 1988, pp 47–76.

Naidich DP, Tarras M, Garay SM, et al. Kaposi's sarcoma: CT-radiographic correlation. Chest 1989; 96:723–728.

O'Brien RF. Pulmonary and pleural Kaposi's sarcoma in AIDS. Semin Respir Med 1989; 10:12–20.

Oldham SAA, Castillo M, Jacobson FL, et al. HIV-associated lymphocytic interstitial pneumonia: radiologic manifestations and pathologic correlation. Radiology 1989; 170:83–87.

Polish LB, Cohn DL, Ryder JW, et al. Pulmonary non-Hodgkin's lymphoma in AIDS. Chest 1989; 96:1321–1326.

Sider L, Horton ES. Pleural effusion as a presentation of AIDS-related lymphoma. Invest Radiol 1989; 24:150–153.

Simberkoff MS, et al. *Streptococcus pneumoniae* infections and bacteremia in patients with AIDS with report of a pneumococcal vaccine failure. Am Rev Respir Dis 1984; 130:1174–1176.

Small PM, et al. Treatment of TB in patients with advanced HIV infection. N Engl J Med 1991; 324:289.

Witt DJ, et al. Bacterial infections in adult patients with AlDS and ARC. Am J Med 1987; 82:900–906.

Yamaguchi E, Reichman LB. Tuberculosis and HIV: keep a high index of suspicion. J Respir Dis 1992; 13:1301.

ALLOPURINOL TOXICITY

Al-Kawas FH, et al. Allopurinol hepatotoxicity. Ann Intern Med 1981; 95:588–590.

Arellano F, Sacristan JA. Allopurinol hypersensitivity syndrome: a review. Ann Pharmacother 1993; 27:337–343.

Hande KR, et al. Severe allopurinol toxicity. Am J Med 1984; 76:47–56.

Singer JZ, Wallace SL. The allopurinol hypersensitivity syndrome. Arthritis Rheum 1986; 29:82–87.

ALPHA$_1$-ANTITRYPSIN

American Thoracic Society. Guidelines for the approach to the patient with severe hereditary alpha$_1$-antitrypsin deficiency. Am Rev Respir Dis 1989; 140:1494–1497.

Burrows B. A clinical trial of efficacy of antiproteolytic therapy: can it be done? Am Rev Respir Dis 1983; 127(2:2); S42–43.

Crystal R. Alpha$_1$-antitrypsin deficiency, emphysema, and liver disease: genetic basis and strategies for therapy. J Clin Invest 1990; 85:1343–1352.

Eriksson S. Alpha$_1$-antitrypsin deficiency: lessons learned from the bedside to the gene and back again. Chest 1989; 95:181–189.

Hubbard RC, Crystal RG. Alpha$_1$-antitrypsin augmentation therapy for alpha$_1$-antitrypsin deficiency. Am J Med 1988; 84(suppl 6A):52–62.

Hutchison DCS. Natural history of alpha$_1$-protease inhibitor deficiency. Am J Med 1988; 84(suppl 6A):3–12.

Lieberman J, Winter B, Sastre A. Alpha$_1$-antitrypsin Pi-types in 965 COPD patients. Chest 1986; 89:370–373.

Kueppers F, Black LF. Alpha$_1$-antitrypsin and its deficiency. Am Rev Respir Dis 1974; 110:176–194.

Laurell CB, Eriksson S. The electrophoretic alpha$_1$-globulin pattern of serum in alpha$_1$-antitrypsin deficiency. Scand J Clin Lab Invest 1963; 15:132–140.

Mittman C. The PiMz phenotype: is it a significant risk factor for the development of chronic obstructive lung disease? (editorial). Am Rev Respir Dis 1978; 118:649–652.

Ostrow DN, Cherniack RM. The mechanical properties of the lungs in intermediate deficiency of alpha$_1$-antitrypsin. Am Rev Respir Dis 1972; 106:377–382.

ALVEOLAR HEMORRHAGE

Bar-On H, Rosenmann E. Schönlein-Henoch syndrome in adults. Isr J Med Sci 1972; 8:1702–1715.

Beirne GJ, Kopp WL, Zimmerman SW. Goodpasture's syndrome dissociation from antibodies to glomerular basement membrane. Arch Intern Med 1973; 132:261–265.

Bell DD, Moffatt SL, Singer M, Munt PW. Antibasement membrane antibody disease without clinical evidence of renal disease. Am Rev Respir Dis 1990; 142:234–237.

Cadman EC, Lundberg WB, Mitcheil MS. Pulmonary manifestations in Behcet's syndrome. Arch Intern Med 1976; 136:944–947.

Chajeck T, Fainaru M. Behcet's disease: report of 41 cases and review of the literature. Medicine 1975; 54:179–196.

Churg A, Franklin W, Chan K, et al. Pulmonary hemorrhage and immune complex deposition in the lung: complications in a patient with systemic lupus erythematosus. Arch Pathol Lab Med 1980; 104:388–391.

Cream JJ, Gumpel JM, Peachey RDG. Schönlein-Henoch purpura in the adult. Q J Med 1978; 9:219–228.

Donaghy M, Rees AJ. Cigarette smoking and lung hemorrhage in glomerulonephritis caused by antibodies to glomerular basement membrane. Lancet 1983; 1:1390–1392.

Efthimiou J, Johnston C, Spiro SG, Turner-Warwick M. Pulmonary disease in Behçet's syndrome. Q J Med 1986; 227:259–280.

Erickson SB, Kurtz SB, Donaldo JV, et al. Use of combined plasmapheresis and immunosuppression in the treatment of Goodpasture's syndrome. Mayo Clin Proc 1979; 54:714–720.

Falk RJ, Jennette JC. Anti-neutrophil cytoplasmic autoantibodies with specificity for myeloperoxidase in patients with systemic vasculitis and idiopathic necrotizing and crescentic glomerulonephritis. N Engl J Med 1988; 318:1651–1657.

Gamble CN, Wiesner KG, Shapiro RF, Boyer WJ. The immune complex pathogenesis of glomerulonephritis and pulmonary vasculitis in Behçet's disease. Am J Med 1979; 6:1031–1039.

Germain MJ, Davidman M. Pulmonary hemorrhage and acute renal failure in a patient with mixed connective tissue disease. Am J Kidney Dis 1984; 3:420–424.

Goeken JA. Antineutrophil cytoplasmic antibody—a useful serologic marker for vasculitis. J Clin Immunol 1991; 2:161–174.

Greening AP, Hughes JMB. Serial estimation of carbon monoxide diffusing capacity in intrapulmonary hemorrhage. Clin Sci 1981; 60:507–512.

Herbert FA, Oxford R. Pulmonary hemorrhage and edema due to inhalation of resins containing trimellitic anhydride. Chest 1979; 76:546–551.

Holdsworth S, Boyce N, Thomson NM, Atkins RC.

The clinical spectrum of acute glomerulonephritis and lung hemorrhage (Goodpasture's syndrome). Q J Med 1985; 216:75–86.

Jennette JC, Wilkman AS, Falk RJ. Anti-neutrophil cytoplasmic antibody associated glomerulonephritis and vasculitis. Am J Pathol 1989; 135:921–930.

Johnson JP, Moore J, Austin HA, et al. Therapy of antiglomerular basement membrane antibody disease: analysis of prognostic significance of clinical, pathologic, and treatment factors. Medicine 1985; 64:219–227.

Leatherman JW, Davies SF, Hoidal JR. Alveolar hemorrhage syndromes: diffuse microvascular lung hemorrhage in immune and idiopathic disorders. Medicine 1984; 63:343–361.

Leatherman JW. The lung in systemic vasculitis. Semin Respir Infect 1988; 3:274–288.

Magee F, Wright JL, Kay JM, et al. Pulmonary capillary hemangiomatosis. Am Rev Respir Dis 1985; 132:922–925.

Mark EJ, Ramierez JF. Pulmonary capillaritis and hemorrhage in patients with systemic vasculitis. Arch Pathol Lab Med 1985; 109:413–418.

Matthay RA, Schwarz MI, Petty TL, et al. Pulmonary manifestations of systemic lupus erythematosus: a review of 12 cases of acute pneumonitis. Medicine 1975; 54:397–409.

Myers JL, Katzenstein M. Microangiitis in lupus-induced pulmonary hemorrhage. Am J Clin Pathol 1986; 85:552–556.

Perl SI, Russell BA, Charlesworth JA, et al. Goodpasture's (anti-GBM) disease and HLA-DRw2. N Engl J Med 1981; 305:463–464.

Rees AJ. Pulmonary injury caused by anti-basement membrane antibodies. Semin Respir Dis 1984; 5:264–272.

Rees AJ, Peters DK, Amos N, et al. The influence of HLA-linked genes on the severity of anti-GBM antibody-mediated nephritis. Kidney Int 1984; 26:444–450.

Schwarz MI, Mortenson RL Colby TV, et al. Systemic necrotizing vasculitis: a new cause of severe irreversible airflow limitation and hyperinflation. Am Rev Respir Dis. 1993; 148:507–511.

Shumak KH, Rock GA. Therapeutic plasma exchange. N Engl J Med 1984; 310:762–771.

Travis WD, Hoffman GS, Leavitt RV, et al. Surgical pathology of the lung in Wegener's granulomatosis: a review of 87 open lung biopsies from 67 patients. Am J Surg Pathol 1991; 15:315–333.

Walker RG, Scheinkestel C, Becker GJ, et al. Clinical and morphological aspects of the management of crescentic anti-glomerular basement membrane antibody (anti-GBM) nephritis/Goodpasture's syndrome. Q J Med 1985; 54:75–89.

Zeiss CR, Wolkonsky P, Chacon R, et al. Syndromes in workers exposed to trimellitic anhydride. Ann Intern Med 1983; 98:8–12.

ALVEOLAR PROTEINOSIS

Andriole VT, Ballas M, Wilson GL. The association of nocardiosis and pulmonary alveolar proteinosis. Ann Intern Med 1964; 60:226–275.

Claypool WD, Rogers RM, Matuschak GM. Update on the clinical diagnosis, management and pathogenesis of pulmonary alveolar proteinosis (phospholipidosis). Chest 1984; 85:550–558.

Kariman K, et al. Pulmonary alveolar proteinosis: prospective clinical experience in 23 patients for 15 years. Lung 1984; 162:223–231.

Lakshminarayan S, Schwarz Ml, Stanford RE. Unsuspected pulmonary alveolar proteinosis complicating acute myelogenous leukemia. Chest 1976; 69:433–435.

Martin RJ, et al. Pulmonary alveolar proteinosis: the diagnosis by segmental lavage. Am Rev Respir Dis 1980; 121:819–825.

Martin RJ, et al. Pulmonary alveolar proteinosis. Shunt fraction and lactic acid dehydrogenase concentration as aids to diagnosis. Am Rev Respir Dis 1978; 117:1059–1062.

Prakash UB, et al. Pulmonary alveolar phospholipoproteinosis: experience with 34 cases and review. Mayo Clin Proc 1987; 62:499–518.

Rogers RM, et al. Physiologic effects of bronchopulmonary lavage in alveolar proteinosis. Am Rev Respir Dis 1978; 118:255–264.

Rosen SH, Castleman B, Liebow AA. Pulmonary alveolar proteinosis. N Engl J Med 1958; 258: 1123–1128.

Selecky PA, Wasserman K, Benfleld JR, Lippman M. The clinical and physiological effect of whole-lung lavage in pulmonary alveolar proteinosis: a ten year experience. Ann Thorac Surg 1977; 24:451–461.

AMYLOIDOSIS

Cohen AS, et al. Survival of patients with primary (AL) amyloidosis. Am J Med 1987; 82:1182–1190.

Cordier JF, et al. Amyloidosis of the lower respiratory tract. Chest 1986; 90:827–831.

Gertz MA, et al. Clinical aspects of pulmonary amyloidosis. Chest 1986; 90:790–791.

Kahn A, et al. Primary pulmonary amyloidosis. Respiration 1984; 45:78–80.

Kline LR, et al. Diagnosis of pulmonary amyloidosis

by transbronchial biopsy. Am Rev Respir Dis 1985; 132:191–194.

Kyke RA, et al. Primary systemic amyloidosis. Am J Med 1985; 79:708–716.

AMYOTROPHIC LATERAL SCLEROSIS

Ellis ER, et al. Treatment of respiratory failure during systemic lupus erythematosus in patients with neuromuscular disease. Am Rev Respir Dis 1987; 135:148.

Kelly BJ, Luce JM. Diagnosis and management of neuromuscular diseases causing respiratory failure. Chest 1991; 99:1485.

Schmidt-Norawa WW, Altman AR. Atelectasis and neuromuscular respiratory failure. Chest 1984; 85:792.

Sivak ED, et al. Long-term management of respiratory failure in ALS. Ann Neurol 1982; 12:18.

ANTICARDIOLIPIN ANTIBODY

Cohen AJ, et al. Circulating coagulant inhibitors in AIDS. Ann Intern Med 1986; 104:175–180.

Gold JE, et al. Lupus anticoagulant in AIDS. N Engl J Med 1986; 314:1252–1253.

Harris EN, et al. Antiphospholipid antibodies-autoantibodies with a difference. Ann Rev Med 1988; 39:261–271.

Hughes GR, et al. The anticardiolipin syndrome. J Rheumatol 1986; 13:486–489.

Lockshin MD. Anticardiolipin antibody. Arthritis Rheum 1987; 30:471–472.

Stimmler MM, et al. Anticardiolipin antibodies in AIDS. Arch Intern Med 1989; 149:1833–1835.

ARTERIOVENOUS FISTULA

Blatchford JW, Bolman RM. Concomitant pulmonary and cerebral arteriovenous fistula. Chest 1985; 88:782–786.

Burke CM, Safai C, Nelson DP, Raffin TA. Pulmonary arteriovenous malformations: a critical update. Am Rev Respir Dis 1986; l34:334–339.

Burke CM, et al. Pulmonary arteriovenous fistula: a critical update. Am Rev Respir Dis 1986; 134:334.

Dines DE, Seward JB, Bernatz PE. Pulmonary arteriovenous fistulas. Mayo Clinic Proc 1983; 58:176–181.

Fishman A. Pulmonary Diseases and Disorders. 2nd ed. Vol. 2. Chapter 64, Pulmonary Hypertension and Cor Pulmonale. McGraw Hill, l988, pp 1043–1045.

Fraser RG, et al. Diagnosis of Diseases of the Chest. 3rd ed. Vol. 11. Chapter 5, Pulmonary Abnormalities of Developmental Origin. Philadelphia, WBSaunders 1990, pp 696–761.

Hatfield DR, Fried AM. Therapeutic embolization of diffuse pulmonary arteriovenous malformations. AJR 1981; 137:861–863.

Lincoln MJ, Shigeoka JW. Pulmonary telangiectasia without hypoxemia. Chest 1988; 193:1097–1098.

Perry WH. Clinical spectrum of hereditary hemorrhagic telangiectasia. Am J Med 1987; 82:989–997.

White RI, Lynch-Nyhan A, et al. Pulmonary arteriovenous malformations: techniques and long-term outcome of embolotherapy. Radiology 1988; 169:663–669.

ASBESTOS

Barrett JC, et al. Multiple mechanisms for the carcinogenic effects of asbestos and other mineral fibers. Environ Health Perspect 1989; 81:81.

Browne K. A threshold for asbestos related lung cancer. Br J Ind Med 1986; 43:556.

Craighead JE. Do silica and asbestos cause lung cancer? Arch Pathol Lab Med 1992; 116:16.

Guillemin B, et al. Role of peptide growth factors in asbestos related lung cancer. Ann N Y Acad Sci 1991; 643:245.

Mossman BT, Gee JB. Asbestos related diseases. N Engl J Med 1989; 320:1721.

Rom WM, et al. Cellular and molecular basis of the asbestos-related diseases. Am Rev Resp Dis 1991; 143:408.

Westerfield T. Asbestos-related lung disease. South J Med 1992; 85:616.

Whitesell PL, Drage CW. Occupational lung cancer. Mayo Clin Proc 1993; 68:183.

ASPERGILLOSIS

Denning DW, Stevens D. Antifungal and surgical treatment of invasive aspergillosis. Rev Infect Dis 1990; 12:1147–1201.

Denning DW, et al. Treatment of invasive aspergillosis with itraconazole. Am J Med 1989; 86:791–800.

Ganer A, Arathoon E, Stevens DA. Initial therapy for progressive mycosis with itraconazole, the first clinically studied triazole. Rev Infect Dis 1987; 95:S77–S86.

Herbert PA, Bayer AS. Fungal pneumonias: invasive aspergillosis. Chest 1981; 80:220–225.

Tomlinson JR, Sahn SA. Aspergilloma in sarcoid and tuberculosis. Chest 1987; 92:505–508.

Weiner H, et al. Antigen detection in the diagnosis of invasive aspergillosis. Ann Intern Med 1983; 99:777–782.

Yu VL, Muder RR, Poorsattar A. Significance of isolation of *Aspergillus* from the respiratory tract in the diagnosis of invasive pulmonary aspergillosis. Am J Med 1986; 81:249–254.

ATROPINE TOXICITY

Neuhaus A, et al. The effects of bronchoscopy with and without atropine premedication on pulmonary function in humans. Ann Thorac Surg 1978; 25:393.

Rumack BH. Anticholinergic poisoning: treatment with physostigmine. Pediatrics 1973; 52:449.

Shutt LE, Bowes JB. Atropine and hyoscine. Anesthesia 1979; 34:476.

AUTO-PEEP

Ashbaugh DG, Petty TL. Positive end-expiratory pressure J Thorac Cardiovasc Surg 1973; 65: 165–170.

Brown DG, Pierson DJ. Auto-PEEP is common in mechanically ventilated patients: a study of incidence, severity, and detection. Respir Care 1986; 31:1069–1074.

Marini J. New concepts in mechanical ventilation. Pulm Perspect 1988; 5:3–8.

Marini JJ, Pepe PE. Occult positive end-expiratory pressure in mechanically ventilated patients with airflow obstruction. The auto-PEEP effect. Am Rev Resp Dis 1982; 126:166–170.

Pepe PE, Marini JJ. Occult positive end-expiratory pressure in mechanically ventilated patients with airflow obstruction. Am Rev Respir Dis 1982; 126:166–170.

Pepe PE, Hudson LD, Carrico CJ. Early application of positive end-expiratory pressure in patients at risk for the adult respiratory distress syndrome. N Engl J Med 1984; 311:281–286.

Scott LR, Benson MS, Pierson DJ. Effect of inspiratory flowrate and circuit compressible volume on auto-PEEP during mechanical ventilation. Respir Care 1986; 31:1075–1079.

Scott LR, Benson MS, Bishop MJ. Relationship of endotracheal tube size to auto-PEEP at high minute ventilation. Respir Care 1986; 31:1080–1082.

Simkovitz P, Brown K, Goldberg P, et al. Interaction between intrinsic and externally applied PEEP during mechanical ventilation. Am Rev Respir Dis 1987; 135:A202.

Tuxen DV, Lane S. The effects of ventilatory, pattern on hyperinflation, airway pressures, and circulation in mechanical ventilation of patients with severe airflow obstruction. Am Rev Respir Dis 1987; 136:872–879.

BCNU TOXICITY

Aronin P, et al. Prediction of BCNU pulmonary toxicity in patients with malignant glioma. N Engl J Med 1980; 303:183–88.

Durant J, et al. Pulmonary toxicity associated with BCNU. Ann Intern Med 1989; 90:191–94.

O'Driscoll B, et al. Active lung fibrosis up to 17 years after chemotherapy with BCNU in childhood. N Engl J Med 1990; 323:378–382.

Selker R, et al. BCNU induced pulmonary fibrosis. Neurosurgery 1980; 7:560–565.

Twokig K, et al. Pulmonary effects of cytotoxic agents other than bleomycin. Clin Chest Med 1990; 11(1):31–54.

Weiss R, et al. The nitrosoureas and pulmonary toxicity. Cancer Treat Rev 1981; 8:25.

BERYLLIOSIS

Fraser, RG et al. Pleuropulmonary disease caused by inhalation of inorganic dust. *In* Fraser RG, et al (eds). Diagnosis of Diseases of the Chest. 3rd ed. Philadelphia, WB Saunders, 1990, pp 2362–2366.

Kreiss K, et al. Screening blood test identifies subclinical beryllium disease. J Occup Med 1989; 31:603–608.

Newman L. Dyspnea with diffuse interstitial infiltrates and hilar adenopathy. *In* Schwarz (ed). Pulmonary Grand Rounds. Toronto, BC Decker, 1990, pp 44–52.

BLASTOMYCOSIS

Dismukes WE, et al. Itraconazole therapy for blastomycosis and histoplasmosis. Am J Med 1992; 93:484–497.

Pappas PG, et al. Blastomycosis in patients with AIDS. Ann Intern Med 1992; 116:847–853.

Recht R, et al. Blastomycosis in immunosuppressed patients. Am Rev Respir Dis 1982; 125:359–362.

Saag M, et al. Treatment of histoplasmosis and blastomycosis. Chest 1988; 93:848–851.

Schwartz J, Baum GL. Blastomycosis. Am J Clin Pathol 1951; 11:999–1029.

BONE MARROW TRANSPLANTATION

Armitage JO. Bone marrow transplantation. N Engl J Med 1994; 330:827–838.

Chan CK, et al. Pulmonary complications following bone marrow transplantation. Clin Chest Med 1990; 11:323–332.

Cordonnier C, et al. Diagnostic yield of bronchoalveolar lavage in pneumonitis occurring after allogeneic bone marrow transplantation. Am Rev Respir Dis 1985; 132:1118–1123.

Clark JG, et al. Idiopathic pneumonia syndrome after bone marrow transplantation. Am Rev Respir Dis 1993; 147:1601–1606.

Ferrara JLM, Deeg HJ. Graft-versus-host disease. N Engl J Med 1991; 324:667–674.

Krowka MJ, et al. Pulmonary complications of bone marrow transplantation. Chest 1985; 87:237–246.

Pecego R, et al. Interstitial pneumonitis following autologous bone marrow transplantation. Transplantation 1986; 42:515–517.

Robbins RA, et al. Diffuse alveolar hemorrhage in autologous bone marrow transplant recipients. Am J Med 1989; 87:511–518.

Rowe JM, et al. Recommended guidelines for the management of autologous and allogeneic bone marrow transplantation. Ann Intern Med 1994; 120:143–158.

Stover DE, et al. Bronchoalveolar lavage in the diagnosis or diffuse pulmonary infiltrates in the immunocompromised host. Ann Intern Med 1984; 101:1–7.

BOTULISM

Benson CA, et al. Acute neurologic infections. Med Clin North Am 1986; 70:987–1011.

Campbell WW, et al. Differential diagnosis of acute weakness. South Med J 1981; 74:1371–1375.

Hatheway G. Toxigenic clostridia. Clin Med Rev 1990; 3:70–76.

Hughes JM, et al. Clinical features of type A and B foodborne botulism. Ann Intern Med 1981; 95:442–444.

Schmidt-Novara WW, et al. Early and late pulmonary complications of botulism. Arch Intern Med 1983; 143:451–456.

Tacket CO, et al. Equine antitoxin use and other factors that predict outcome in type A foodborne botulism. Am J Med 1984; 76:794–798.

Wilcox PG. Long-term follow-up of symptoms, pulmonary function, respiratory muscle strength and exercise performance after botulism. Am Rev Respir Dis 1989; 139:157–163.

BRONCHIECTASIS

Barker AF, Bardana EJ. Bronchiectasis: update of an orphan disease. Am Rev Respir Dis 1988; 137:969–978.

Barker AF, Craig S, Bardana EJ. Humoral immunity in bronchiectasis. Ann Allergy 1987; 59:179–182.

Cunningham-Rundles C, Siegal FP, Smithwick EM, et al. Efficacy of intravenous immunoglobulin in primary humoral immunodeficiency disease. Ann Intern Med 1984; 101:435–439.

Pirovsky B. Intravenous immune globulin therapy in hypogammaglobulinemia. A review. Am J Med 1984; 76(suppl 3A):53–60J.

Roifman CM, Lederman HM, Lavi S, et al. Benefit of intravenous IgG replacement in hypogammaglobulinemic patients with chronic sinopulmonary disease. Am J Med 1985; 79:171–174.

BRONCHIOLITIS OBLITERANS

Burke CM, et al. Post-transplant obliterative bronchiolitis and other late lung sequellae in human heart-lung transplantation. Chest 1984; 86:824.

Dorinsky PM, Davis WB, Lucas JG, et al. Adult bronchiolitis: evaluation by bronchoalveolar lavage and response to prednisone therapy. Chest 1985; 88:58–63.

Epler GR, Colby T. The spectrum of bronchiolitis obliterans. Chest 1983; 83:161.

Geddes DM, Corrin B, Brewerton DA, et al. Progressive airway obliteration in adults and its association with rheumatoid arthritis. Q J Med 1977; 184:427–444.

Gosink BB, Friedman PJ, Liebow AA. Bronchiolitis obliterans roentgenographic-pathologic correlation. AJR 1973; 117:816–832.

King TE. Bronchiolitis obliterans. Lung 1989; 167:69–93.

Milne JH. Nitrogen dioxide inhalation and bronchiolitis obliterans. J Occup Med 1969; 11:538–547.

Ostrow D, et al. Bronchiolitis obliterans complicating bone marrow transplantation. Chest 1985; 87:8–28.

Schwarz MI, King TE Jr (eds). Interstitial Lung Disease. 2nd Ed. St. Louis, Mosby Year Book, 1993.

Wohl MEB, Chernick V. Bronchiolitis. Am Rev Respir Dis 1978; 118:759.

BRONCHIOLITIS OBLITERANS ORGANIZING PNEUMONIA

Colby TV. Pathologic aspects of bronchiolitis obliterans organizing pneumonia. Chest 1992; 102(1): 38S–43S.

Costabel U, Guzman J. BOOP: What is old? What is new? Eur Respir J 1991; 4:771.

Epler GR, et al. Bronchiolitis obliterans organizing pneumonia. N Engl J Med 1985; 312:152–158.

Epler GR, Colby TV, McLoud TC, et al. Systemic lupus erythematosus and bronchiolitis obliterans organizing pneumonia. N Engl J Med 1985; 312:152–158.

Flowers JR, et al. BOOP: clinical and radiologic features. Clin Radiol 1992; 45:371.

Guerry-Force ML, et al. A comparison of BOOP, UIP, and small airway disease. Am Rev Respir Dis 1987; 135:705–712.

King TE, Mortenson RL. Syndromes that mimic idiopathic pulmonary fibrosis. Immun Allerg Clin North Am 1992; 12:489.

Kitaichi M. Differential diagnosis of BOOP. Chest 1992; 102(1):45S–49S.

Myers JL, Katzenstein AL. Ultrastructural evidence of alveolar epithelial injury in idiopathic bronchiolitis obliterans organizing pneumonia. Am J Pathol 1988; 132:102–109.

Nishimura K, Itoh HR. CT features of BOOP. Chest 1992; 102:26s.

Schwarz MI, King TE Jr (eds). Interstitial Lung Disease. 2nd Ed. St. Louis, Mosby Year Book, 1993.

Turton CW, Williams G, Green M. Cryptogenic obliterative bronchiolitis in adults. Thorax 1981; 36:805.

BRONCHIOLOALVEOLAR CARCINOMA

Dunn D, et al. Bronchioloalveolar cell carcinoma of the lung: a clinicopathological study. Ann Thorac Surg 1978; 26:241.

Edwards CW. Alveolar carcinoma: a review. Thorax 1984; 39:166.

Ludington LG, et al. Bronchiolar carcinoma (alveolar cell), another great imitator: a review of 41 cases. Chest 1972; 61:622–628.

Munnell ER, Lawson RC, Keller DF. Solitary bronchiolar (alveolar cell), carcinoma of the lung. J Thorac Cardiovasc Surg 1966; 52:261–270.

Schraufnagel D, Peloquin A, Pare JAP, Wang N. Differentiating bronchiolo-alveolar carcinoma from adenocarcinoma. Am Rev Respir Dis 1982; 125:74–79.

Sestini P, et al. Bronchoalveolar lavage diagnosis of bronchioloalveolar carcinoma. Eur J Respir Dis 1985; 66:55–58.

BRONCHOGENIC CARCINOMA

Bishop JM. Oncogenes. Sci Am 1982; 246:80–92.

Bishop JM. Cellular oncogenes and retroviruses. Ann Rev Biochem 1983; 52:301–354.

Doyle A, Martin J, Funa K, et al. Markedly decreased expression of class I histocompatibility antigens, protein, and mRNA in human small cell lung cancer. J Exp Med 1985; 161:1135–1151.

Hopkins JM, Evans HJ. Cigarette smoke-induced DNA damage and lung cancer risks. Nature 1980; 298:388–390.

Kolata G. Cell biology yields clues to lung cancer. Science 1982; 218:38–39.

Little CD, Nau MM, Carney DN, et al. Amplification and expression of the c-myconcogene in human lung cancer cell lines. Nature 1983; 306:194–196.

Moody TW, Pert C, Gazdar A, et al. High levels of intracellular bombesin characterize human small cell carcinoma. Science 1981; 214:1246–1248.

Sporn M, Todaro G. Autocrine secretion and malignant transformation of cells. N Engl J Med 1980; 303:878–880.

Whang-Peng J, Kao-Shan CS, Lee EC. Specific chromosome defect associated with human small cell lung cancer: Deletion 3p (14–23). Science 1982; 215:181–182.

BRONCHOGENIC CYST

Bolton, JW, Shahian DM. Asymptomatic bronchogenic cysts: What is the best management? Ann Thorac Surg 1992; 53:1134–1137.

Haddon J, Bowen A. Bronchopulmonary and neurenteric forms of foregut anomalies. Imaging for diagnosis and management. Radiol Clin North Am 1991; 29:241–254.

Marks, C, Marks P. The embryologic basis of tracheobronchopulmonary maldevelopment. Int Surg 1987; 72:109–114.

St. George R, et al. Clinical spectrum of bronchogenic cysts of the mediastinum and lung in the adult. Ann Thorac Surg 1991; 52(1):6–13.

BRONCHIAL TRAUMA

Alber JE, Rath RK, et al. Severity of intrathoracic injuries associated with first rib fractures. Ann Thorac Surg 1982; 33:614.

Ecker RR, Libertini RV, Rea WJ, et al. Injuries of the trachea and bronchi. Ann Thorac Surg 1971; 11:289.

Hara KS, Prakash UBS. Fiberoptic bronchoscopy in the evaluation of acute chest and upper airway trauma. Chest: 1989; 93:627-630.

Kelly JP, et al. Management of airway trauma I: tracheobronchial injuries. Ann Thorac Surg 1985; 40:551-555.

Mattox L, Moore EE, Feliciano DV. Trauma. Norwalk, Conn, Appleton & Lange, 1988, pp 335–347.

BRONCHOPLEURAL FISTULA

Baumann M, Sahn S. Medical management and therapy of bronchopleural fistulas in the mechanically ventilated patient. Chest 1990; 97:721.

Jones D, David I. Gelfoam occlusion of peripheral bronchopleural fistulas. Ann Thorac Surg 1986; 42:334.

Martin W, et al. Closure of a BPF with bronchoscopic instillation of tetracycline. Chest 1991; 99:1040.

Opie JC, et al. Endobronchial closure of a postpneumonectomy bronchopleural fistula. Ann Thorac Surg 1992; 53:686.

Regel G, et al. Occlusion of bronchopleural fistula after lung injury; a new treatment by bronchoscopy. J Trauma 1989; 29:223.

York E, et al. Endoscopic diagnosis and treatment of post-op bronchopleural fistula. Chest 1990; 97:1390.

BURNS

Bingham HG, et al. Early bronchoscopy as a predictor of ventilatory support for burned patients. J Trauma 1987; 27:1286–1288.

Haponik EF, et al. Upper airway function in burn patients. Am Rev Respir Dis 1984; 129:251–257.

Haponik EF, et al. Acute upper airway injury in burn patients. Am Rev Respir Dis 1987; 135:360–366.

Heimbach DM. Inhalation injuries. Ann Emerg Med 1988; 17:1316–1320.

Herndon DN, et al. Pulmonary injury in burned patients. Surg Clin North Am 1987; 67:31–46.

CANCER

Cuttitta F, Carney D, Mulshine J, et al. Bombesin-like peptides can function as autocrine growth factors in human small cell lung cancer. Nature 1985; 316:823–826.

Doyle A, Martin J, Funa K, et al. Markedly decreased expression of class I histocompatibility antigens, protein, and mRNA in human small cell lung cancer. J Exp Med 1985; 161:1135–1151.

Karp J, et al. Lung cancer in patients with AIDS. Chest 1993; 103:410–413.

Heitzman ER. Pulmonary neoplastic and lymphoproliferative disease in AIDS: a review. Radiology 1990; 177:347–357.

Monfardini S, et al. Unusual malignant tumors in 49 patients with HIV infection. AIDS 1989; 3:449–453.

Naidich DP, et al. Pulmonary manifestations of AIDS: CT and radiographic correlations. Radiol Clin North Am 1991; 29:999–1017.

CARCINOID

Attar S, Miller JE, Hankins J, et al. Bronchial adenoma: a review of 51 patients. Ann Thorac Surg 1985; 40:126–132.

Lima RD. Bronchial adenoma, clinicopathologic study and results of treatment. Chest 1980; 77:81–84.

DeCaro LF, Paladagu R, Benfield JR, et al. Typical and atypical carcinoids within the pulmonary APUD tumor spectrum. J Thorac Cardiovasc Surg 1983; 86:528–536.

Higgins G, et al. The solitary pulmonary nodule: ten year follow-up of V.A. Armed Forces Cooperative Study. Arch Surg 1975; 110:5705.

Harpole DH, et al. Bronchial carcinoid tumors: a retrospective analysis of 126 patients. Ann Thorac Surg 1992; 54:50.

Hurt R, Bates M. Carcinoid tumors of the bronchus: a 33 year experience. Thorax 1984; 39:617.

McCaughan BC, Bains MS. Bronchial carcinoids. J Thorac Surg 1985; 89:8–17.

McCaughan BC, et al. Bronchial carcinoids: review of 124 cases. J Thorac Cardiovasc Surg 1985; 89:8.

Norheim I, Oberg K, Theodorsson-Norheim E, et al. Malignant carcinoid tumors. Ann Surg 1987; 206:115–126.

Rea F, et al. Bronchial carcinoids: a review of 60 patients. Ann Thorac Surg 1989; 47:412.

Torre M, et al. Typical and atypical bronchial carcinoids. Respir Med 1989; 83:305.

Wilkins E, Grillo HC, Moncure AC, Scannell JG. Changing times in surgical management of bronchopulmonary carcinoid tumor. Ann Thorac Surg 1984; 38:339–345.

CHILDHOOD BRONCHOPULMONARY INFECTION

Hardy K, et al. Obliterative bronchiolitis in children. Chest 1988; 93:3.

Milner AD. Acute bronchiolitis in infancy: treatment and prognosis. Thorax 1989; 44:1–5.

Northway W, et al. Pulmonary disease following respiratory therapy of hyaline membrane disease. N Engl J Med 1967; 276: 357–368.

CHURG-STRAUSS SYNDROME

American College of Rheumatology. 1990 criteria for the classification of Churg-Strauss syndrome. Arthritis Rheum 1990; 338:1094–1100.

Churg J, Strauss L. Allergic granulomatosis, allergic angiitis, and polyarteritis nodosa. Am J Pathol 1951; 27:277–301.

Lanham JG, Elkon KB, Pusey CD, Hughes CR. Systemic vasculitis with asthma and eosinophilia: a clinical approach to the Churg-Strauss syndrome. Medicine (Baltimore) 1984; 63:65–81.

CHYLOTHORAX

Fairfax AJ, et al. Chylothorax: a review of 18 cases. Thorax 1986; 41:880–885.

Sahn SA. State of the art: the pleura. Am Rev Respir Dis 1988; 138:184–234.

Sasson CS, Light RW. Chylothorax and pseudochylothorax. Clin Chest Med 1985; 6:163–171.

Staats BA, et al. The lipoprotein profile of chylous and nonchylous pleural effusions. Mayo Clin Proc 1980; 55:700–704.

Vennera MC, et al. Chylothorax and tuberculosis. Thorax 1983; 38:694–695.

COCAINE TOXICITY

Cregler LL, Mark H. Medical complications of cocaine abuse. N Engl J Med 1986; 315: 1495–1500.

Cucco RA, Yoo OH, Cregler L, Chang JC. Nonfatal pulmonary edema after "freebase" cocaine smoking. Am Rev Respir Dis 1987; 136:179–181.

Forrester JM, Steele AW, Waldron JA, Parsons PE. Crack lung: an acute pulmonary syndrome with a spectrum of clinical and histopathologic findings. Am Rev Respir Dis 1990; 142:462–467.

Itkonen J, Schnoll S, Glassroth J. Pulmonary dysfunction in "freebase" cocaine users. Arch Intern Med 1984; 144:2195–2197.

Murray RJ, et al. Diffuse alveolar hemorrhage temporally related to cocaine smoking. Chest 1988; 93:427–429.

Patel RC, Dutta D, Schonfeld SA. Free-base cocaine use associated with bronchiolitis obliterans organizing pneumonia. Ann Intern Med 1987; 107:186–187.

COCCIDIOIDOMYCOSIS

Ampel NM, et al. Coccidioidomycosis during HIV infection. Am J Med 1993; 94:235–240.

Bronnimann DA, et al. Coccidioidomycosis in AlDS. Ann Intern Med 1987; 106:372–379.

Einstein HE, et al. Coccidioidomycosis: new aspects of epidemiology and therapy. Clin Infect Dis 1993; 16:349–356.

Fish DG, et al. Coccidioidomycosis during HIV infection. Medicine 1990; 69:384–390.

COLCHICINE POISONING

Rovan IG, et al. Reversal of colchicine-induced toxicity by monoclonal antibody. Am J Pathol 1990; 137:779–787.

Sauder PH, et al. Hemodynamic studies in eight cases of acute colchicine poisoning. Hum Toxicol 1983; 2:169–173.

Wallace SL. Review: systemic toxicity associated with the intravenous use of colchicine—guidelines for use. J Rheum 1988; 153:495–498.

CYSTIC FIBROSIS

Davis PB. Cystic fibrosis. Clinical manifestations in older patients. Clin Notes Respir Dis 1983; 21:3–12.

Knowltoll RG, et al. A polymorphic DNA marker linked to cystic fibrosis is located on chromosome 7. Nature 1985; 318:380–382.

Nadler HC, Ben-Joseph Y. Genetics. *In* Taussig LM (ed). Cystic Fibrosis. New York, Thieme-Stratton, 1984, pp 10–24.

Tsui LC, et al. Progress in mapping thc cystic fibrosis gene. Am J Hum Genet 1095; 37:179A.

Wainwright BL, et al. Localization of cystic fibrosis locus to human chromosome 7 cen-q22. Nature 1985; 318:384–385.

White R, et al. A closely linked genetic marker for cystic fibrosis. Nature 1985; 318:382–384.

DIABETIC KETOACIDOSIS

Basran GS, Ramasubrarnanian R, Verma R. Intrathoracic complications of acute pancreatitis. Br J Dis Chest 1987; 81:326.

Brun-Buisson CJL, Bonnet F, Bergeret S, et al. Recurrent high-permeability pulmonary edema associated with diabetic ketoacidosis. Crit Care Med 1985; 13:56.

Carrol P, Matz R. Adult respiratory distress syndrome complicating severely uncontrolled diabetes mellitus: report of nine cases and a review of the literature. Diabetes Care 1982; 5:574.

Guice KS, Oldharn KT, Wolfe RR, et al. Lung injury in acute pancreatitis: primary inhibition of pulmonary phospholipid synthesis. Am J Surg 1987; 153:54.

Lee BC, Malik AB, Minnear FL. Effect of acute pancreatitis on pulmonary transvascular fluid and protein exchange. Am Rev Respir Dis 1981; 123:618.

Russell J, Follansbee S, Matthay M. Adult respiratory distress syndrome complicating diabetic ketoacidosis. West J Med 1981; 135:148.

Sprung CL, Rackow EC, Fein A. Pulmonary edema: a complication of diabetic ketoacidosis. Chest 1980; 77:687.

DOWN SYNDROME

Chi TL, et al. The pulmonary vascular bed in children with Down syndrome. J Pediatr 1975; 86: 533–538.

Cooney TP, Thurlbeck MB. Pulmonary hypoplasia in Down's syndrome. N Engl J Med 1982; 307: 1170–1173.

Hayes A, Batshaw ML. Down syndrome. Pediatr Clin North Am 1993; 40:523–535.

Loughlin GM, et al. Sleep apnea as a possible cause of pulmonary hypertension in Down syndrome. J Pediatr 1981; 98:435–437.

Southall DP, et al. Upper airway obstruction with hypoxemia and sleep disruption in Down syndrome. Dev Med Child Neurol 1987; 29:734–742.

EMBOLISM

Anderson E, Simon G, Reid L. Primary and thromboembolic hypertension: a quantitative pathological study. J Pathol 1973; 110:4:273–293.

Bell WR, et al. The clinical features of massive and submassive pulmonary embolism. Am J Med 1977; 62:355–360.

Dalen JE, et al. Resolution rate of acute pulmonary embolism in man. N Engl J Med 1969; 280: 1194–1198.

D'Alanzo C, Bower J, Dantzker D. Differentiation of patients with primary and thromboembolic pulmonary hypertension. Chest 1984; 85:4:457–461.

D'Alonzo GE, et al. The mechanisms of abnormal gas exchange in acute massive pulmonary embolism. Am Rev Respir Dis 1983; 128:170.

Dantzker DR, Bower JS. Alterations in gas exchange following pulmonary thromboembolism. Chest 1982; 81:495.

Dantzker D, Bower J. Mechanisms of gas exchange abnormality in patients with chronic obliterative pulmonary vascular disease. J Clin Invest 1979; 64:1050–1055.

Hull RD, et al. Diagnostic value of ventilation/perfusion scanning in patients with suspected pulmonary emboli. Chest 1985; 88:819–828.

Iber C, Sirr S. Diagnosis of pulmonary embolism. Semin Respir Infect 1988; 3:203–215.

International Multicenter Trial: Prevention of fatal postoperative pulmonary embolism by low doses of heparin. Lancet 1975; 2:45–51.

Libby LS, King TE, LaForce FM, Schwarz MI. Pulmonary cavitation following pulmonary infarction. Medicine 1985; 64:342–348.

Moser K. Pulmonary embolism: state of the art. Am Rev Respir Dis 1977; 115:829.

Moser KM, Auger WR, Fedullo PF. Chronic major vessel thromboembolic pulmonary hypertension. Circulation 1990; 81:1735–1743.

Moser KM, et. al. Thromboendarterectomy for chronic, major-vessel thromboembolic pulmonary hypertension. Ann Intern Med 1987; 107: 560–565.

Nicol P, et al. Pulmonary angiography in severe chronic pulmonary hypertension. Ann Intern Med 1987; 107:565–568.

Powers PJ, et al. A randomized trial of less intense postoperative warfarin or aspirin therapy in the prevention of venous thromboembolism after surgery for fractured hip. Arch Intern Med 1989; 149:771–774.

Urokinase Pulmonary Embolism Trial: Phase 1 results. JAMA 1970; 214:2163–2172.

Wagenvoort C. Pulmonary hypertension: a pathological study of the lung vessels in 156 clinically diagnosed cases. Circulation 1970; 42:1163–1184.

EMPYEMA

Bergh N, et al. Intrapleural streptokinase in the treatment of haemothorax and empyema. Scand J Thorac Cardiovasc Surg 1977; 11:265–268.

Lee K, et al. Treatment of thoracic multiloculated empyemas with intracavitary urokinase: a prospective study. Radiology 1991; 179:771–775.

Lemmer J, et al. Modern management of adult thoracic empyema. J Thorac Cardiovasc Surg 1985; 90: 849–855.

Moulton J, et al. Treatment of loculated pleural effusions with transcatheter intracavitary urokinase. Am J Radiol 1989; 153:941–945.

Neff C, et al. CT follow-up of empyema: pleural peels resolve after percutaneous catheter drainage. Radiology 1990; 176:195–197.

Light R. Parapneumonic effusions and empyema. Clin Chest Med 1985; 5:55–62.

EOSINOPHILIC GRANULOMA

Aguayo SM, Schwarz MI, Mortenson RL, et al. The role of chest radiograph in the evaluation of disease severity and clinical course in eosinophilic granuloma. Am Rev Respir Dis 1990; 141:A61.

Banks DA, Salvaggio JE, Goetzl EJ. Eosinophilic syndromes and eosinophilic granuloma. *In* Murray JF, Nadel JA (eds). Textbook of respiratory medicine. Philadelphia, WB Saunders, 1988.

Friedman PJ, Liebow AA, Sokoloff J. Eosinophilic granuloma of lung: clinical aspects of primary pulmonary histiocytosis in the adult. Medicine 1981; 60:385.

King TE, Mortenson RL. Syndromes that mimic idiopathic pulmonary fibrosis. Immunol Allerg Clin North Am 1992; 12:461.

Marcy TW, Reynolds HY. Pulmonary histiocytosis X. Lung 1985; 163:129.

Stern EJ, Webb WR, Golden JA, Gamsu, G. Cystic lung disease associated with eosinophilic granuloma and tuberous sclerosis: air trapping at dynamic ultrafast high–resolution CT. Radiology 1992; 182:325.

EOSINOPHILIC PNEUMONIA

Carrington CB, Addington WW, Goff AM, et al. Chronic eosinophilic pneumonia. N Engl J Med 1969; 280:787–798.

Dejaegher P, Demedts M. Bronchoalveolar lavage in eosinophilic pneumonia before and during corticosteroid therapy. Am Rev Respir Dis 1984; 129:631–632.

Leibow AA, Carrington CB. The eosinophilic pneumonias. Medicine 1969; 48:251–285.

Middleton WG, Paterson IC, Grant WB, Douglas AC. Asthmatic pulmonary eosinophilia: a review of 65 cases. Br J Dis Chest 1977; 71:115–122.

EPIGLOTTITIS

Mayo Smith F, et al. Acute epiglottis in adults. N Engl J Med 1986; 314:1135–1139.

Franz T, et al. Acute epiglottitis in adults. JAMA 1994; 272:1358–1360.

Aboussoan L, et al. Diagnosis and management of upper airway obstruction. Clin Chest Med 1994; 15:35–53.

EPSTEIN-BARR VIRUS

Kaplan ME, Tan EM. Antinuclear antibodies in infectious mononucleosis. Lancet 1968; 16:561–563.

Lander P, Palayew MJ. Infectious mononucleosis—a review of chest roentgenographic manifestations. J Can Assoc Radiol 1974; 25:303–306.

Tosata G, Blaese RM. Epstein-Barr virus infections. Adv Immunol 1985; 37:102–128.

ETHYLENE GLYCOL

Galliot M, et al. Treatment of ethylene glycol poisoning with intravenous 4-methylpyrazole. N Engl J Med 1988; 319:97–100.

Haupt M, et al. Massive ethylene glycol poisoning without evidence of crystalluria: a case for early intervention. J Emerg Med 1988; 6:295.

Jacobsen D, et al. Ethylene glycol intoxication: evaluation of kinetics and crystalluria. Am J Med 1988; 84:145.

Jacobsen D, et al. Methanol and ethylene glycol poisonings: mechanism of toxicity, clinical course, diagnosis, and treatment. Med Toxicol 1986; 1:309.

Parry M, Wallach R. Ethylene glycol poisoning. Am J Med 1974; 57:143.

EXERCISE

Jones N L. Exercise testing in pulmonary evaluation: rationale, methods and the normal respiratory response to exercise. N Engl J Med 1975; 293:541.

Jones NL. Exercise testing in pulmonary evaluation. Clinical applications. N Engl J Med 1975; 293:647.

Wasserman K, Hansen J. *In* Principles of Exercise Testing and Interpretation. Philadelphia, Lea & Febiger, 1987, p 326.

Weber K, Janicki J. *In* Jeff AR (ed). Cardiopulmonary Exercise Testing. New York, Grune & Stratton, 1986, p 3.

Whipp BJ, Ward SA. The normal respiratory response to exercise. *In* Jeff AR (ed). Cardiopulmonary

Exercise Testing. New York, Grune & Stratton, 1986.

Younes M. Interpretation of clinical exercise testing in respiratory disease. Clin Chest Med 1984; 5:189.

FAT EMBOLI

Ashbaugh DG, Petty TL. The use of corticosteroid in treatment of respiratory failure associated with massive fat embolism. Surg Gynecol Obstet 1966; 123:493–500.

Dines DE, Linscheid RL, Didier EP. Fat embolism syndrome. Mayo Clin Proc 1972; 47:237–240.

Jones JP Jr. Fat embolism and osteonecrosis. Orthoped Clin North Am 1985; 16:595–633.

Oh WH, Mital MA. Fat embolism: current concepts of pathogenesis, diagnosis, and treatment. Orthoped Clin North Am 1978; 9:769–779.

Schonfeld SA, et al. Fat embolism prophylaxis with corticosteroids. A prospective study in high-risk patients. Ann Intern Med 1983; 99:438–443.

GUILLAIN-BARRÉ SYNDROME

Gracey DR, et al. Respiratory failure in Guillain-Barré syndrome. Mayo Clin Proc 1982; 57: 742–746.

Huvwitz ES, et al. national Surveyance for Guillain-Barré syndrome. Neurology 1983; 33:150.

McKawnn G. Plasmapheresis and acute Guillain-Barré syndrome. Neurology 1985; 35:10–46.

HAMARTOMA

Bateson EM. So-called hamartoma of the lung—a true neoplasm of fibrous connective tissue of the bronchi. Cancer 1972; 31:1458.

Hamper UM, et al. Pulmonary hamartoma: diagnosis by transthoracic needle aspiration biopsy. Radiology 1985; 155:15.

Madani MA, et al. Multiple hamartomata of the lung. Thorax 1966; 21:468.

Sagel SS, Ablow RC. Hamartoma: on occasion a rapidly growing tumor of the lung. Radiology 1968; 91:971.

Van Den Bosch JM, et al. Mesenchymoma of the lung (so-called hamartoma): a review of 154 parenchymal and endobronchial cases. Thorax 1987; 42:790.

HEPATIC ARTERIOVENOUS SHUNTS

Berthelot P, Walker JG, Sherlock S, Reid L. Arterial changes in the lungs in cirrhosis of the liver — lung spider nevi. N Engl J Med 1966; 274:291–298.

Edell ES, Cortese DA, Krowka MJ, Rehder K. Severe hypoxemia and liver disease. Am Rev Respir Dis 1989; 140:1631–1635.

Eriksson LS, et al. Is hypoxemia in cirrhotic patients due to a functional hepatopulmonary syndrome? J Hepatology 1988; 7(suppl):529.

Krowka MJ, Cortese DA. Pulmonary aspects of liver disease and liver transplantation. Clin Chest Med 1989; 10:593–616.

Krowka MJ, Cortese DA. Hepatopulmonary syndrome. Chest 1990; 98:1053–1054. (Editorial)

HEPATIC PLEURAL EFFUSION

Frothingham JR. Cirrhosis of the liver complicated by persistent right hydrothorax and ascites. N Engl J Med 1942; 226:679–682.

Morrow CS, Kantor M, Arrnen NA. Hepatic hydrothorax. Ann Intern Med 1958; 49:193–203.

Johnston RF, Loo RV. Hepatic hydrothorax. Studies to determine the source of the fluid and report of thirteen cases. Ann Intern Med 1964; 61: 385–400.

Lieberman FL, Hidemura R, Peters RL, et al. Pathogenesis and treatment of hydrothorax complicating cirrhosis with ascites. Ann Intern Med 1966; 64:341–351.

HIGH-FREQUENCY JET VENTILATION

Branson RD, Hurst JM, Dehaven CB. Use of high frequency jet ventilation during mechanical ventilation for control of elevated intracranial pressure. Respir Care 1984; 29:l221–1225.

Froese AB, Bryan AC. High frequency ventilation. Am Rev Respir Dis 1987; 135:1363–1374.

Gillespie DJ. High frequency ventilation: a new concept in mechanical ventilation. Mayo Clin Proc 1983; 58:187–196.

Hurst JM, Dehaven CB. Adult respiratory distress syndrome: improved oxygenation during high frequency jet ventilation/continuous positive airway pressure. Surgery 1984; 96:764–769.

Rougby JJ, Fusciardi J, Bourgain JL, Viars P. High frequency jet ventilation in postoperative respiratory failure: determinants of oxygenation. Anesthesiology 1983; 59:281–287.

HODGKIN'S DISEASE

Ball DG, et al. Primary pulmonary Hodgkin's disease: a case report. Arch Intern Med 1982; 142: 1941–1943.

Kern WH, et al. Primary Hodgkin's Disease of the Lung. Cancer 1961;14:1151–1165.

MacDonald IB, et al. Lung involvement in Hodgkin's disease. Thorax 1977; 32:664–667.

Pik A, et al. Primary pulmonary Hodgkin's disease with air bronchogram. Respiration 1986; 50:226–229.

Pinson P, et al. Primary pulmonary Hodgkin's disease. Respiration 1992; 59:314–316.

Radin AI, et al. Primary pulmonary Hodgkin's disease. Cancer 1990; 65:550–563.

van der Schee AC, et al. Primary pulmonary manifestation of Hodgkin's disease. Respiration 1990; 57:127–128.

Yousem SA, et al. Primary pulmonary Hodgkin's disease. Cancer 1986; 57:1217–1224.

HYDROCARBON POISONINGS

Brander PE, et al. Fire-eater's lung. Eur Respir J 1992; 5:112–114.

Kizer KW. Toxic inhalations. Emerg Med Clin North Am 1984; 2(3):649–666.

Klein BL, et al. Hydrocarbon poisonings. Ped Clin North Am 1986; 33(2):411–419.

Perrot IJ, et al. Fatal hydrocarbon lipoid pneumonia and pneumonitis secondary to automatic transmission fluid ingestion. J Forensic Sci 1992; 37(5):1422–1427.

Scott PP. Hydrocarbon ingestion: an unusual cause of multiple pulmonary pseudotumors. South Med J 1989; 82(8): 1032–1033.

HYPEREOSINOPHILIA

Fauci AS, et al. The idiopathic hypereosinophilic syndrome: clinical, pathophysiologic, and therapeutic considerations. Ann Intern Med 1982; 97:78–92.

Flaum MA, et al. A clinicopathologic correlation of the idiopathic hypereosinophilic syndrome. I. Hematologic manifestations. II. Clinical manifestations. Blood 1981; 58(5):1012–1026.

Jameson MD, Segraves SS. Idiopathic hypereosinophilic syndrome. Postgrad Med 1988; 84(8): 93–101.

HYPERLEUKOCYTOSIS

Engler R. Granulocytes and oxidative injury in myocardial ischemia and reperfusion. Fed Proc 1987; 46:2395.

Lichtman R. Hyperleukocytic leukemia: rheologic, clinical, and therapeutic considerations. Blood 1982; 650:279–283.

Shelhamer J, et al. Respiratory disease in the immunosuppressed patient. Ann Intern Med 1992; 117:415.

Tenholder H. Pulmonary infiltrates in leukemia. Chest 1980; 78:468.

HYPOPHOSPHATEMIA

Bourke E, Yanagawa N. Assessment of hyperphosphatemia and hypophosphatemia. Clin Lab Med 1993; 13(1):183–207.

Camp MA, Allon M. Severe hypophosphatemia and hospitalized patients. Mineral Electrolyte Metab 1990; 16:365–368.

Knochel JP. Hypophosphatemia and rhabdomyolysis. Am J Med 1992; 92:455–457.

Knochel JP. The pathophysiology and clinical characterstics of severe hypophosphatemia. Arch Intern Med 1977; 137:203–220.

Newman J, Neff T, Ziporin P. Acute respiratory failure associated with hypophosphatemia. N Engl J Med 1977; 296:1101–1103.

Peppers MP, et al. Hypophosphatemia and hyperphosphatemia. Crit Care Clin 1991; 7(1):201–214.

HYPERSENSITIVITY PNEUMONITIS

Bourke SJ, et al. Longitudinal course of extrinsic allergic alveolitis in pigeon breeders. Thorax 1989; 44:415–418.

Braun SR, et al. Farmer's lung disease: long-term clinical and physiologic outcome. Am Rev Respir Disease 1979; 119:185–191.

Greenberger PA, et al. End-stage lung and ultimately fatal disease in a bird fancier. Am J Med 1989; 86:119–122.

Murayama J, et al. Lung fibrosis in hypersensitivity pneumonitis. Chest 1993; 104(1):38–43.

Perez-Padilla R, et al. Mortality in Mexican patients with chronic pigeon breeder's lung compared with those with usual interstitial pneumonia. Am Rev Respir Dis 1993; 148:49–53.

Schmidt CD, et al. Longitudinal pulmonary function changes in pigeon breeders. Chest 1988; 93(2):359–363.

HYPOGAMMAGLOBULINEMIA

Barker AF, Bardana EJ. Bronchiectasis: update of an orphan disease. Am Rev Respir Dis 1988; 137; 969–978.

Barker AF, Craig S, Bardana EJ. Humoral immunity in bronchiectasis. Ann Allergy 1987; 59:179–182.

Cunningham-Rundles C, Siegal FP, Smithwick EM, et al. Efficacy of intravenous immunoglobulin in primary humoral immunodeficiency disease. Ann Intern Med 1984; 101:435–439.

Pirovsky B. Intravenous immune globulin therapy in hypogammaglobulinemia. A review. Am J Med 1984; 76(suppl 3A):53–60.

Roifman CM, Lederman HM, Lavi S, et al. Benefit of intravenous IgG replacement in hypogammaglobulinemic patients with chronic sinopulmonary disease. Am J Med 1985; 79:171–174.

IDIOPATHIC PULMONARY FIBROSIS

Crystal RG et al. Interstitial lung diseases of unknown cause: disorders characterized by chronic inflammation of the lower respiratory tract. N Engl J Med 1984; 310:154–156.

King TE Jr. Idiopathic pulmonary fibrosis. *In* Schwarz MI, King TE Jr (eds). Interstitial Lung Disease. 2nd Ed. St Louis, Mosby Year Book, 1993.

King TE Jr, Cherniack RM, Schwarz MI. Idiopathic pulmonary fibrosis and other interstitial lung diseases of unknown etiology. *In* Murray JF, Nadel JA (eds). Textbook of Respiratory Medicine. 2nd Ed. Philadelphia, WB Saunders Co, 1994, p 1827.

McLeod TC, et al. Diffuse infiltrative lung disease: a new scheme for description. Radiology 1983; 149:353–363.

Mueller N, et al. Disease activity in idiopathic pulmonary fibrosis: CT and pathologic correlation. Radiology 1987; 165:731–734.

Scadding JG, Hinson KFW. Diffuse fibrosing alveolotis (diffuse interstitial fibrosis of the lungs). Thorax 1967; 22:291–304.

Schwarz MI, King TE Jr, Cherniack RM. General principles and diagnostic approach to the interstitial lung diseases. *In* (Murray JF, Nadel JA (eds). Textbook of Respiratory Medicine. 2nd Ed. Philadelphia, WB Saunders Co, 1994, p 1803.

Turner-Warwick M. et al. Cryptogenic fibrosing alveolitis: clinical features and their influence on survival. Thorax 1980; 35:171–180.

IMMUNOCOMPROMISED HOST

Martin WJ. Role of BAL in the assessment of opportunistic pulmonary infection. Mayo Clin Proc 1987; 62:549–557.

Springmeyer SC. Use of bronchoalveolar lavage to diagnose acute diffuse pneumonia in the immunocompromised host. J Infect Dis 1986; 154:604–610.

Wilson WR. Pulmonary disease in the immunocompromised host. Mayo Clin Proc 1985; 60:473–487, 610–631.

Young JA, Pulmonary infiltrates in the immunocompromised patients diagnosis by BAL. J Clin Pathol 1984; 37:390–397.

IMMUNOLOGY

Brain JD, Proctor DF, Reid LM. Respiratory defense mechanisms. Parts I and II. *In* Lenfant C (ed). Lung Biology in Health and Disease. Vol. 5. New York, Marcel Dekker, 1977.

Brain JD, Godleski JJ, Sorokin SP. Quantification, origin, and fate of pulmonary macrophages. *In* Defense Mechanisms. New York, Marcel Dekker, 1977, pp 849–892.

Huber GL, Johanson WG, Jr, LaForce FM. Experimental models and pulmonary antimicrobial defenses. *In* Brain JD, Proctor DF, Reid LM (eds). Respiratory Defense Mechanisms. New York, Marcel Dekker, 1977.

Kaltreider HB. Immune defenses of the lung. *In* Sande MA, Root RK, Hudson LD (eds). Respiratory Infections. Contemporary Issues in Infectious Diseases. Vol. 5. New York, Churchill Livingstone, 1986.

Kaltreider HB. Phagocytic, antibody and cell-mediated immune mechanisms. *In* Murray JF, Nadel JA (eds). Textbook of Respiratory Medicine. Philadelphia, WB Saunders, 1988.

Kaltreider HB. Local immunity. *In* Bienenstock J (ed). Immunology of the Lung and Upper Respiratory Tract. New York, McGraw-Hill, 1984.

McDermott MR, Befus AD, Bienenstock J. The structural basis for immunity in the respiratory tract. Int Rev Exp Pathol 1982; 23:47–112.

Reynolds HY, Merrill WW. Lung immunology: the inflammatory response in lung parenchyma. *In* Simmons DH (ed). Current Pulmonology. Vol. 2. Boston, Houghton Mifflin, 1980.

KAPOSI'S SARCOMA

Garay SM, et al. Pulmonary manifestations of Kaposi's sarcoma. Chest 1987; 91:39–43.

O'Brien RF. Pulmonary and pleural Kaposi's sarcoma in AIDS. Semin Respir Med 1989; 10(1):12–20.

LACTIC ACIDOSIS

Astiz ME, et al. Relationship of oxygen delivery and mixed venous oxygenation to lactic acidosis in patients with sepsis and acute myocardial infarction. Crit Care Med 1989; 16:655–658.

Bakker J, et al. Blood lactate levels are superior to oxygen derived variables in predicting outcome in human septic shock. Chest 1991; 99:956–963.

Edwards JD, et al. Use of survivor's cardiorespiratory values as therapeutic goals in septic shock. Crit Care Med 1989; 17:1093–1099.

Fenwick JC, et al. Increased concentrations of plasma lactate predict pathologic dependence of oxygen consumption on oxygen delivery in patients with ARDS. J Crit Care 1990; 5:81–87.

Hotchkiss RS, Karl IE. Reevaluation of the role of cellular hypoxia and bioenergetic failure in sepsis. JAMA 1992: 267:1503–1510.

Rashkin MC, et al. Oxygen delivery in critically ill patients: relationship to blood lactate and survival. Chest 1985; 87:580–584.

LEGIONNAIRES' DISEASE

Chastre J. Pulmonary fibrosis following pneumonia due to acute legionnaires' disease: clinical, ultrastructural, and immunofluorescent study. Chest 1987; 91:57–62.

Edelstein PH, Meyer RD. Legionnaires' disease. A review. Chest 1984; 85:114–120.

Fain JS, Bryan RN, Cheng L, et al. Rapid diagnosis of *Legionella* infection by a nonisotopic in situ hybridization method. Am J Clin Pathol 1991; 95:719–724.

Kohler RB, Zimmerman SE, Wilson E, et al. Rapid radioimmunoassay diagnosis of legionnaires' disease by detection of urinary antigen and partial characterization of the antigen. Ann Intern Med 1981; 94:601–605.

Moiraghi A, et al. Nosocomial legionellosis associated with use of oxygen bubble humidifiers and underwater chest drains. J Hosp Infect 1987; 10:47–50.

Winn WC, Jr. *Legionella* and legionnaires' disease: a review with emphasis on environmental studies and laboratory diagnosis. CRC Crit Rev and Lab Sci 1985; 21:323–338.

Yu VL, Nguyen MLT. Legionnaires' disease: new insights. Contemp Intern Med 1992; 6:49–59.

Zuravleff JJ, Yu VL, Shonnard JW, et al. Diagnosis of legionnaires' disease. An update of laboratory methods with new emphasis on isolation by culture. JAMA 1983; 250:1981–1985.

LYMPHANGIOLEIOMYOMATOSIS

Appelbaum FA. Introduction and overview of interferon alfa in myeloproliferative and hemangiomatous diseases. Semin Hematol 1990; 27(3):1–5.

Brentani MM, et al. Steroid receptors in pulmonary LAM. Chest 1984; 85(1):96–99.

Burger CD, et al. Pulmonary mechanics in lymphangioleiomyomatosis. Am Rev Respir Dis 1991; 143(5):1030–1033.

Carrington CB, et al. Lymphangioleiomyomatosis. Physiologic-pathologic-radiologic correlations. Am Rev Respir Dis 1977; 116(6):977–995.

Eliasson AH, et al. Treatment of LAM: a meta-analysis. Chest 1989; 96(6):1352–1355.

Taylor JR. Lymphangioleiomyomatosis. N Engl J Med 1990; 323(18):1254–1260.

LYMPHANGITIC CARCINOMATOSIS

Aranda C, et al. Transbronchial lung biopsy in the diagnosis of lymphangitic carcinomatosis. Cancer 1978; 42:1995–1998.

Janower ML, Blennerhassett JB. Lymphangitic spread of metastatic cancer to the lung. Radiology 1971; 101:267–273.

Levy H, et al. The value of bronchial washings and bronchoalveolar lavage in the diagnosis of lymphangitic carcinomatosis. Chest 1988; 94: 1028–1030.

Masson RG, et al. Pulmonary microvascular cytology in the diagnosis of lymphangitic carcinomatosis. N Engl J Med 1989; 321:71.

Munk PL, et al. Pulmonary lymphangitic carcinomatosis: CT and pathologic findings. Radiology 1988; 166:705–709.

LYMPHOCYTIC INTERSTITIAL PNEUMONITIS

Banerjee D, Ahmad D. Malignant lymphoma complicating lymphocytic interstitial pneumonia: a monoclonal B-cell neoplasm arising in a polyclonal lymphoproliferative disorder. Hum Pathol 1982; 13:780–782.

Carrington CB, Liebow AA. Lymphocytic interstitial pneumonia. Am J Pathol 19 6; 48:36a.

Farber HW, Mathers JAL, Glauser FL. Gallium scans and serum angiotensin converting enzyme levels in talc granulomatosis and lymphocytic interstitial pneumonitis. South Med J 1980; 73:1663–1667.

Glickstein M, et al. Nonlymphomatous lymphoid disorders of the lung. Am J Radiol 1986; 147:227–237.

Grieco MH, Chinoy-Acharya P. Lymphocytic interstitial pneumonia associated with the acquired immune deficiency syndrome. Am Rev Respir Dis 1985; 131:952–955.

Ishizaki T, et al. Lymphoid interstitial pneumonia: findings at bronchoalveolar lavage. Eur J Respir Dis 1985; 67:128–132.

Morris JC, et al. Lymphocytic interstitial pneumonia in patients at risk for the acquired immune deficiency syndrome. Chest 1987; 91:63–67.

Solal-Celigny P, et al. Lymphoid interstitial pneumonitis in acquired immunodeficiency syndrome-related complex. Am Rev Respir Dis 1985; 131:956–960.

Strimlan CV, Rosenow EC, Weiland LH. Lymphocytic interstitial pneumonitis: review of 13 cases. Ann Intern Med 1978; 88:616–621.

LYMPHOMA

Kennedy JL, et al. Pulmonary lymphomas and other pulmonary lymphoid lesions. Cancer 1985; 56:539–552.

L'Hoste RJ, et al. Primary pulmonary lymphomas: a clinicopathologic analysis of 36 cases. Cancer 1984; 54:1397–1406.

LYMPHOMATOID GRANULOMATOSIS

DeRemee RA, Weiland LH, McDonald TJ. Polymorphic reticulosis, lymphomatoid granulomatosis. Two diseases or one? Mayo Clin Proc 1978; 53:634–640.

Fauci AS, Haynes BF Costa J, et al. Lymphomatoid granulomatosis, prospective clinical and therapeutic experience over ten years. N Engl J Med 1982; 306:68–74.

Katzenstein A, Carrington CB, Liebow AA. Lymphomatoid granulomatosis: a clinicopathologic study of 152 cases. Cancer 1979; 43:360–373.

Liebow AA, Carrington CB, Friedman RJ. Lymphomatoid granulomatosis. Hum Pathol 1972; 3:457–558.

Saldana MJ, Patchefsky AS, Israel H, et al. Pulmonary angiitis and granulomatosis. The relationship between histological features, organ involvement and response to treatment. Hum Pathol 1977; 8:391–409.

MEDIASTINAL MASS

Davis RD, Oldham HN, et al. Primary cysts and neoplasms of the mediastinum: recent changes in clinical presentation, methods of diagnosis, management, and results. Ann Thorac Surg 1987; 44:229–237.

Oldham HN Jr, et al. Primary tumors and cysts of the mediastinum. Monogr Surg Sci 1967; 4:243.

MENINGITIS

Bohr VA. Neurological sequela and fatality as prognostic measures in 875 cases of bacterial meningitis. Dan Med Bull 1988; 35:92.

Callahan M. Fulminant bacterial meningitis without meningeal signs. Ann Emerg Med 1989; 18(1):90.

Niemoller UM, et al. Brain edema and increased intracranial pressure in the pathophysiology of bacterial meningitis. Eur J Clin Microbiol Infect Dis 1989; 8(2):109.

Roos KL, et al. The management of fulminant meningitis in the intensive care unit. Crit Care Clin 1988; 4(2):375.

Tunkel AR, et al. Bacterial meningitis: recent advances in pathophysiology and treatment. Ann Intern Med 1990; 112:610.

MESOTHELIOMA

Antman K. Natural history and staging of malignant mesothelioma. Chest 1989; 96:93S.

Antman K, Corson J. Benign and malignant pleural mesothelioma. Clin Chest Med 1985; 6(1):127.

Ball D, et al. The treatment of malignant mesothelioma of the pleura: review of a 5-year experience, with special reference to radiotherapy. Am J Clin Oncol 1990; 13(1):4.

Hillerdal G. Asbestos related pleural disease. Semin Respir Med 1987; 9:65.

Pisani RJ, et al. Malignant mesothelioma of the pleura. Mayo Clin Proc 1988; 63:1234.

Peterson JT, et al. Non-asbestos related malignant mesothelioma. Cancer 1984; 54:951.

Shepherd KE, et al. Diffuse malignant pleural mesothelioma in an urban hospital: clinical spectrum and trend in incidence over time. Am J Indust Med 1989; 16:373.

METHEMOGLOBINEMIA

Caudill L, et al. Methemoglobinemia as a cause of coma. Ann Emerg Med 1990; 19:677–779.

Curry S. Methemoglobinemia. Ann Emerg Med 1982; 11:214–221.

Kotler R, et al. Severe methemoglobinemia after flexible fiberoptic bronchoscopy. Thorax 1988; 44:234–235.

Mansouri A, Lurie A. Concise review: methemoglobinemia. Am J Hematol 1993; 42:7–12.

MOUNIER-KUHN SYNDROME

Johnston RF, Green RA. Tracheobronchomegaly: report of 5 cases and demonstration of familial occurrence. Am Rev Respir Dis 1965; 91:35–50.

Sane AC, et al. Tracheobronchomegaly. Chest 1992; 102:618–619.

Shin MS, et al. Tracheobronchomegaly: CT diagnosis. AJR 1988; 150:777–779.

Woodring JH, et al. Congenital tracheobronchomegaly: a report of 10 cases and review of the literature. J Thorac Imaging 1991; 2:1–10.

MYXEDEMA

Bagdade JD. Endocrine emergencies. Med Clin North Am 1986; 70:1111.

Blum M. Myxedema coma. Am J Med 1972; 264:432.

Nicoloff JT. Thyroid storm and myxedema coma. Med Clin North Am 1985; 69(5):1005–1017.

Zwillich CW, et al. Ventilatory control in myxedema and hypothyroidism. N Engl J Med 1975; 292:662–665.

NEUROGENIC TUMORS

Harjula A, Mattila S, Luosto R, Kostiainen S, Mattila I. Mediastinal neurogenic tumors: early and late results of treatment. Scand J Thorac Cardiovasc Surg 1986; 20:115–118.

Ikezoe J, Sone S, et al. CT of intrathoracic neurogenic tumors. Eur J Radiol 1986; 6:266–269.

NEUROMUSCULAR BLOCKADE

Douglass JA, et al. Myopathy in severe asthma. Am Rev Respir Dis 1992; 146:517–519.

Griffin D, et al. Acute myopathy during treatment of asthma with corticosteroids and steroidal muscle relaxants. Chest 1992; 102:510–514.

Hansen Flascher JH, et al. Neuromuscular blockade in the ICU. Am Rev Respir Dis 1993; 147:234–236.

Kupfer Y, et al. Prolonged weakness after long term infusion of vecuronium bromide. Ann Intern Med 1992; 117:484–486.

Segredo V, et al. Persistent paralysis in critically ill patients after long term administration of vecuronium. N Engl J Med 1992; 327:524–528.

Witt NJ, et al. Peripheral nerve function in sepsis and multiple organ failure. Chest 1991; 99:176–184.

Zochodne DW, et al. Critical illness polyneuropathy. Brain 1987; 110:819–842.

NITRIC OXIDE

Kinsella JP, et al. Low-dose inhalation nitric oxide in persistent pulmonary hypertension of the newborn. Lancet 1992; 340:819–820.

Pearl RG. Inhaled nitric oxide. The past, the present, and the future. Anesthesiology 1993; 78:413–416.

Pepke-Zaba J, et al. Inhaled nitric oxide as a cause of selective pulmonary vasodilatation in pulmonary hypertension. Lancet 1991; 338:1173–1174.

Rossaint R, et al. Inhaled nitric oxide for the adult respiratory distress syndrome. N Engl J Med 1993; 328:399–405.

Snyder S, Bredt DS. Biological roles of nitric oxide. Sci Am 1992; 5:68–77.

NITROFURANTOIN

Chudnofsky CR, Otten EJ. Acute pulmonary toxicity to nitrofurantoin. J Emerg Med 1989; 7:15–19.

Hailey FJ, et al. Pleuropneumonic reactions to nitrofurantoin. N Engl J Med 1969; 281(20):1087–1090.

Holmberg L, et al. Adverse reactions to nitrofurantoin. Analysis of 921 reports. Am J Med 1980; 69:733–738.

Witten CM. Pulmonary toxicity of nitrofurantoin. Arch Phys Med Rehabil 1989; 70:55.

NOCARDIOSIS

Balikian JP, et al. Pulmonary nocardiosis. Radiology 1978; 126:569–573.

Presant CA, et al. Factors affecting survival in nocardiosis. Am Rev Respir Dis 1973; 108:1444–1448.

PANCOAST'S TUMOR

Ahmad K, Fayos J, Kirsh M. Apical lung carcinoma. Cancer 1984; 54:913–917.

Byers T, Vena J, Rzepka T. Predilection of lung cancer for the upper lobes: an epidemiologic inquiry. JNCI 1984; 72:6:1271–1275.

Murray J, Nadel J. Textbook of respiratory medicine. Philadelphia, WB Saunders, 1994, pp 1528–1596.

Stanford R, et al. Influence of staging in superior sulcus (pancoast) tumors of the lung. Ann Thorac Surg 1980; 29:5:406–409.

Van Houtte P, et al. External radiation in the management of superior sulcus tumor. Cancer 1984; 54:223–227.

PHYSIOLOGY

American Thoracic Society. Standardization of spirometry–1987 update. Am Rev Respir Dis 1987; 136:1285.

Boren H, Kory RC, Syner JC. The Veterans Administration Army cooperative study of pulmonary function. II. The lung volume and its subdivisions in normal men. Am J Med 1966; 41:96.

Briscoe WA, Dubois AB. The relationship between airway resistance, airway conductance and lung volume in subjects of different age and body size. J Clin Invest 1958; 37:1279.

Cherniack RM. Pulmonary Function Testing. 2nd Ed. Philadelphia, WB Saunders, 1992.

Cherniack RM, Cherniack L. Respiration in Health and Disease. 3rd Ed. Philadelphia, WB Saunders, 1983.

Cherniack RM, Raber MB. Normal standards for ventilatory function using an automated wedge spirometer. Am Rev Respir Dis 1972; 106:38.

Goldman HI, Becklake MR. Respiratory function tests. Normal values at medium altitudes and the prediction of normal results. Am Rev Tuberc 1959; 79:457.

Kory RC, Callahan R, Boren HG, Syner JC. The Veterans Administration-Army cooperative study of pulmonary function. I. Clinical spirometry in normal men. Am J Med 1961; 30:243.

Macklem PT. Tests of lung mechanics. N Engl J Med 1975; 293:339.

Manfreda J, Nelson N, Cherniack RM. Prevalence of respiratory abnormalities in a rural and an urban community. Am Rev Respir Dis 1978; 117:215.

Raine JM, Bishop JM. A-a difference in O_2 tension and physiologic dead space in normal man. J Appl Physiol 1963; 18:284.

PLEURAL EFFUSION

Good JT Jr, Antony VB, Reller LB, et al. The pathogenesis of the low pleural fluid pH in esophageal rupture. Am Rev Respir Dis 1983; 127:702–704.

Good JT Jr, Taryle DA, Maulitz RM, et al. The diagnostic value of pleural fluid pH. Chest 1980; 78:55–59.

Good IT Jr, King TE, Antony VB, Sahn SA: Lupus pleuritis: Clinical features and pleural fluid characteristics with special reference to pleural fluid antinuclear antibody titers. Chest 1983; 84: 714–718.

Light RW, Ball WC. Lactate dehydrogenase isoenzymes in pleural effusions. Am Rev Respir Dis 1973; 108:660–664.

Light RW, Ball WC Jr. Glucose and amylase in pleural effusions. JAMA 1973; 225:257–259.

Light RW, MacGregor Ml, Luchsinger PV, Ball WC. Pleural effusions: the diagnostic separation of transudates and exudates. Ann Intern Med 1972; 77:507–513.

Sahn SA. Pathogenesis and clinical features of diseases associated with a low pleural fluid glucose. *In* Chretien J, Bignon J, Hirsch A (eds). The Pleura in Health and Disease. New York, Marcel Dekker, 1985, pp 267–285.

Sahn SA. Pleural fluid pH in the normal state and in diseases affecting thc pleural space. *In* Chretien J, Bignon J, Hirsch A (eds). The Pleura in Health and Disease. New York, Marcel Dekker, 1985, pp 253–266.

Stark DD, Shanes JG, Baron RL, Loch DD. Biochemical features of urinothorax. Arch Intern Med 1982; 142:1509–1511.

PLEURAL EFFUSION WITH ASCITES

Datta N, et al. Radionucleotide demonstration of peritoneal-pleural communication as a cause for pleural fluid. JAMA 1984; 252:210.

Frazer IH, et al. Pleuroperitoneal effusion without ascites. Med J Aust 1983; 2:520.

Hartz RS, et al. Pleural ascites without abdominal fluid: surgical considerations. J Thorac Cardiovasc Surg 1984; 87:141.

PLEURAL EFFUSION WITH HEPATIC DISEASE

Frothingham JR. Cirrhosis of the liver complicated by persistent right hydrothorax and ascites. N Engl J Med 1942; 226:679–682.

Johnston RF, Loo RV. Hepatic hydrothorax. Studies to determine the source of the fluid and report of thirteen cases. Ann Intern Med 1964; 61:385–400.

Lieberman FL, Hidemura R, Peters RL, et al. Pathogenesis and treatment of hydrothorax complicating cirrhosis with ascites. Ann Intern Med 1966; 64:341–351.

Llaneza PP, et al. Unilateral pleural effusion without clinical ascites in Laennec's cirrhosis. Dig Dis Sci 1985; 30:88.

Morrow CS, Kantor M, Arrnen NA. Hepatic hydrothorax. Ann Intern Med 1958; 49:193–203.

PLEURAL EFFUSION WITH KAPOSI'S SARCOMA

Fouret PJ, et al. Pulmonary Kaposi's sarcoma in patients with AIDS: a clinicopathological study. Thorax 1987; 42:262–268.

Meduri GU, et al. Pulmonary Kaposi's sarcoma in the acquired immunodeficiency syndrome. Am J Med 1986; 81:18.

O'Brien RF, Cohn DL. Serosanguinous pleural effusions in AIDS-associated Kaposi's sarcoma. Chest 1989; 96:460–466.

Sivit CH, et al. Kaposi's sarcoma of the lung in AIDS: radiographic-pathologic analysis. AJR 1987; 148:25–28.

PLEURAL EFFUSION WITH MALIGNANCY

Hartman D, et al. Comparison of insufflated talc under thoracoscopic guidance with standard tetracycline and bleomycin pleurodesis for control of malignant pleural effusions. J Thorac Carciovasc Surg 1993; 105:743–747.

Hausheer F, et al. Diagnosis and treatment of malignant pleural effusions. Semin Oncol 1985; 12:54–75.

PLEURAL EFFUSION WITH PANCREATIC DISEASE

Dewan NA, et al. Chronic massive pancreatic pleural effusion. Chest 1984; 85:497–501.

Gertsch P, et al. Chronic pancreatic pleural effusions and ascites. Int Surg 1984; 69:145–147.

Roseman DM, et al. Pulmonary manifestations of pancreatitis. N Engl J Med 1968; 263:294–296.

PLEURAL EFFUSION WITH TUBERCULOSIS

Banales JL, et al. Adenosine deaminase in the diagnosis of tuberculous pleural effusions. Chest 1991; 99:355–357.

Barbas CSV, et al. The relationship between pleural fluid findings and the development of pleural thickening in patients with pleural tuberculosis. Chest 1991; 100:1264–1267.

Epstein DM, et al. Tuberculous pleural effusions. Chest 1987; 91:106–109.

Soubrette AF, et al. Tuberculous pleural effusion: twenty year experience. Chest 1991; 99:883–886.

Yam LT. Diagnostic significance of lymphocytes in pleural effusions. Ann Intern Med 1967; 66:972.

PNEUMOCOCCAL INFECTION

Brewin A. High-dose penicillin therapy and pneumococcal pneumonia. JAMA 1974; 230:409.

Fruchtman SM, et al. Adult respiratory distress syndrome as a cause of death in pneumococcal pneumonia. Chest 1983; 83:598.

Mannes GPM, et al. Adult respiratory distress syndrome due to bacteremic pneumococcal pneumonia. Eur J Respir Dis 1991; 4:503.

Mufson MA. Pneumococcal infections. JAMA 1981; 246:1942.

Mandell GL, et al (eds). *Streptococcus pneumoniae. In* Principles and Practice of Infectious Diseases. 3rd ed. New York, Churchill Livingstone, 1990,

PNEUMOCYSTIS

Barrio JL, et al. *Pneumocystis carinii* pneumonia presenting as cavitating and noncavitating solitary pulmonary nodules in patients with AIDS. Am Rev Respir Dis 1986; 134:1094–1096.

Chaffey MH, Klein JS, Gamsu G, et al. Radiographic distribution of *Pneumocystis carinii* pneumonia in patients with AIDS treated with prophylactic inhaled pentamidine. Radiology 1990; 175: 715–719.

Feuerstein IM, Archer A, Pluda JM, et al. Thin-walled cavities, cysts and pneumothorax in *Pneumocystis carinii* pneumonia: further observations with histopatholic correlation. Radiology 1990; 174: 697–702.

Hartz JW, et al. Granulomatous *Pneumocystosis* presenting as a solitary pulmonary nodule. Arch Pathol Lab Med 1985; 109:466–469.

PNEUMOTHORAX

Hnatiuk OW, Dillard TA, Oster CN. Bleomycin sclerotherapy for bilateral pneumothoraces in a patient with AIDS. Ann Intern Med 1990; 113:998–990.

Macoviac MA, Stephenson LW, Ochs R, Edmunds HE. Tetracycline pleurodesis during active pulmonary-pleural air leak for prevention of recurrent pneumothorax. Chest 1982; 81:78–81.

POLYMYOSITIS

Colby TV, et al. ILD in polymyositis and dermatomyositis. Am Rev Respir Dis 1990; 141:727–733.

PRIMARY PULMONARY HYPERTENSION

Anderson E, Simon G, Reid L. Primary and thromboembolic hypertension: a quantitative pathological study. J Pathol 1973; 110:4:273–293.

D'Alanzo C, Bower J, Dantzker D. Differentiation of patients with primary and thromboembolic pulmonary hypertension. Chest 1984; 85:4:457–461.

Dantzker D, Bower J. Mechanisms of gas exchange abnormality in patients with chronic obliterative pulmonary vascular disease. J Clin Invest 1979; 64:1050–1055.

Edwards WD, Edwards JE. Clinical primary pulmonary hypertension: three pathologic types. Circulation 1977; 56:884.

Goldsmith C, et al. Primary pulmonary hypertension in classical hemophilia. Ann Intern Med 1988; 108:797.

Rich S, et al. Primary pulmonary hypertension: Ntional Pospective Study. Ann Intern Med 1987; 107:216–223.

Wagenvoort CS. Lung biopsy specimens in the evaluation of pulmonary vascular disease. Chest 1980; 77:5:614–625.

Wilson A, Harris C, Lavender J, Oakley C. Perfusion lung scanning in obliterative pulmonary hypertension. Br Heart J 1973; 35:917–930.

Legioux B, et al. Primary pulmonary hypertension and HIV. Am J Med 1990; 89:122.

PULMONARY HEMORRHAGE

Bradley JD. The pulmonary hemorrhage syndromes. Clin Chest Med 1982; 3:593–605.

RESPIRATORY BRONCHIOLITIS

Myers JL. Respiratory bronchiolitis with interstitial lung disease. Semin Respir Med 1992; 3: 134–139.

Myers, JL. et al. Respiratory bronchiolitis causing interstitial lung disease. Am Rev Respir Dis 1987; 135: 880–884.

Wright J. Small airways disease: its role in chronic airflow obstruction. Semin Respir Med 1992; 3:72–84.

RETROPHARYNGEAL ABSCESS

Barratt GE, et al. Retropharyngeal abscess—a ten-year experience. Laryngoscope 1984; 94:455–463.

Haug RH, et al. Diagnosis and treatment of the retropharyngeal abscess in adults. Br J Oral Maxill Surg 1990; 28:34–38.

"SABER-SHEATH" TRACHEA

Callan E, Karandy EJ, Hilsinger RL. "Saber-sheath" trachea. Ann Otol Rhinol Laryngol 1988; 97:512–515.

Greene R, Lechner GL. "Saber-sheath" trachea: a clinical and functional study of marked coronal narrowing of the intrathoracic trachea. Radiology 1975; 115:265–268.

Greene R. "Saber-sheath" trachea: relation to chronic obstructive pulmonary disease. Am J Radiol 1978; 130:441–445.

SALICYLATE INTOXICATION

Anderson RJ, et al. Unrecognized adult salicylate intoxication. Ann Intern Med 1976; 85:745–748.

Heffner J, et al. Salicylate-induced noncardiogenic pulmonary edema. West J Med 1979; 130:263–266.

Hill JB. Salicylate intoxication. N Engl J Med 1973; 288:110–113.

Sallis RE. Management of salicylate toxicity. Am Fam Physician 1989; 39:265–270.

Temple AR. Acute and chronic effects of aspirin toxicity and their treatment. Arch Intern Med 1981; 141:364–369.

Walters JS, et al. Salicylate-induced pulmonary edema. Radiology 1983; 146:289–293.

SARCOID

Carrington CB, Gainsler EA, Mikus JP, et al: Structure and function in sarcoidosis. Ann N Y Acad Sci 1976; 278:265–282.

Churg A, Carrington CB, Gupta R: Necrotizing sarcoid granulomatosis. Chest 1979; 76:406–413.

Cooper SD, et al. Neurosarcoidosis: evaluation using computed tomography and magnetic resonance imaging. J Comput Assist Tomogr 1991; 12:90–99.

Daniele RP, et al. Pathogenesis of sarcoidosis. Chest 1986; 89(S):174S.

Daniele RP, et al. Immunologic abnormalities in sarcoidosis. Ann Intern Med 1980; 92:406.

Delaney P. Neurologic manifestations in sarcoidosis, review of the literature, with a report of 23 cases. Ann Intern Med 1977; 87:336–345.

Hudspith B, et al. Lack of immune deficiency in sarcoidosis: compartmentalization of the immune response. Thorax 1987; 42:250.

Hunninghake GW, et al. Pathogenesis of granulomatous lung disease. Am Rev Respir Dis 1984: 130:476.

Israel HL, Sones M. Sarcoidosis, tuberculosis, and tuberculin anergy. Am Rev Respir Dis 1966; 94:887–895.

Koss MN, Hochholzer L, Feigin DS, et al: Necrotizing sarcoid-like granulomatosis: clinical, pathologic, and immunopathologic findings. Hum Pathol 1980; 11(suppl):510–519.

Mayock RL, Bertrand P, Morrison CE, Scott JA. Manifestations of sarcoidosis. Analysis of 145 patients with a review of nine series selected from the literature. Am J Med 1963; 35:67–89.

Oksanen V. Neurosarcoidosis: clinical presentation and course in 50 patients. 1986; 73:283–290.

Rosen Y, Moon S, Huang CT, et al. Granulomatous pulmonary angiitis in sarcoidosis. Arch Pathol Lab Med 1977; 101:170–174.

Sharma OP, Sharma AM. Sarcoidosis of the nervous system. A clinical approach. Arch Intern Med 1991; 151:1317–1321.

Schwartz M, King TE Jr. Interstitial Lung Disease. St. Louis, Mosby Year Book, 1992, pp 165–172.

Thomas PD, Hunninghake GW. Current concepts of the pathogenesis of sarcoidosis. Am Rev Respir Dis 1987; 135:747.

SMALL CELL CARCINOMA

Frank, Chauvin, Trillet, et al: Pretreament staging evaluation in small cell lung carcinoma. Chest 1992; 102:497.

Irving, Kron, Harman, et al: A reappraisal of limited-stage undifferentiated carcinoma of the lung. J Thorac Cardiovasc Surg 1982; 84:734–737.

Robinson, Baker, Ettinger, et al: The role of surgery in the management of selected patients with small cell carcinoma of the lung. J Clin Oncol 1987; 5:697–802.

SWYER-JAMES SYNDROME

Gold RE, et al. Adenoviral pneumonia and its complications in infancy and childhood. J Can Assoc Radiol 1969; 20:218.

Howk VN, et al. Unilateral hyperlucent lung. A study in pathophysiology and etiology. Am J Med Sci 1967; 253:406–416.

MacLeod WM. Abnormal transradiancy of one lung. Thorax 1954; 9:147–153.

MacPherson RI, et al. Unilateral hyperlucent lung: a complication of viral pneumonia. J Can Assoc Radiol 1969; 20:225.

O'Dell CE, et al. Ventilation-perfusion lung images in the Swyer-James syndrome. Radiology 1976; 212:423–426.

Swyer PR, James G. A case of unilateral pulmonary emphysema. Thorax 1954; 8:133–136.

SYSTEMIC LUPUS ERYTHEMATOSUS

Carr W. Plasmapheresis and pulse cyclophosphamide in systemic lupus erythematosus. Ann Intern Med 1988; 108:152–153.

Lewis E, et al. A Controlled trial of plasmaphoresis

therapy in severe lupus nephritis. N Engl J Med 1992; 326:1373–1379.

Pines A, et al. Pleuropulmonary manifestations of systemic lupus erythematosus: clinical features of its subgroups. Chest 1985; 88:129–135.

Matthay R, et al. Pulmonary manifestations of systemic lupus erythematosus: review of twelve cases of acute lupus pneumonitis. Medicine 1975; 54:397–409.

Schroeder J, et al. Synchronization of plasmapheresis and pulse cyclophosphamide in severe systemic lupus erythematosus. Ann Intern Med 1987; 107:344–346.

TALCOSIS

Crouch E, Churg A. Progressive massive fibrosis of the lung secondary to IV injection of talc. Am J Clin Pathol 1983; 80(4):520–526.

Heffner J, et al. Pulmonary reactions from illicit substance abuse. Clin Chest Med 1990; 11(1):151–162.

Hind C. Pulmonary complications of IV drug misuse. Thorax 1990: 45(1):891–898.

Overland ES, et al. Alterations of pulmonary function in IV drug abusers: prevalence, severity and characterization of gas exchange abnormalities. Am J Med 1980; 68:231–237.

Pare JP, et al. Long-term follow up of drug abusers with IV talcosis. Am Rev Respir Dis 1989; 139:233–241.

Pare JP, et al. Pulmonary "mainline" granulomatosis: talcosis of IV methadone abuse. Medicine 1979; 58(3):229–239.

THYMOMA

Ellis K, Austin JHM, Jaretski A. Radiologic detection of thymoma in patients with myasthenia gravis. AJR 1988; 151:873–881.

Goldel N, et al. Chemotherapy of invasive thymoma: a retrospective study of 22 cases. Cancer 1989; 63:1493–1500.

Kaye AD, Janss BR, Arger PH, et al. Mediastinal computed tomography in myasthenia gravis. J Comput Assist Tomogr 1983; 7:273–279.

Loehrer PJ, et al. Chemotherapy for advanced thymoma: preliminary results of an intergroup study. Ann Intern Med 1990; 113:520–524.

McCurran WJ, et al. Invasive thymoma—the role of mediastinal irradiation following complete or incomplete surgical resection. J Clin Oncol 1988; 6:1722–1727.

Nakata HI, Nakayama C, Nobe T, Koga M. Computed tomography characterization of anterior mediastinal tumors. J Comput Assist Tomogr 1985; 9:161–166.

Pescarmora E, et al. Analysis of prognostic factors and clinicopathological staging of thymoma. Ann Thorac Surg 1990; 50:534–538.

THYROID CARCINOMA

Cady B. An expanded view of risk-group definition in differentiated thyroid carcinoma. Surgery 1988; 104(6):947–953.

Massin JP. Pulmonary metastases in differentiated thyroid carcinoma. Cancer 1984; 53:982–992.

Mizukami Y. Distant metastases in differentiated thyroid carcinomas. Hum Pathol 1990; 21:283–290.

Smith S. Mortality from papillary thyroid carcinoma. Cancer 1988; 62:1381–1388.

TOXOPLASMA

Catterall JR, et al. Pulmonary toxoplasmosis. Am Rev Respir Dis 1986; 133:704.

Derouin F, et al. Laboratory diagnosis of pulmonary toxoplasmosis in patients with AIDS. J Clin Microbiol 1989; 27:1661.

Goodman PC, et al. Pulmonary toxoplasmosis in AIDS. Radiology 1992; 184:791.

Pugin J, et al. Extreme elevations of LDH differentiating pulmonary toxoplasmosis from *Pneumocystis* pneumonia. N Engl J Med 1992; 326:1226.

Schnapp LM, et al. *T. gondii* pneumonitis in patients infected with the HIV. Arch Int Med 1992; 152:1073.

TRACHEOESOPHAGEAL FISTULA

Burt M, et al. Malignant esophagorespiratory fistula: management options and survival. Ann Thorac Surg 1991; 52(6):122–128.

Hilgenberg AD, Grillo HC. Acquired nonmalignant tracheoesophageal fistula. J Thorac Cardiovasc Surg 1983; 85(4):492–498.

Little AG, et al. Esophageal carcinoma with respiratory tract fistula. Cancer 1984; 53(6):1322–1328.

Thomas AN. Management of tracheoesophageal fistula caused by cuffed tracheal tubes. Am J Surg 1972; 124(2):181–189.

TUBERCULOSIS

Bertelsen S, et al. Isolated middle lobe atelectasis: etiology, pathogenesis, and treatment of the so-called middle lobe syndrome. Thorax 1980; 35:449–452.

British Thoracic Society Research Committee. Short-course chemotherapy for tuberculosis of lymph nodes: a controlled trial. Br Med J 1985; 290: 1106–1113.

Caligiuri PA, et al. Tuberculous main-stem bronchial stenosis treated with Sleeve resection. Arch Intern Med 1984; 144:1302–1303.

Chaisson RE, et al. Tuberculosis in patients with the acquired immunodeficiency syndrome. Am Rev Respir Dis 1987; 136:570–574.

Chan HS, et al. Effect of corticosteroids on deterioration of endobronchial tuberculosis during chemotherapy. Chest 1989; 96(5):1195.

Dutt A, Moers D, Stead W. Short-course chemotherapy for extrapulmonary tuberculosis. Ann Intern Med 1986; 104:7–12.

Medical Research Council Working Party on Tuberculosis of the Spine. A controlled trial of six-month and nine-month regimens of chemotherapy in patients undergoing radical surgery for tuberculosis of the spine in Hong Kong. Tubercle 1986; 67:243–259.

Prout S, Benatar SR. Disseminated tuberculosis. South Afr Med J 1980; 22:835–839.

Sagrista-Sauleda J, et al. Tuberculous pericarditis-ten year experience with a prospective protocol for diagnosis and treatment. J Am Coll Cardiol 1988; 11:724–728.

Smith LS, et al. Endobronchial tuberculosis. Chest 1987; 91(5):644.

Tse CY, et al. Serious sequelae of delayed diagnosis of endobronchial tuberculosis. Tubercle 1988; 69:213.

Van den Brande PM, et al. Clinical spectrum of endobronchial tuberculosis in elderly patients. Arch Intern Med 1990; 150:2105.

Williams DJ, et al. Endobronchial tuberculosis presenting as asthma. Chest 1988; 93(4):836.

UPPER EXTREMITY DEEP VENOUS THROMBOSIS

Aburahma AF, et al. Axillary-subclavian vein thrombosis. Changing patterns of etiology, diagnostic, and therapeutic modalities. Am Surg 1991; 57:101–107.

Becker GJ, et al. Local thrombolytic therapy for subclavian and axillary vein thrombosis. Radiology 1983; 149:419–423.

Bolgiano EB, et al. Deep venous thrombosis of the upper extremity: diagnosis and treatment. J Emerg Med 1990; 8:85–91.

Lisse JR, et al. Upper extremity deep venous thrombosis: increased prevalence due to cocaine abuse. Am J Med 1989; 87:457–458.

Monreal M, et al. Upper extremity deep venous thrombosis and pulmonary embolism. Chest 1991; 99:280–283.

Tilney NL, et al. Natural history of major venous thrombosis of the upper extremity. Arch Surg 1970; 101:792–796.

VENTILATORS

Abraham E, Yoshihara G. Cardiorespiratory effects of pressure-controlled inverse-ratio ventilation in severe respiratory failure. Chest 1989; 96: 1356–1359.

Al-Saady N, Bennett E. Decelerating inspiratory flow waveform improves lung mechanics and gas exchange in patients on intermittent positive pressure ventilation. Intensive Care Med 1985; 11:68–75.

Berman L, Downs J, Van Eeden A, Delhagen D. Inspiration:expiration ratio: is mean airway pressure the difference? Crit Care Med 1981; 9:775–777.

Cole A, Weller S, Sykes M. Inverse-ratio ventilation compared with PEEP in adult respiratory failure. Intensive Care Med 1984; 10: 227–232.

Coggeshall JW, Marini JJ, Nevman JH. Improved oxygenation after muscle relaxation in adult respiratory distress syndrome. Arch Intern Med 1985; 145:17–18.

Corbridge T, Wood L, Crawford G, et al. Adverse effects of large tidal volume and low PEEP in canine acid aspiration. Am Rev Respir Dis 1990; 142:311–315.

Dreyfuss D, Basset G, Soler P, Saumon G. Intermittent positive-pressure hyperventilation with high inflation pressures produces microvascular injury in rats. Am Rev Respir Dis 1985; 132:880–884.

Dreyfuss D, Soler P, Basset G, Saumon G. High-inflation pressure pulmonary edema: respective effects of high airway pressure, high tidal volume and positive end-expiratory pressure. Am Rev Respir Dis 1988; 137:1159–1164.

Gattinoni L, Presenti A, Mascheroni D, et al. Low-frequency positive-pressure ventilation with extracorporeal CO_2 removal in severe acute respiratory failure. JAMA 1986; 256:881–886.

Haake R, Schlichtig R, Ulstad D, Henschen R. Barotrauma: pathophysiology risk factors and prevention. Chest 1987 91:608–613.

Holzapfel L, Robert D, Perrin FPLB, et al. Static pressure-volume curves and effect of positive end-expiratory pressure on gas exchange in adult respiratory distress syndrome. Crit Care Med 1983; 11: 591–597.

Hudson L. Ventilatory management of patients with adult respiratory distress syndrome. Semin Respir Med 1981; 2:128–139.

Jardin F, Farcot J-C, Boisante L, et al. Influence of positive end-expiratory pressure on left ventricular performance. N Engl J Med 1981; 304:387–392.

Kolton M, Cattran C, Kent G, et al. Oxygenation during high-frequency ventilation compared with conventional mechanical ventilation in two models of lung injury. Anesth Analg 1982; 61:323–332.

Lain D, DiBenedetto R, Morris S, et al. Pressure control inverse ratio ventilation as a method to reduce peak inspiratory pressure and provide adequate ventilation and oxygenation. Chest 1989; 95:1081–1088.

MacIntyre N, Follet J, Deitz J. Jet ventilation at 100 breaths per minute in adult respiratory failure. Am Rev Respir Dis 1986; 134:897.

Marini J. Lung mechanics in adult respiratory distress syndrome: recent conceptual advances and implications for management. Clin Chest Med 1990; 11:1–18.

Marini J. Paying the piper. The linkage of alveolar ventilation to alveolar pressure. Intensive Care Med 1990; 16:734–745.

Marini J, Crooke P, Truwit J. Determinants and limits of pressure preset ventilation: a mathematical model of pressure control. J Appl Physiol 1989; 67:1081–1092.

Marini J. Should PEEP be used in airflow obstruction? Am Rev Respir Dis 1989; 140:1–3.

Pepe P, Marini J. Occult positive end expiratory pressure in mechanically ventilated patients with airflow obstruction: the auto-PEEP effect. Am Rev Respir Dis 1982; 126:166–170.

Perel A. Newer ventilation modes temptations and pitfalls. Crit Care Med 1987;15:707–709.

Peterson G, Baier H. Incidence of pulmonary barotrauma in a medical ICU. J Crit Care Med 1983; 11:67–69.

Pierson D. Alveolar rupture during mechanical ventilation: role of PEEP, peak airway pressure and distending volume. Respir Care 1988; 33:472–486.

Ralph D, Robertson H, Weaver L, er al. Distribution of ventilation and perfusion during positive end-expiratory pressure in the adult respiratory distress syndrome. Am Rev Respir Dis 1985; 131:54–60.

Tharratt R, Allen R, Albertson T. Pressure-controlled inverse-ratio ventilation in severe adult respiratory failure. Chest 1988; 94:755–762.

WEGENER'S GRANULOMATOSIS

DeRemee RA, McDonald TJ, Harrison EG Jr, et al. Wegener's granulomatosis: anatomic correlates, a proposed classification. Mayo Clin Proc 1976; 51:777–781.

Falk RJ, Jennette JC. Anti-neutrophil cytoplasmic autoantibodies with specificity for myeloperoxidase in patients with systemic vasculitis and idiopathic necrotizing and crescentic glomerulonephritis. N Engl J Med 1988; 318:1651.

Jennette JC, Falk RJ. Antineutrophil cytoplasmic autoantibodies and associated diseases. A review. Am J Kidney Dis 1990; 15:517–529.

Specks U, Wheatley CL, et al. Anticytoplasmic autoantibodies in the diagnosis and follow-up of Wegener's granulomatosis. Mayo Clin Proc 1989; 64:28–36.

Specks U, et al. Granulomatous vasculitis, Wegener's and Churg-Strauss. Rheum Dis Clin North Am 1990; 162:377–397.

Van der Woude FJ, Lobatto S, et al. Autoantibodies against neutrophils and monocytes: tool for diagnosis and marker of disease activity in Wegener's granulomatosis. Lancet 1985; 1:425–429.

Yoshikawa Y, Watanabe T. Pulmonary lesions in Wegener's granulomatosis. A clinicopathologic study of 22 autopsy cases. Hum Pathol 1986; 17:401–410.

WILLIAMS-CAMPBELL SYNDROME

Mitchel R, Bury RG. Congenital bronchiectasis due to deficiency of bronchial cartilage (Williams-Campbell syndrome). J Pediatr 1975; 87:230–234.

Watanabe T, et al. Congenital bronchiectasis due to cartilage deficiency: CT demonstration. J Comput Assist Tomogr 1987; 11:70–103.

Wayne KS, Taussig LM. Probable familial congenital bronchiectasis due to cartilage deficiency (Williams-Campbell syndrome). Am Rev Respir Dis 1976; 114(1):15–22.

Williams H, Campbell P. Generalized bronchiectasis associated with deficiency of cartilage in the bronchial tree. Arch Dis Child 1960; 35:182–191.

YELLOW NAIL SYNDROME

Angelillo VA, O'Donohue WJ. Yellow nail syndrome with reduced glucose in pleural fluid. Chest 1979; 75:83.

Emerson, PA. Yellow nails, lymphedema, and pleural effusions. Thorax 1966; 21:247–253.

Guin JD, Elleman JH. Yellow nail syndrome. Possible association with malignancy. Arch Dermatol 1979; 115:734.

Runyon BA, Forker EL, Sopko JA. Pleural-fluid kinetics in a patient with primary lymphedema, pleural effusions, and yellow nails. Am Rev Respir Dis 1979; 119:821.

Samman PD, White WF. The "yellow nail syndrome." Br J Dermatol 1964; 76:153–157.